PULMONARY FUNCTION
IN
HEALTHY, EXERCISING AND DISEASED ANIMALS

PIERRE LEKEUX

Flemish Veterinary Journal

Vlaams Diergeneeskundig Tijdschrift

Special issue

General Editor

P. SIMOENS

University of Ghent

The Flemish Veterinary Journal "Vlaams Diergeneeskundig Tijdschrift" is published in 6 issues per year and is edited by the Faculty of Veterinary Medicine, State University of Ghent. Subscription (outside Belgium) : 1.000 BEF net (yearly) on postal account 000-0135379-64 with reference "Vlaams Diergeneeskundig Tijdschrift, B-9000 Gent, Belgium".

ISBN 90-74070-02-7
ISSN 0303 - 9021 (series)
Wettelijk depot D/1991/2796/1

UNIVERSITEIT GENT

Printed in Belgium

PULMONARY FUNCTION
IN
HEALTHY, EXERCISING AND DISEASED
ANIMALS

Pierre Lekeux, DVM, PhD,
Professor of Physiology and
Head of the Laboratory for Functional Investigation
Faculty of Veterinary Medicine
University of Liege
Liege, Belgium

1993
VLAAMS DIERGENEESKUNDIG TIJDSCHRIFT
GENT, BELGIUM

PREFACE

In the beginning of this century, Emile FRANCQUI claimed that *'a country without scientific activity remains as a body without brain and spirit'*. It was under his influence, and with the support of King Albert - who served an old tradition of all members of the Belgian court, that is the permanent interest for Sciences and Arts - that a new scientific foundation was established in 1932.
The aim of the FRANCQUI-Foundation was to promote scientific research and help scientists regardless of their political and philosophical convictions, language and institution. The Foundation had to facilitate the scientists' free development of thinking by supporting them on a moral and financial basis. Consequently, a FRANCQUI-Award and a FRANCQUI-Chair were created.
Every year, in Belgium, each University has the opportunity to select two Academic staff members from Belgian Universities for the conferment of the FRANCQUI-Chair, on the basis on their outstanding scientific qualification. The titular is invited to present his scientific work in a series of lectures.
The Rector of the University of Ghent conferred one of the FRANCQUI-Chairs 1992-1993 to Prof. Pierre LEKEUX because of his major contribution to the understanding of animal pulmonary function and dysfunction.
Prof. LEKEUX graduated in 1978 as Doctor in Veterinary Medicine at the University of Liege. His research work on bovine pulmonary function started at the University of Utrecht-The Netherlands, and resulted in a Ph.D.-degree in 1984. After post-doctoral studies in several European and North-American Universities, he has been nominated head of the Department of Veterinary Physiology in the University of Liege.
In the Veterinary Faculty of Liege, he established the Laboratory for Functional Investigation in Large Animals which today competes with the most prominent Research Centres all over the world. Among the three academic tasks which are entrusted to this Laboratory, that are teaching, research and service, fundamental researches in the area of bovine pulmonary dysfunction and equine exercise intolerance are very important.

The numerous basic research studies performed in this Laboratory which resulted in the publication of many papers in different international scientific journals, the many invitations he received to present state-of-the-art lectures at several specialized scientific congresses, and the conferment of three important international scientific awards reflect the general acceptance of Prof. LEKEUX as an international well known expert in his research area.
With rather wide divarication, the lectures of Prof. LEKEUX set out the scientific knowledge of yesterday and the experimental facts of today. As his lectures proceeded, and with his well-known enthusiasm, the focus cleared. Though, in his conclusion by no means agreement was claimed, he innovated some potential strategies to improve pulmonary function.
The contributions of Prof. LEKEUX to the FRANCQUI-Chair resulted in this unique volume of the Flemish Veterinary Journal. The publication of this book serves three purposes. At first, in this way the Veterinary Faculty symbolizes the importance it attributes to the scientific educational basis and training of its students, which is the result of personal experience in fundamental research of its academic staff members. Secondly, the Flemish Veterinary Journal has now the opportunity to share with veterinarians, researchers and students many recently acquired scientific data dealing with the physiology and the pathophysiology of respiration in several animal species. Finally, by this publication, which is the written expression of scientific research at a University as it has been originally defined by Emile FRANCQUI, it is hoped that the permanent splitting of minds, cultures and regions within Europe, which is so conspicuous during periods of recession, will never destroy the fundamental and primary human sense and scope which have to be experienced between and within all academic members of different Veterinary Faculties : high-quality veterinary education, research and practice.

C. BURVENICH
Department of Physiology,
Biochemistry and Biometrics

H. LAUWERS
Dean of the Veterinary Faculty
University of Ghent

CONTRIBUTORS

Tatiana Art, DVM, PhD, Equine Sport Medicine Unit, Faculty of Veterinary Medicine, University of Liege (ULg), Bât. B42, Sart Tilman, B-4000 Liege

Cecile Clercx, DVM, PhD, Department of Small Animal Medicine, Faculty of Veterinary Medicine, ULg, Bât. B44, Sart Tilman, B-4000 Liege

Roland Close, Ir, Laboratory for Functional Investigation, Faculty of Veterinary Medicine, ULg, Bât. B42, Sart Tilman, B-4000 Liege

Daniel Desmecht, DVM, Laboratory for Functional Investigation, Faculty of Veterinary Medicine, ULg, Bât. B42, Sart Tilman, B-4000 Liege

Bruno Genicot, DVM, Laboratory for Functional Investigation, Faculty of Veterinary Medicine, ULg, Bât. B42, Sart Tilman, B-4000 Liege

Pascal Gustin, DVM, PhD, Laboratory of Pharmacology and Toxicology, Faculty of Veterinary Medicine, ULg, Bât. B41, Sart Tilman, B-4000 Liege

Pierre Lekeux, DVM, PhD, Laboratory for Functional Investigation, Faculty of Veterinary Medicine, ULg, Bât. B42, Sart Tilman, B-4000 Liege

Annick Linden, DVM, Laboratory for Functional Investigation, Faculty of Veterinary Medicine, ULg, Bât. B42, Sart Tilman, B-4000 Liege

Frederic Rollin, DVM, Department of Large Animal Medicine, Faculty of Veterinary Medicine, ULg, Bât. B42, Sart Tilman, B-4000 Liege

ACKNOWLEDGEMENTS

The authors thank :

-) Prof. L. De Meyer, Rector of the University of Ghent, Prof. H. Lauwers, Dean of the Faculty of Veterinary Medicine, and Prof. C. Burvenich, Chairman of the Department of Veterinary Physiology, for their welcome in the University of Ghent,

-) Prof. P. Simoens, General Editor of the Vlaams Diergeneeskundig Tijdschrift, for his assistance and helpfulness in the publication of this book,

-) Prof. E. Muylle, Prof. N.E. Robinson and Prof. R. Rose for their advice,

-) C. Gresse, M. Leblond, M. Motkin and I. Sbaï for their technical assistance.

CONTENTS

CHAPTER I

PULMONARY FUNCTION AS A POTENTIAL LIMITING FACTOR FOR HEALTH, PRODUCTION AND EXERCISE

P. Lekeux

Laboratory for Functional Investigation
Faculty of Veterinary Medicine
University of Liege

SUMMARY

After a description of the various links of the oxygen line and a definition of the notion "limiting factor", this paper describes why the pulmonary function can become a limiting factor in some domestic animals which have been selected for improved economic or athletic performances.

KEY WORDS

Respiratory system - Pulmonary function - Limiting factor.

1. INTRODUCTION

In order to ensure its metabolic functions, each cell consummes oxygen and produces carbon dioxide. In small unicellular organisms, the cellular surface allows sufficient gas exchange by simple diffusion between extra- and intracellular contents.

However, this highly simple mechanism is only effective in organisms with a diameter lower than one millimeter. Pluricellular organisms need more sophisticated structures in order to ensure sufficient gas exchange for the requirements the cells. Two mean systems for the transport of gas between the athmospheric air and the mitochondria are necessary in these organisms. The respiratory and the circulatory systems ensure the transfer of oxygen and carbon dioxide between air and blood and between the lung and the cells, respectively.

This specialization has contributed to considerably increase the possibilities for gas exchange between the organism and his outside environment and therefore his ability to transform energy. Unfortunately, because of this specialization, the gas exchange mechanisms have become much more complex. This has resulted into an "oxygen line" in which each link works in a context of solidarity following the principle "one for all and all for one". In such a system, each deficient link becomes a limiting factor for the whole line, i.e. for the gas exchange and for the energy transformation.

2. SIGNIFICANCE OF THE LIMITING FACTOR

This concept of a work line based on solidarity is not without functional consequences. Indeed, the efficiency of each link is less important in term of absolute value than of relative one. The weakest link of the line will always determine the work level of the other units, independently of their own potential. Therefore, one of the transport's systems of gas between air and the mitochondria may become the limiting factor because either it shows a functional deficiency, or its potential did not improve enough when compared to the other links of the line, or the organism is living in an environment which

is hostile or inappropriate for this particular species.
Fortunately, the line for the transport of respiratory gas is most of the time able to ensure the gas exchange requirements of the cells. Indeed, each link has reached a sufficient potential in order to avoid to become a limiting factor in physiological conditions, following the principle of symmorphosis (Weibel et al, 1987). This equilibrium, which is specific for each group of living creatures, results from an evolution that is either adaptative (for instance due to natural selection), allometric (for instance due to somatic growth) or induced (for instance due to training).

3. OXYGEN LINE

Oxygen transfert between air and mitochondria occurs mainly by convection and diffusion. In this process, five steps are described :
- pulmonary ventilation which allows the transport of oxygen to the alveoli by convection;
- alveolo-capillary diffusion which allows the transfer of oxygen from air to blood by diffusion;
- blood circulation which allows the transport of oxygen to the tissues by convection;
- capillary-cell diffusion which allows the gas transfer from capillaries to mitochondria;
- oxygen combustion in the mitochondria.

4. RELATIVE IMPORTANCE OF THE DIFFERENT STEPS IN MAXIMAL OXYGEN CONSUMPTION

Oxygen is essential for the aerobic transformation of energy required for metabolisms, growth, thermoregulation, physical exertion and all animal productions in general. Of course, oxygen consumption is related to the need of the organism. For instance, a heavy exercise can induce a 40 times increase of the resting oxygen consumption. Therefore, each link of the oxygen line must adapt its working level to the gas exchange requirements of the tissues.

4.1. Oxydative capacity of skeletal muscles

The maximal oxygen consumption of the body can never exceed the capacity of the mitochondria to utilize oxygen. Indeed, it has been demonstrated that one ml of mitochondria consumes approximately four ml of oxygen per minute (Kayar et al, 1989). In domestic animals, there is a linear relation between the mitochondrial volume and the maximal oxygen consumption (Fig. 1-1.) (Wagner et al, 1991). Therefore this last factor is related not only to the global lean body mass of an organism but also to the relative volume and the oxidative enzyme concentration of its mitochondria. This explains why, with identical body weight, the maximal oxygen consumption is about three times larger in horses and dogs than in cattle and goats, respectively (Taylor et al, 1991).

4.2. Oxygen supply by the capillaries of the skeletal muscles

This supply depends on the total capillary length which is obtained by multiplying muscle volume with capillary density. This one is significantly higher in athletic species than in sedentary ones (Hoppeler et al, 1981) and in conventional cattle than in double-muscled ones (Stavaux et al, 1993). Therefore, the oxygen extraction will mainly depend on two aspects of this peripheral perfusion, i.e. vascular resistance to blood flow and capillary transit time which is the ratio between capillary blood volume and muscle blood flow.

4.3. Oxygen transport by hemoglobin

Because of the low amount of dissolved oxygen in blood and tissues, the oxygen transport by hemoglobin is an important link in the oxygen line. This explains both the negative effect of anemia on gas exchange and the positive effect of hemoconcentration induced by exercise in athletic species (Weibel et al, 1987).

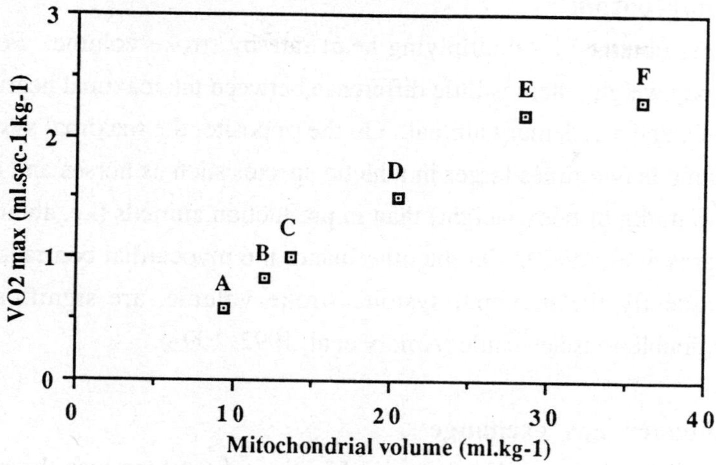

Fig. 1-1. Relation between mitochondrial volume and maximal oxygen consumption (Wagner et al, 1991). A : Calf, B : Goat, C : Steer, D : Pony, E : Horse, F : Dog.

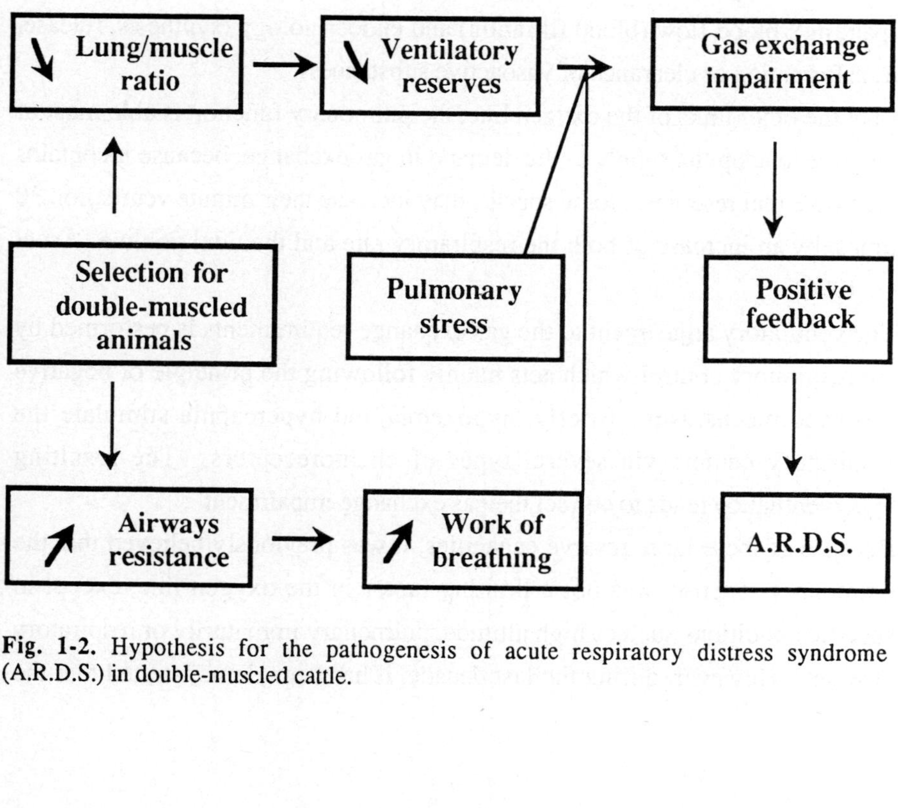

Fig. 1-2. Hypothesis for the pathogenesis of acute respiratory distress syndrome (A.R.D.S.) in double-muscled cattle.

4.4. Cardiac output

This value is obtained by multiplying heart rate by stroke volume. For an identical body weight, there is little difference between the maximal heart rate of an athletic and a sedentary animal. On the opposite, the maximal systolic stroke volume is two times larger in athletic species such as horses and dogs (i.e. about 3 ml/kg of body weight) than in production animals (i.e. about 1.5 ml/kg) (Karas et al, 1987). On the other hand, the myocardial contractility, and consequently the maximal systolic stroke volume, are significantly reduced in double-muscled cattle (Amory et al, 1992; 1993).

4.5. Pulmonary gas exchange

It was previously believed that the main function of the lung was the blood cooling. Since Lavoisier, however, the crucial role of the lung in gas exchanges has been definitely recognized. Since then, other functions of the respiratory system have been described, dealing with thermoregulation (panting), blood flow (blood filtration) and endocrinology (synthesis, release, transformation or clearance of vasoactive substances).

Like the other links of the oxygen line, the pulmonary function is able most of the time to adapt its supply to the demand in gas exchange, because it contains high potential reserves. Some species may increase their minute ventilation 30 times, by an increase of both the respiratory rate and the tidal volume (Art et al, 1990).

The ventilatory adjustment to the gas exchange requirements is performed by the respiratory control which acts mainly following the principle of negative feedback mechanism. Briefly, hypoxemia and hypercapnia stimulate the respiratory centers via several types of chemoreceptors. The resulting hyperventilation tends to correct the gas exchange impairment.

Because of these large reserve capacities, it was previously believed that the pulmonary function was not a limiting factor in the oxygen line, except in specific conditions such as high altitude, pulmonary immaturity or respiratory diseases. However, during the last decade, it has been demonstrated that the respiratory system is not always able to fulfill its physiological function, during some specific but not exceptional conditions. This is for instance the case in some domestic animals which have been selected for high performances. As a result of this, the pulmonary function may be a potential limiting factor of the oxygen line, which can be illustrated by several examples described below.

5. ACUTE RESPIRATORY DISTRESS SYNDROME IN HYPER-MUSCLED CATTLE

The selection for the double-muscled character in cattle has induced a significant increase in the ratio between their skeletal muscle volume and pulmonary volume (Hanset et al, 1982) and a significant decrease in the cross-sectional area of their airways (Gustin et al, 1987). Although in physiological conditions the pulmonary gas exchange is proportional to the demand, the specific energetic cost of breathing is higher and the ventilatory reserves are lower in these animals than in conventional cattle. This explains why an identical respiratory infection may induce a moderate and quickly reversible pulmonary dysfunction in conventional cattle and a severe and sometimes irreversible dysfunction in some double-muscled cattle.

Indeed, when the ventilatory reserves are small and the inflammatory reaction is too acute, the deficiencies of the pulmonary function can be so important that they may be responsible for an aggravation of the clinical condition, by positive feedback mechanisms (Fig. 1-2.) (Lekeux et al, 1985). Briefly, the severe gas exchange impairment and the resulting acidosis induce several reactions of the organism (i.e. vasoconstriction, decreased mucociliar clearance, decreased clearance of the autacoids by the pulmonary endothelium, ...), which aggravate the pulmonary gas exchange impairment via the principle of vicious circle.

This lack of sufficient ventilatory reserve is particularly crucial in young cattle which do not reach pulmonary functional maturity before one year of age (Lekeux et al, 1984).

6. EXERCISE-INDUCED HYPOXEMIA AND HEMORRHAGE IN THOROUGHBRED HORSES

In healthy race horses, heavy short term exercise induces hypoxemia and hypercapnia (Bayly et al, 1983; Thornton et al, 1983), despite pulmonary ventilation may increase 30 times in these animals (Art et al, 1990). The pulmonary function in these horses which are selected mainly on the basis of their athletic performances, has thus become a limiting factor in the oxygen line during maximal exercise. This is aggravated by the fact that training induces in the horse an improvement of all the links of the oxygen line (Evans et al, 1988), except for the pulmonary function (Fig. 1-3.) (Art et al, 1992).
This extreme situation may affect the integrity of the lung. Indeed, 75 % of the thouroughbred horses show hemorrhages in the caudodorsal part of their lungs during heavy exercise (Raphel et al, 1982; Sweeney et al, 1983). Although many hypotheses have been proposed to explain this phenomenon, it seems likely that these hemorrhages are due to disruption of pulmonary vessels secondary to pulmonary overstreching and to sudden and important changes in transmural pressure inside the lung (Fig. 1-4.) (Lekeux et al, 1993). Indeed, intense exercise induces a large increase in the pulmonary blood pressure (Erickson et al, 1990) together with highly negative pressures in the airways (Art et al, 1988). Sudden changes in this transmural pressure in a lung overstreched by the hyperventilation represent a stress which could damage the vessel walls (Fu et al, 1992).

7. EXERCISE-INDUCED HYPERTHERMIA IN RACE GREYHOUNDS

Some dogs have been selected for their ability to perform short distance races. Their skeletal muscle mass has reached about 60 % of their body mass, compared to the 40 % recorded in conventional breeds (Gunn et al, 1978).
Despite the high exercise intensity, the pulmonary gas exchange function does not seem to be a limiting factor during this athletic discipline in which the required metabolism is mainly anaerobic (Osnes et al, 1972). However, this

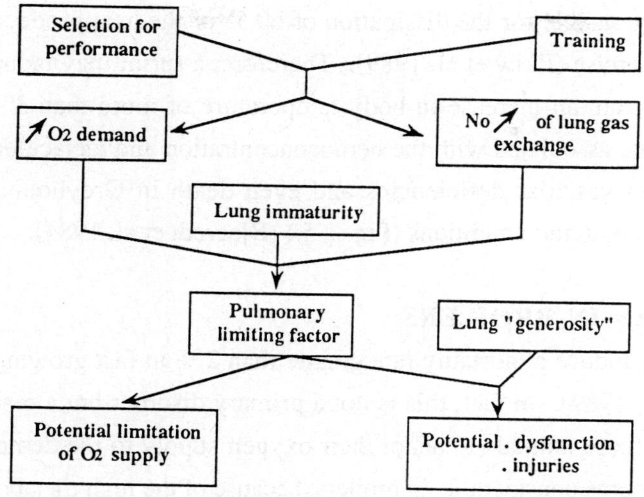

Fig. 1-3. Hypothesis for exercise-induced hypoxemia and hypercapnia in the racehorse.

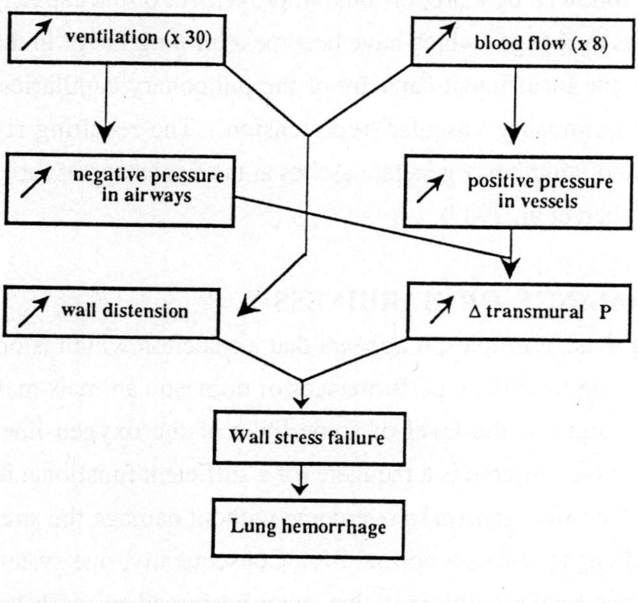

Fig. 1-4. Hypothesis for exercise-induced pulmonary hemorrhage in thoroughbred horses.

is not the case for the thermoregulatory function of the respiratory system which is responsible for the dissipation of 60 % of the heat produced by the muscular exercise (Ilkiw et al, 1989). Therefore, a sprint may induce in less than one minute an increase in body temperature of more than 3° C. This hyperthermia, associated with the hemoconcentration and lactacidemia, may contribute to vascular deficiencies and even death in Greyhounds racing during hot and humid conditions (Fig. 1-5.) (Bjotvedt et al, 1984).

8. ASCITES IN BROILERS

Ascites may induce a mortality rate greater than 2 % in fast growing broilers (Julian et al, 1989). In fact, this is not a primary disorder but a result of the inability of these animals to adapt their oxygen supply to the demand. The latter has become considerable in broilers, because of the high metabolic needs required by the rapid growth, the thermoregulation and the stress.
Unfortunately, the improvement of the production performances of broilers has not been followed by a proportional improvement of the capacity of their pulmonary gas exchanges which have become a limiting factor in the oxygen line. Indeed, the insufficient capacity of the pulmonary capillaries of these birds induce pulmonary vascular hypertension. The resulting right heart hypertrophy and failure may generate ascites at the final stage of the syndrome (Fig. 1-6.) (Julian et al, 1987).

9. PERFORMANCE OR HARDINESS ?

By analyzing these exemples, it appears that a selection which is only based on the production or athletic performances of domestic animals may abolish the security margin at the level of some links of the oxygen line. Yet, a sufficient functional reserve is a requisite for a sufficient functional hardiness, i.e. the ability for an organism to overcome without damage the stress which has to be challenged during a normal life. Consequently, one system, which has become the weakest link in a line, may be forced to work beyond its physiological limits, which may result in inappropriate functioning or even in

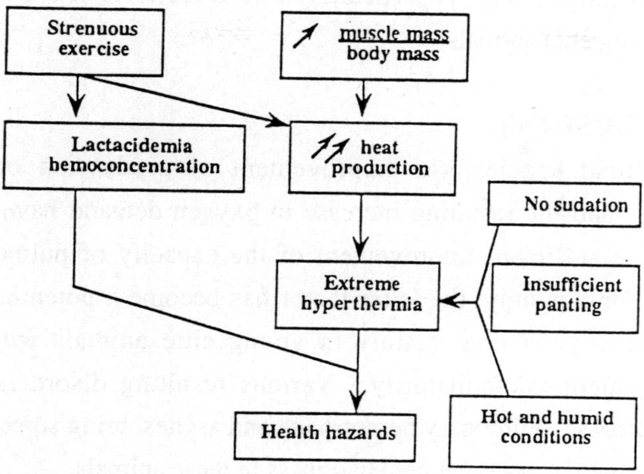

Fig. 1-5. Hypothesis for the pathogenesis of some exercise-induced health hazards in Greyhounds.

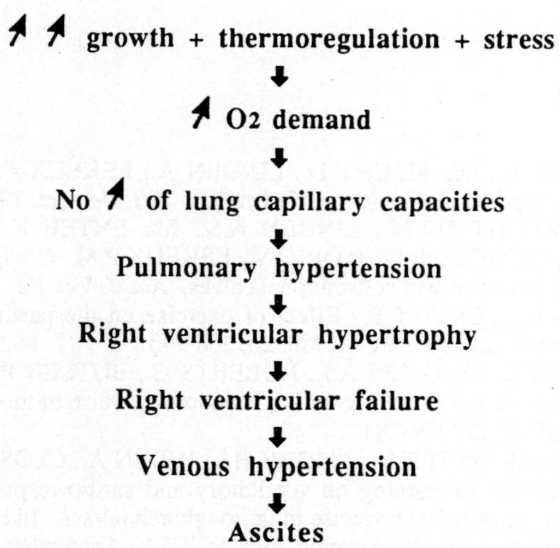

Fig. 1-6. Hypothesis for the pathogenesis of ascites in fast growing Broilers.

irreversible damages. This is particularly true at the level of the respiratory system in young elite animals.

10. CONCLUSIONS

In some animal species, the improvement of production or athletic performances and the resulting increase in oxygen demand have not been followed by a sufficient improvement of the capacity of pulmonary gas exchange. Consequently, the latter factor has become a potential limiting factor in the oxygen line, mainly in young elite animals which show pulmonary functional immaturity. Various resulting disorders such as respiratory distress, pulmonary hemorrhage and ascites, bring some evidence of the lack of pulmonary functional hardiness in these animals.

The limiting factors of the aerobic metabolism should be taken into consideration in selection programs, in order to avoid that the increasing frequency of these predictable injuries becomes inacceptable from an economical and ethical point of view.

REFERENCES

AMORY H., ROLLIN F., DESMECHT D., LINDEN A., LEKEUX P. Cardiovascular response to acute hypoxia in double-muscled calves. *Res. Vet. Sci.* 1992, 52, 316-324.

AMORY H., DESMECHT D.J.M., LINDEN A.S., Mc ENTEE K., ROLLIN F.A., BEDUIN J.M.L., GENICOT B.C., D'ORIO V., LEKEUX P.M. Comparison of cardiac function in double-muscled and conventional calves. *Am. J. Vet. Res.*, 1993, in press.

ART T., SERTEYN D., LEKEUX P. Effect of exercise on the partitioning of equine respiratory resistance. *Equine Vet. J.* 1988, 20, 268-273.

ART T., ANDERSON L., WOAKES A.J., ROBERTS C., BUTLER P.J., SNOW D.H., LEKEUX P. Mechanics of breathing during strenuous exercise in thoroughbred horses. *Respir. Physiol.* 1990, 82, 279-284.

ART T., VOTION D., Mc ENTEE K., AMORY H., LINDEN A., CLOSE R., LEROY P., LEKEUX P. Influence of training on ventilatory and cardio-respiratory parameters measured during a standardized exercise in thoroughbred horses. In Proceedings : 11th Comparative Respiratory Society Meeting, Urbana (USA), September 1992, P1.

BAYLY W.M., GRANT B.D., BREEZE R.G. The effects of maximal exercise on acid-base balance and arterial blood gas tension in thoroughbred horses. In : *Equine Exercise Physiology*, Snow, D.H., Persson, S.G.B., Rose, R.J. (Eds), Granta Editions, Cambridge, 1983, pp 400-407.

BJOTVEDT G., WEEMS C.W., FOLEY K. Strenuous exercise may cause health hazards

for racing Greyhounds. *Vet. Med.* 1984, 79, 1481-1487.
ERICKSON B.K., ERICKSON H.H., COFFMAN J.R. Pulmonary artery, aortic and oesophageal pressure changes during high intensity treadmill exercise in the horse: a possible relation to exercise-induced pulmonary hemorrhage. *Equine Vet. J.* 1990, suppl 9, 47-52.
EVANS D.L., ROSE R.J. Cardiovascular and respiratory responses to submaximal exercise training in the thoroughbred horse. *Pflügers Arch.* 1988, 411, 316-321.
FU Z., COSTELLO M.L., TSUKIMOTO K., PREDILETTO R., ELLIOT A.R., MATHIEU-COSTELLO O., WEST J.B. High lung volume increases stress failure in pulmonary capillaries. *J. Appl. Physiol.* 1992, 73, 123-133.
GUNN, H.M. The proportions of muscle, bone and fat in two different types of dogs. *Res. Vet. Sci.* 1978, 24, 277-282.
GUSTIN P., LOMBA F., BAKIMA M., LEKEUX P., VAN DE WOESTIJNE K.P. Partitioning of pulmonary resistance in Friesian and double-muscled calves. *J. Appl. Physiol.* 1987, 62, 1826-1832.
HANSET R. Muscular hypertrophy as a racial characteristic: the case of the Belgian Blue breed. In : *Muscle Hypertrophy of Genetic Origin and its Use to improve Beef Production*, King, J.W.B., Menissier, F. (Eds), Martinus Nijhoff, The Hague, 1982, pp 437-449.
HOPPELER H., MATHIEU O., KRAUER R., CLAASSEN H., ARMSTRONG R.B., WEIBEL E.R. Design of the mammalian respiratory system. VI. Distribution of mitochondria and capillaries in various muscles. *Respir. Physiol.* 1981, 44, 87-111.
ILKIW J.E., DAVIS P.E., CHURCH D.B. Hematologic, biochemical, blood-gas, and acid-base values in Greyhounds before and after exercise. *Am. J. Vet. Res.* 1989, 50, 583-586.
JULIAN R.J., FRIARS G.W., FRENCH H., QUINTON M. The relationship of right ventricular hypertrophy, right ventricular failure, and ascites to weight gain in broiler and roaster chickens. *Avian Dis.* 1987, 31, 130-315.
JULIAN R.J., McMILLAN I., QUINTON M. The effect of cold and dietary energy on right ventricular hypertrophy, right ventricular failure and ascites in meat-type chickens. *Avian Pathol.* 1989, 18, 675-684.
KARAS R.H., TAYLOR C.R., RÖSLER K., HOPPELER H. Adaptive variation in the mammalian respiratory system in relation to energetic demand. V. Limits to oxygen transport by the circulation. *Respir. Physiol.* 1987, 69, 65-79.
KAYAR S.R., HOPPELER H., LINDSTEDT S.L., CLAASSEN H., JONES J.H., ESSEN-GUSTAVSSON B., TAYLOR C.R. Total muscle mitochondrial volume in relation to aerobic capacity of horses and steers. *Pflügers Arch.* 1989, 413, 343-347.
LEKEUX P., HAJER R., BREUKINK H.J. Effect of somatic growth on pulmonary function values in healthy Friesian cattle. *Am. J. Vet. Res.* 1984, 45, 2003-2007.
LEKEUX P., HAJER R., VAN DEN INGH T.S.G.A.M., BREUKINK H.J. Pathophysiologic study of 3-methylindole-induced pulmonary toxicosis in immature cattle. *Am. J. Vet. Res.* 1985, 46, 1629-1631.
LEKEUX P., ART T. The respiratory system: anatomy, physiology, adaptation to exercise and training. In : *The Athletic Horse*, Hodgson, D.R., Rose, R.J. (Eds), W.B. Saunders, Philadelphia, 1993, in press.
OSNES J.B., HERMANSEN L. Acid-base balance after maximal exercise of short duration. *J. Appl. Physiol.* 1972, 31, 59-63.
RAPHEL C.F., SOMA L.R. Exercise-induced pulmonary hemorrhage in thoroughbreds after racing and breezing. *Am. J. Vet. Res.* 1982, 43, 1123-1127.
STAVAUX D., Mc ENTEE K., ART T., REZNIK M., LEKEUX P. Effect of age and breed on muscle fibers type and capillary density in cattle. Submitted for publication.

SWEENEY C.R., SOMA L.R. Exercise induced pulmonary haemorrhage in horses. In : *Equine Exercise Physiology*, Snow, D.H., Persson, S.G.B., Rose, R.J. (Eds), Granta Editions, Cambridge, 1983, pp 51-56.

TAYLOR C.R., WEIBEL E.R. Learning from comparative physiology. In : *The Lung: Scientific Foundations*, Crystal, R.G., West, J.B. (Eds), Raven Press, New York, 1991, pp 1595-1607.

THORNTON J.R., ESSEN-GUSTAVSSON B., LINDHOLM A. Effects of training and detraining on oxygen uptake, cardiac output, blood gas tensions, pH and lactate concentrations during and after exercise in the horse. In : *Equine Exercise Physiology*, Snow, D.H., Persson, S.G.B., Rose, R.J. (Eds), Granta Editions, Cambridge, 1983, pp 470-486.

WAGNER P.D., HOPPELER H., SALTIN B. Determinants of maximal oxygen uptake. In : *The Lung: Scientific Foundations*, Crystal, R.G., West, J.B. (Eds), Raven Press, New York, 1991, pp 1585-1593.

WEIBEL E.R., TAYLOR C.R., KARAS R.H., HOPPELER H. Adaptive variation in the mammalian respiratory system in relation to energetic demand. I. Introduction to problem and strategy. *Respir. Physiol.* 1987, 69, 1-6.

CHAPTER II

PULMONARY FUNCTION TESTING IN VETERINARY MEDICINE

P. Lekeux[1], R. Close[1], T. Art[2]

[1] Laboratory for Functional Investigation
[2] Equine Sport Medicine Unit
Faculty of Veterinary Medicine
University of Liege

SUMMARY

This paper describes the material and methods used for pulmonary function tests in unsedated domestic animals. The usefulness and clinical significance of these techniques are also analyzed.

KEY WORDS

Respiratory system - Pulmonary function testing - Functional investigation.

1. INTRODUCTION

During the two last decades, pulmonary function testing has been intensively used in domestic animals for research purposes. More recently, some of these tests have been proposed for clinical purposes and introduced in specialized equine and companion animal hospitals.

Pulmonary function testing does not provide specific diagnoses : this is the job of the clinician who must evaluate all the available information. These tests are mainly helpful for quantifying the degree of physiologic abnormality in patients and the degree of functional recovery after treatment.

Until now, heavy equipment located in an air-conditioned laboratory is often necessary in order to obtain accurate and useful information on the pulmonary function. However, in the future, it could be possible to fasten a small device onto the patient under field conditions in order to record, store and analyze several useful functional parameters.

Errors may be important when some technical and methodological requirements are not met. Therefore, the results of a functional test must be analyzed carefully. Physiological variability is often important for functional parameters and comparison between tests may only be done if they are performed in standardized conditions.

The horse is the first and most intensively investigated domestic animal as far as pulmonary function is concerned. Therefore this paper will firstly describe the tests available for unsedated horses and, subsequently, somes technical peculiarities of the other domestic species.

This paper does not approach the clinical examination which remains essential in each case.

2. MEASUREMENT OF THE PULMONARY FUNCTION IN THE UNSEDATED HORSE

2.1. Gas exchange

2.1.1. Blood gases

An overal evaluation of the pulmonary gas exchange can be provided by the measurement of *arterial blood gases tensions*, i.e. PaO_2 and $PaCO_2$. Hypoxemia (PaO_2 lower than 80-84 mmHg) may be the result of limitation at the level of ventilation, perfusion, diffusion or ventilation-perfusion matching. Hypercapnia ($PaCO_2$ higher than 46-50 mmHg) is considered as a good indicator of alveolar hypoventilation. The interpretation of these data is complicated in the exercising horse because heavy exercise induces hypoxemia and hypercapnia. However, most healthy horses show normal blood gas values at moderate exercise (up to 50 % of their maximal O_2 consumption), which seems not to be the case in horses with respiratory dysfunctions (Littlejohn and Bowles, 1981; Bayly et al, 1984). Arterial blood must be sampled anaerobically in a heparinized seringue from the carotid or facial artery and stored in ice if the measurements cannot be performed immediately. Sampling in glass syringes is recommanded when the measurements cannot be done within one hour. The presence of air in the syringe will induce an overestimation and underestimation of O_2 and CO_2 tensions, respectively. Blood gas values may also be underestimated if they are not corrected for body temperature (Table 1-1.). This is of critical importance in heavy exercising or diseased horses which can reach body temperatures higher than 41° C, while the apparatus is calibrated for measuring at 37° C. Most computerized blood gas analyzers calculate the corrected values by using appropriate equations (Kelman and Nunn, 1966).

An increase in the *alveolar-arterial O_2 gradient* ($A\text{-}aDO_2$ higher than 10 mmHg) is also an indicator of impaired O_2 exchange due to diffusion impairment, ventilation-perfusion mismatching or right-to-left vascular shunt.

Table 1-1. Comparison of blood gas values from a similar sample measured at 37° C and corrected for several body temperatures.

Value	Unit	Body temperature			
		37° C	38.5° C	40° C	41.5° C
PaO_2	mmHg	85.6	92.8	100.6	109.0
$PaCO_2$	mmHg	42.5	45.0	48.0	51.2
pH	-	7.384	7.362	7.341	7.319

Alveolar partial pressure in O_2 can be evaluated by measuring the end-tidal fraction of O_2 in the expired gas with a mass spectrometer or by using the equation : $PAO_2 = [(PB - PH_2O) \times FIO_2] - PACO_2$
or its simplified version : $PAO_2 = 150 - PaCO_2$.
PB is the ambient barometric pressure (around 760 mmHg at sea level) and PH_2O is the water vapor pressure which varies with the temperature (for example 47.1 and 58.3 mmHg at 37 and 41° C respectively) and FIO_2 is the fractional concentration of O_2 in inspired air (0.21).
The measurement of *hemoglobin blood concentration* (Hb) and venous blood gas tensions (PvO_2 and $PvCO_2$) is useful in order to calculate the *arterial O_2 content* ($CtaO_2$) and the arterio-venous gradient in the O_2 content ($Cta\text{-}vO_2$). In contrast with arterial O_2 partial pressure, these parameters are directely correlated with the intensity of the exercise in healthy horses. Arterial O_2 content can be calculated from the following equation :
$CtaO_2 \text{ (vol \%)} = (1.39 \times Hb \times SaO_2/100) + (0.003 \times PaO_2)$
The *arterial hemoglobin O_2 saturation* (SaO_2) can be evaluated by continuous and non invasive monitoring, using the pulse oximetry (Powers et al, 1989). However, from our experience, this technique provides accurate data only in sedated horses. Hemoglobin O_2 saturation data are often provided by automatic blood gas analyzer. However, these data are calculated on the basis of human blood and need to be corrected for the horse by using appropriate algorithms (Clerbaux et al, 1986).

Some equipments for collecting blood samples by *radiotelemetry* from horses running on the field have also been described (De Waal et al, 1986).

2.1.2. O_2 uptake, CO_2 output and respiratory quotient

These parameters are of critical importance in sport medicine and must be recorded during heavy exercise in order to reach maximal values. Three different techniques have been described for measuring VO_2max and VCO_2max in horses.

The *bag-collection technique* requires the use of an airtight face mask connected to a non-rebreathing valve which allows the collection and analysis of expired gases in a large balloon (Persson et al, 1980; Evans and Rose, 1987). The main disadvantages of this reference technique are the discomfort induced by the high resistance and dead space of the equipment and the impossibility to measure transient changes in the data.

The *open flow technique* requires the use of a loose-fitting face mask connected to a 3 meter long flexible tubing, an airflow indicator, a high velocity centrifugal blower and a gas sampling device (Bayly et al, 1987; Rose et al, 1988; Seeherman and Morris, 1990). This technique allows accurate measurements of O_2 uptake and CO_2 output with a minimal discomfort for the horse (Fig. 2-1.).

The *breath-by-breath technique* requires the use of airflow sensors placed on a tight face mask, the entry of which is connected via a narrow catheter to a mass spectrometer which allows *on line* measurements of the concentration of the gases (Beaver et al, 1973; Art et al, 1990a). This technique provides a continuous and simultaneous recording of all transient changes, not only in gas exchange data (O_2 uptake, CO_2 output and the respiratory quotient) but also in ventilatory data (inspiratory and expiratory flows, volumes, times) (Fig. 2-2.).

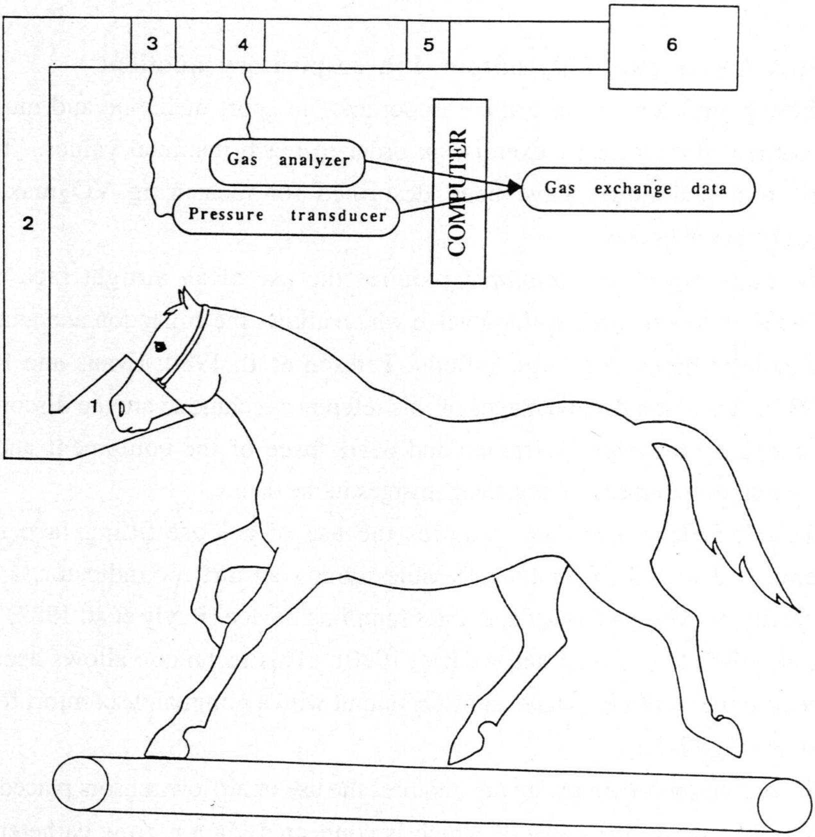

Fig. 2-1. Open flow technique for gas exchange measurements. 1. : Face mask; 2 : Flexible tubing; 3 : Venturi tube; 4 : Flow control; 5 : Valve; 6 : Blower (Seeherman and Morris, 1990).

2.2. Ventilatory data

Airflow is usually measured with a pneumotachograph connected to a tight confortable face mask whith low dead space and as limited effects as possible on the pulmonary function (Art and Lekeux, 1988a). Volume is calculated by integration of the flow signal. This integration is preferably performed by a computer program in order to avoid the traditional drift problems due to the electronic integrators.

Several systems have been proposed for use in the horse. *Fleisch and Lilly pneumotachographs* are reference techniques (Spörri and Leeman, 1964; Gillespie et al, 1966) but, because of their limited flow ranges, they are more suitable for measuring resting than exercising flows which can reach 100 l/sec in the horse.

Ultrasonic phase-shift flowmeters are particularly well adapted for flow measurements both in resting and highly exercising horses because of their low weight, low dead space, low resistance, high range of linearity and low sensitivity to contamination by condensation and nasal discharge (Woakes et al, 1987; Art et al, 1990a).

Calibration of these pneumotachographs concerns both flow and volume. Flow can be calibrated with a rotameter adapted to the appropriate flow range. However, from our experience, the use of an air velocity transducer (TSI, St Paul, USA) connected to a high flow modulable generator is particularly appropriate for an accurate calibration of high flow ranges. Volume is controled with calibrated syringes. For accuracy, it is always preferable to calibrate the equipment within the ranges of flows and volumes which are expected to be measured during the real test.

Most computer softwares associated with the flowmeters allow direct calculation of the ventilatory data.

Flow-volume loops can be obtained by using an XY recorder or an appropriate software in resting horses (Koterba et al, 1988) and in exercising horses (Art and Lekeux, 1988b).

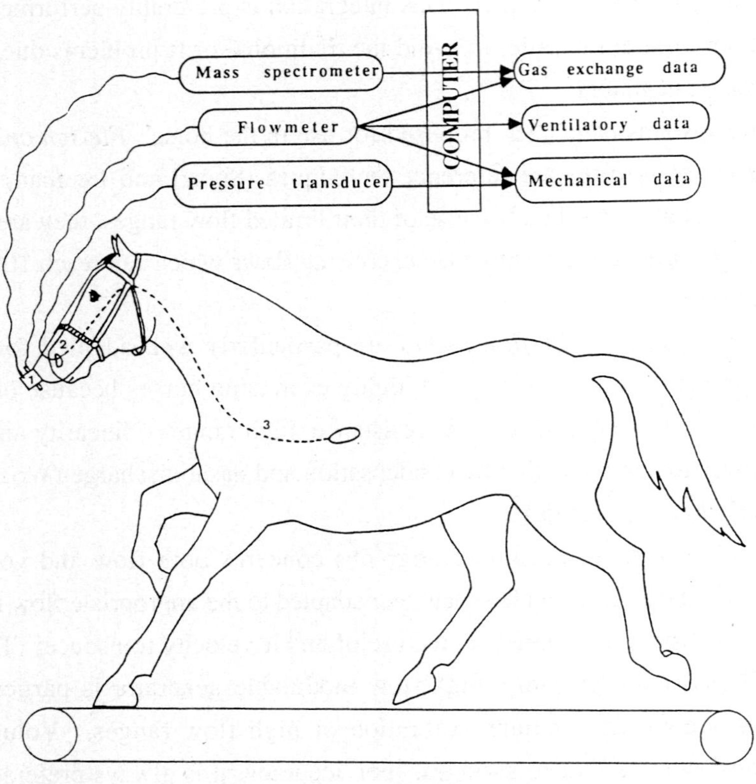

Fig. 2-2. Breath-by-breath technique for gas exchange measurement. 1 : Ultrasonic sensor; 2 : Face mask; 3 : esophageal balloon-catheter system (Art et al, 1990a).

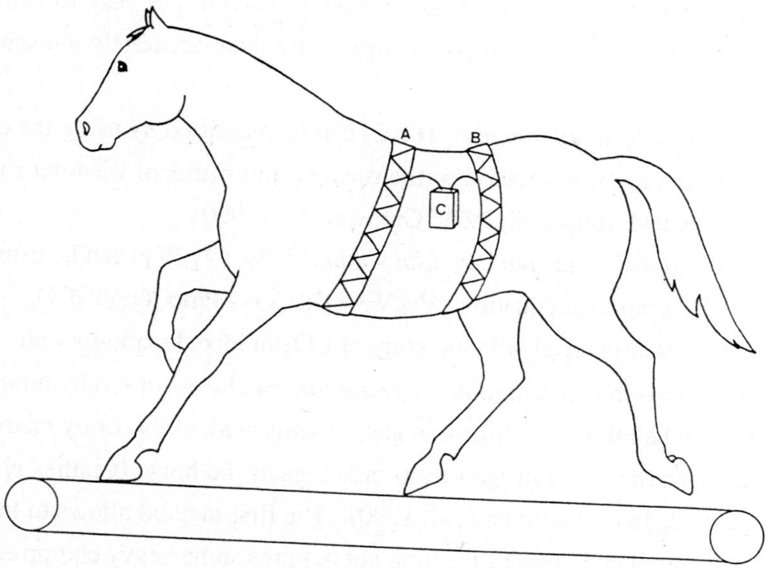

Fig. 2-3. Inductance plethysmography for measurement of respiratory volumes. A : Thoracic band; B : Abdominal band; C : Oscillation and demodulation units.

Analysis of these loops may bring interesting information about uncommon patterns of breathing (Amis and Kurpershoek, 1986).
Lung volume changes can also be evaluated without any face mask by using other technologies. The *inductance plethysmography* requires the use of respibands applied to the rib cage and abdomen, frequency oscillators and a calibrator-demodulator unit (Fig. 2-3.) (Respitrace, Ambulatory Monitoring, Ardsley, USA). The sum of the rib cage and abdominal displacement gives a signal proportional to the tidal volume (Koterba et al, 1988).
The *impedance plethysmography* requires the use of current and voltage electrodes applied to the thorax, a phase sensitive detector and a voltage-controlled oscillator. This system provides impedance changes across the thorax which are proportional to the pulmonary volume changes (Attenburrow et al, 1990a).

Both last techniques are non-invasive, easy to use but not easy to calibrate. Several problems need to be solved before to use them accurately in exercising horses.

The *functional residual capacity* (FRC) can be measured by using the closed circuit helium dilution method or the open circuit nitrogen washout method (Willoughby and McDonell, 1979; Gallivan et al, 1990).

The *physiological dead space to tidal volume ratio* (V_D/V_T) can be estimated by using the simplified equation : $V_D/V_T = (PaCO_2 - PmeCO_2)/PaCO_2$ in which $PmeCO_2$ is the partial pressure of CO_2 in mixed expiratory air.

The *adequacy of the distribution of ventilation* can be evaluated by lung scans during the inhalation of radioactive gases (Amis et al, 1984) or by examining the rate of washout of nitrogen from the lungs as the horse breathes pure O_2 (Muylle et al, 1972; Gallivan et al, 1990). The first method allows to localize the poorly ventilated areas of the lung but requires some heavy equipment like a gamma camera. The second method allows to quantify the ventilatory asynchronism which may be present in subclinical lower airway problems but requires a regular tidal volume during the measurement.

2.3. Intrapleural pressure measurements

Intrapleural pressure can be measured by direct puncture of the pleural cavity but this is not recommended. The most appropriate technique is to measure the pressure changes in the medial thoracic part of the esophagus, which provides accurate measurements both in resting (Derksen and Robinson, 1980) and exercising horses (Art and Lekeux, 1988a). From our experience, the best results are obtained when a condom containing 0.5 ml of air is tighly fixed on the distal part of a semi-rigid polyethylene catheter (internal diameter : 4 mm; external diameter : 6 mm). Before introducing the balloon-catheter system in the esophagus via the nose, the proximal part of the catheter must be tightly connected to a pressure transducer in order to avoid an excess of air in the balloon. Indeed a balloon distended too much induces abnormally positive and damped pressure recordings.

The balloon-catheter-transducer system must be calibrated by means of a water manometer.
Some interesting information about the respiratory system can be obtained by the mere measurement of intrapleural pressures changes (Ventigraph, Boehringer, Germany) (Deegen and Klein, 1987). However, in the absence of simultaneous flow and volume recordings, it is rather hazardous to conclude whether an increase in pleural pressure change is due either to a pathological increase of the pulmonary resistance, or a physiological increase of the airflow, or both.

2.4. Mechanics of breathing

The simultaneous recording of flow, volume and intrapleural pressure changes allows the measurement of several parameters of the mechanics of breathing in unsedated resting or exercising horses. When the resistance of the flowmeter is high, the mask pressure is no longer equal to atmospheric pressure and must be recorded in order to calculate the transpulmonary pressure, i.e. the gradient between intrapleural and mask pressures.
The *dynamic lung compliance* is the volume change per unit of intrapleural pressure change measured at the 2 points of zero flow. A decrease in resting dynamic lung compliance can be due to an increased rigidity of the lung parenchyma or, much more frequently, to a ventilatory asynchronism resulting from partial obstruction of small airways (Robinson et al, 1983). During exercise, dynamic lung compliance is overestimated and may even become negative. This is due to the fact that the inertial factors are usually neglected in its calculation. This may not be tolerated in the exercising horse because of the high air acceleration and therefore high inertial pressure changes (Art et al, 1989).
The *total pulmonary resistance* is the intrapleural pressure change per unit of flow change recorded at isovolume, for example at 50 % of inspiratory and expiratory volumes. An increase in total pulmonary resistance can be due to excessive intra-airways materials, contraction of airway smooth muscles,

inflammation of the mucosa, dynamic collapse due to a compressive transmural pressure or dysfunction at the level of the upper airways. Because of the partitioning of the airway resistance to airflow, total pulmonary resistance is more sensitive to changes in large than in small airways (Art et al, 1988). In contrast with dynamic lung compliance, total pulmonary resistance can be accurately measured in exercising horses because this parameter is measured at 2 points (isovolume 50 %) where accelerations and consequently inertial pressure changes are negligible (Art et al, 1989) .

The *work of breathing* can be estimated from the measurement of the area of the transpulmonary pressure-volume loop (Art and Lekeux, 1988c). An increase in the work of breathing can be due to both an increase in total pulmonary resistance or a decrease in dynamic lung compliance.

In order to obtain accurate information, the phase compatibility between the flow and pressure signals must be tested up to 10 and better 20 Hz. Any dephasage must be corrected either by adapting the length of the tubings of the measuring equipment or by using an appropriate software. The measurements of the data must be performed on at least 10 breathing cycles. The most appropriate method is therefore a computerized system which provides continuous calculation of required data (for example ACEC, Charleroi, Belgium and Buxco Electronics, Sharon, USA). Another non-expensive method is to adapt a highly powerful data storing and processing software like Superscope (GW Instruments, Somerville, USA).

Some techniques allow to evaluate the resistance to airflow without recording the intrapleural pressure.

The *flow interruptor method* is based on the fact that alveolar pressure can be evaluated at the level of the nose during repeated short term flow interruptions. Associated with a flow measurement, this allows evaluation of the resistance of the respiratory system (Mead and Whittenberger, 1954; Grobet, 1989).

The *forced oscillation method* has been adapted for the equine species (Gustin et al, 1988c; Art et al, 1989; Young and Hall, 1989). This method requires a loud speaker as generator of pressure waves, a flow and pressure meter and a

fast Fourrier analyzer in order to measure the resistance and the reactance (i.e. the sum of compliance and inertance) of the respiratory system at several frequencies from 2 to 30 Hz.
The *mono-frequency forced oscillation method* is a simplified technique which allows the evaluation of the resistance of the respiratory system by using a small portable equipment connected to a face mask. This method is easy to use in field conditions (Le Ninivin et al, 1991).

2.5. Pulmonary hemodynamics

Pulmonary vascular resistance is directly proportional to the pulmonary driving pressure (i.e. the difference between the pulmonary artery pressure and the pulmonary artery wedge pressure) and inversely proportional to the pulmonary blood flow. Pulmonary artery pressures can be measured by means of a balloon-tipped flow-directed catheter (Swan-Ganz) connected to a pressure transducer levelled at the scapulohumeral joint or a catheter-tip micromanometer (Millar, Houston, USA) introduced in the pulmonary artery via the left jugular vein and the right heart.
A vasoconstriction at the level of the pulmonary arterioles will induce a pulmonary artery hypertension and an increase in pulmonary vascular resistance. This may happen during alveolar hypoxia or be secondary to the action of vasoconstrictive agents (Dixon, 1978; Muylle et al, 1982).
The interpretation of these measurements is complicated in the exercising horse. Indeed, exercise induces an increase in pulmonary artery and capillary pressures (Manohar, 1992) and a decrease in pulmonary vascular resistance due to the large increase in blood flow and to the recruitment and enlargement of pulmonary vessels. Furthermore, pressure measurements in these vessels are highly influenced by the high pleural pressure changes occurring during hyperpnea (Amory et al, 1990).

2.6. Ventilation-perfusion matching

Measurement of the ventilation to perfusion matching can help to diagnose pulmonary dysfunctions in the horse. Two elaborate techniques can be used in the horse.

The *radioactive isotope gas method* analyzes the topographic distribution of the ventilation/perfusion ratio by measuring the lung radioactivity by nuclear scintigraphy during a steady-state inhalation and intravenous infusion of the radioactive gas ^{81m}Krypton or ^{99m}Technetium (Amis et al, 1984; O'Callaghan et al, 1987).

The *multiple inert gas elimination method* allows the determination of pulmonary dead space and shunt as well as a continuous description of the ventilation/perfusion ratio both at rest (Hedenstierna et al, 1987) or during exercise (Wagner et al, 1989). This technique measures, with a gas chromatograph, the steady-state concentration of 6 infused inert gases in pulmonary arterial and carotid arterial blood and in mixed expiratory gas.

2.7. Diffusion capacity

The pulmonary diffusing capacity for O_2 can be evaluated by measuring the diffusing capacity for carbon monoxide with the single breath or the steady-state method (Gillespie and Tyler, 1969). This requires the measurement of the inspired and expired concentration of carbon monoxide by an infra-red analyzer after inhalation of air containing 0.1 % of carbon monoxide.

2.8. Mucociliar clearance rate

The tracheal mucociliar clearance rate may be impaired by viral infections or by excessive ammonium concentration in inspired air. This clearance rate can be determined in the horse from endoscopic examinations, by measuring Carbon movement (Sweeney, 1989) or India Ink in sirup movement (Turgut and Sasse, 1989), or from scintigraphic examinations, by measuring ^{99m}Technetium sulphide colloid movement with scintillation probes (Nelson and Hampe, 1983; Coombs and Webbon, 1987) or with a gamma camera

(Willoughby et al, 1991).

2.9. Upper airway function

Upper respiratory tract dysfunctions are frequently responsible for poor performance by increasing the resistance to airflow. It is therefore of crucial interest to make an early and precise diagnose of these dysfunctions, to analyze whether they are responsible for the poor performance by impairing the pulmonary gas exchange, and to analyze the functional efficiency of the treatment.

Answers to these questions may be partly provided by videoscopic examination and resistance measurement of the upper airways at rest and during strenuous exercise (Derksen et al, 1986; Morris and Seeherman, 1990). Some other techniques such as laryngeal palpation (Cook, 1989), laryngeal muscles electromyography (Moore et al, 1988) and electrolaryngography (Cook, 1991), allow to detect some laryngeal abnormalities, including subclinical dysfunctions. However, they cannot definitely assess whether these abnormalities are responsible for gas exchange limitation and poor performance in the investigated horse.

Upper airway endoscopy can be carried out by using a flexible fiberendoscope or videoendoscope. The latter technique provides a better visualization on a large monitor and allows the storage of the recording on videotapes.

Endoscopic examination in the resting and post-exercising horse is usually performed in an unsedated horse using a twitch as restraint and a 180 cm long endoscope with a diameter of 12 mm. This allows to detect the visible abnormalities, from the nasal passages up to the tracheobronchial tree, which could decrease the permeability of upper airways to airflow. This includes intraluminal abnormalities such as excessive secretion or blood, intramural abnormalities such as severe lymphoid hyperplasia or narrowing of the airway, and extramural abnormalities such as compressing retropharyngeal lymph nodes.

Pharyngeal and laryngeal functions are not always easy to interpret in the quietly breathing horse. A momentarily dorsal displacement of the soft palate which disappears by flushing this area may be due to a gag reflex induced by the introduction of the endoscope. A laryngeal asynchronism may be suspected by an endoscope introduced via the right but not the left nare. Some specific manipulations may therefore be required. The thoraco-laryngeal reflex, i.e. the slap test, consists of a unilateral laryngeal adduction generated by a hand slap on the heterolateral thoracic wall. This reflex is supposed to be partly or totally inhibited by recurrent laryngeal neuropathy. Laryngeal movements can also be accentuated by nasal occlusion, the rebreathing bag technique or the injection of a ventilatory stimulant like doxapram (40 mg/kg of body weight) or lobeline (0.2 mg/kg) (Archer et al, 1991; Art et al, 1991). On the other hand, sedation is suspected to alter the coordination, the synchronism and the response of pharyngeal and laryngeal movements.

Endoscopy in the exercising horse is performed on a high speed treadmill when the horse is outfitted with its usual gear with a 100 cm long, 9 mm diameter endoscope introduced in the nasopharynx and fastened to the bridle with adhesive tape. This allows to determine the adequacy of physiological adjustments to exercise, such as complete laryngeal abduction, and the occurrence of exercise-induced obstruction of the upper airways, such as dorsal displacement of the soft palate or collapse of the pharyngeal mucosa.

Upper airway resistance can be evaluated by the simultaneous recording of flow and lateral tracheal pressure changes recorded with a side-hole catheter connected to a pressure transducer (Derksen et al, 1986; Art et al, 1988). Inspiratory and expiratory impedances are calculated as the ratio of peak tracheal pressure and flow during inspiration and expiration, respectively. A simplified technique based only on the recording of intratracheal pressure may also provide useful information (Funkquist et al, 1988; Williams et al, 1990), but the lack of simultaneous flow measurement makes the conclusions more hazardous.

These techniques allow to evaluate the dysfunction generated by an upper

airway abnormality and the efficiency of its treatment at a functional level.
Electromyographic examination of some laryngeal muscles may help to detect abnormal electrical activity associated with denervation injuries (Moore et al, 1988). Indeed, electromyograms performed with transcutaneous needles on the dorsal cricoarytenoid muscle showed abnormalities such as fibrillation potentials, positive sharp waves, bizarre high frequency discharges or reduced insertional activity in horses suspected of having laryngeal neuropathy.
Electrolaryngography allows to measure the latency of the thoraco-laryngeal reflex on the right and left sides (Cook, 1991). The reflex is elicitated by a hand slap on the thorax, close to the spine. The hand carries a switch to trigger a storage oscilloscope. The motor end-point of the reflex is recorded using surface and subdermal electrodes placed lateral to the larynx (Fig. 2-4.). Latency periods, calculated by a computer, greater than 45 and 90 milliseconds are considered by the author to be pathognomonic of a laryngeal hemiparesis and hemiplegia, respectively.
It must be emphasized that abnormalities recorded by these two last tests in resting horses are not always correlated with clinical symptoms nor with exercise-induced functional abnormalities.
The *airway occlusion test* may be useful in order to test the possibility of oral breathing, which can be the result of a dorsal displacement of the soft palate. However, from our experience, this must always be confirmed by an endoscopic examination. Indeed, in some horses, this forced oral breathing can be due to a lack of airtightness of the palato-laryngeal junction without dorsal displacement of the soft palate.

2.10. Respiratory sound analysis

The respiratory sound intensity can be recorded by using a calibrated radiostethoscope placed upon the trachea and connected to sound transducer, transmission and recording systems (Attenburrow et al, 1983; 1990b). Peak expiratory sound intensity was showed to be linearly correlated with the stride frequency and the peak expiratory flow, and was considered by the author as

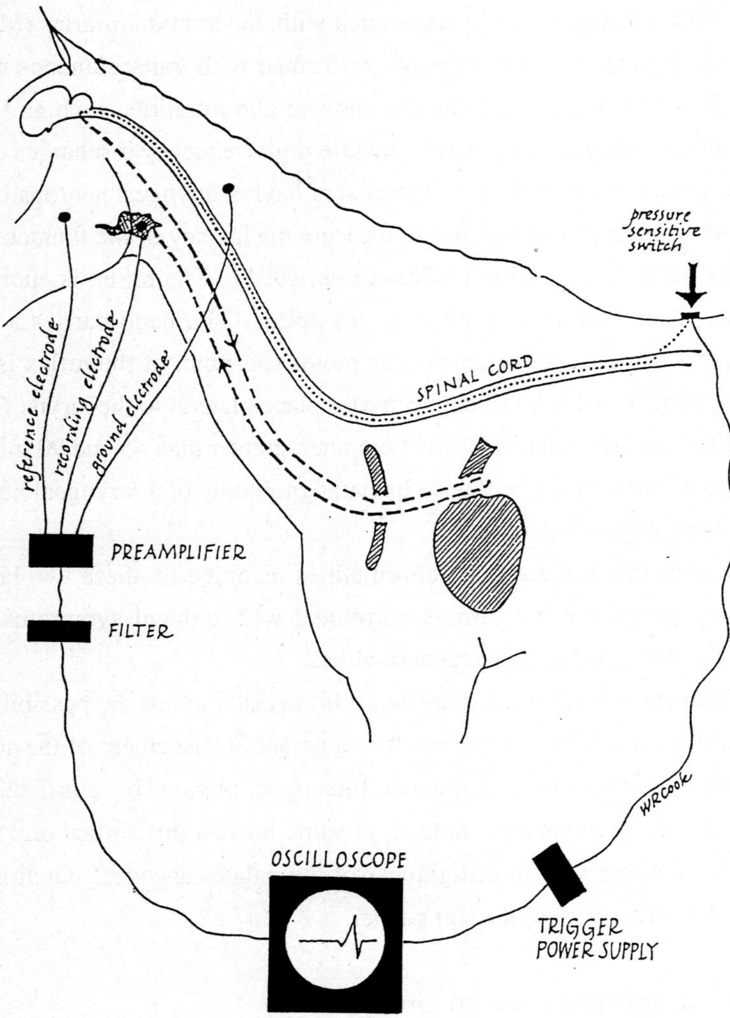

Fig. 2-4. Electromyography for the measurement of the latency of the thoraco-laryngeal reflex (Cook, 1991).

an useful and easy-to-measure parameter for the detection and recognition of certain abnormalities in the upper airways.

The *real time stethacoustic analyzer* provides interesting information about the wheezing in human patients (Lens et al, 1987) but it is not applicable in its present form in horses.

2.11. Fatigue of the ventilatory muscles

Diaphragmatic fatigue may induce specific changes in the spectral analysis of the electromyographic signals (i.e. a shift of the power spectrum towards low frequencies) (Cohen et al, 1982) and in the shape of the transdiaphragmatic pressure curves (Esau et al, 1983). This was demonstrated in human but not yet in horse.

Transdiaphragmatic pressure can be evaluated in the resting (Koterba et al, 1988) or exercising horse (Art et al, 1990b; Slocombe et al, 1991) by subtraction of gastric pressure from esophageal pressure, both being measured with a balloon-catheter-transducer system.

The *electromyographic signals* from the diaphragm can be measured in the horse by using paired silver electrodes built into a hollow catheter and placed in the lower esophagus close to the stomach (Koterba et al, 1988).

2.12. Control of breathing

In order to test the ability of the respiratory centers to induce a hyperventilation in response to hypercapnia and hypoxemia, the rebreathing method can be used (Muir et al, 1975). However, abnormalities in the control of breathing are uncommon, except in the neonatal foal, and this test does not differenciate central from peripheral problems.

2.13. Other tests

Some diagnostical procedures do not really test the pulmonary function but may bring some interesting information in horses with poor performance syndrome or with clinical diseases.

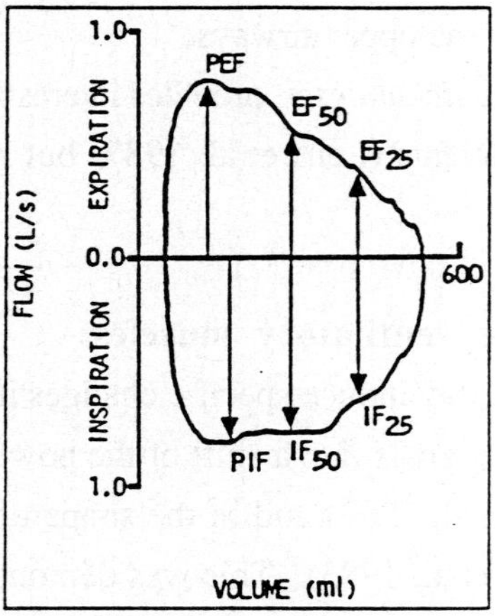

Fig. 2-5. Flow-volume loop analyzis in a dog. PEF : Peak expiratory flow; PIF : Peak inspiratory flow (Amis and Kurpershoek, 1986).

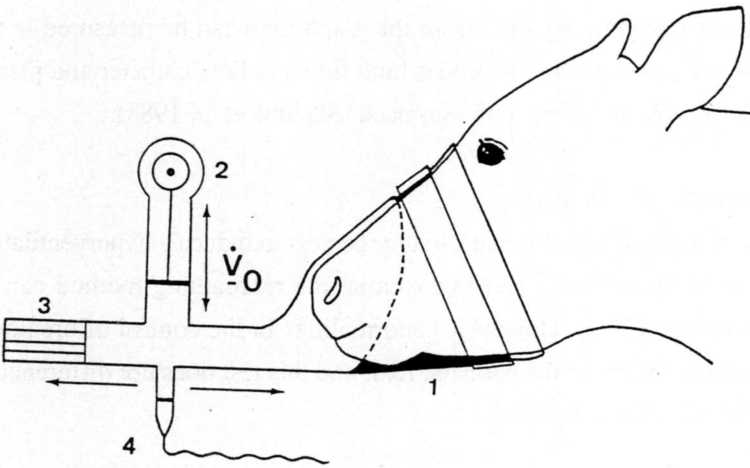

Fig. 2-6. Monofrequency oscillation technique for measurement of mechanics of breathing in unsedated cattle. 1 : Face mask; 2 : Oscillatory pump; 3 : Reference tubing with a known impedance; 4 : Pressure transducer (Reinhold et al, 1992).

Radiographic examination of the airways may reveal abnormalities with functional impact such as shortening of the epiglottis (Lindford et al, 1983), hypoplasia of the soft palate (Bertone et al, 1986), or narrowing of the airways (O'Callaghan and Goulden, 1982).

Information about subclinical lower airway problems and pulmonary allergic problems can also be provided by tracheobronchial aspiration (Beech, 1981), bronchoalveolar lavage (Viel, 1983; Derksen et al, 1985a), dosage of serum precipiting antibodies (Lawson et al, 1979), and intradermal or bronchial provocation tests (McPherson et al, 1979; Derksen et al, 1985b; Klein and Deegen, 1986; Doucet et al, 1991; Evans et al, 1992).

3. TECHNICAL PECULIARITIES OF PULMONARY FUNCTION TESTING IN DOGS AND CATS

Most of the tests described above are adaptable and useful in small animals. This is for example the case for measurement of the mechanics of breathing (Clark et al, 1977; McKiernan et al, 1989; King and Hendricks, 1990), ventilation perfusion matching (Amis et al, 1982; Clercx, 1988), and upper airway function (Smith et al, 1986).

Unfortunately, many of these techniques require general anesthesia or at least sedation in companion animals, which limits their clinical application. This is not the case for arterial blood gas measurement (McKiernan, 1991), tidal breathing flow-volume loop analysis (Fig. 2-5.) (Amis and Kurpershoek, 1986; McKiernan, 1991), measurement of total respiratory impedance by the forced oscillation method (Clercx et al, 1989; 1991) and bronchoreactivity test (Clercx et al, 1992). These tests are practical, safe and non-invasive and have been adapted for being used in unsedated patients.

4. TECHNICAL PECULIARITIES OF PULMONARY FUNCTION TESTING IN PRODUCTION ANIMALS

Measurement of the pulmonary function has little value in the clinical examination of production animals. However, these techniques are essential at a research point of view, in order to study the physiology, pathophysiology and pharmacology of the respiratory system of these animals.

Specific tests have been adapted for sheep (Mitchell and Williams, 1975; Abraham et al, 1981; Sauder et al, 1986; Collie et al, 1992), goats (Chapman et al, 1979; Bisgard et al, 1982; Messina et al, 1984; Bakima et al, 1988), pigs (Hannon et al, 1990) and cattle (Kiorpes et al, 1978; Slocombe et al, 1982; Lekeux et al, 1984a,b,c; 1988a). The latter species has been intensively investigated because of the high frequency and severity of its respiratory disorders. Partitioning of airway resistance (Lekeux et al, 1985; Gustin et al, 1987), tidal breathing flow-volume loops (Lekeux et al, 1988b), lung scintigraphy (Gustin et al, 1988a; Verhoeff et al, 1988), pulmonary hemodynamics (Slocombe et al, 1984; Gustin et al, 1988b; Amory et al, 1990), forced oscillation technique (Gustin et al, 1988c), gas exchange (Gustin et al, 1988d), multiple breath nitrogen washout (Gallivan and McDonell, 1989), monofrequency oscillation technique (Fig. 2-6.) (Close et al, 1992; Reinhold et al, 1992) and diaphragmatic fatigue measurement (Desmecht et al, 1991; 1992a) have been adapted in unsedated calves. Analysis of the data must take into account some peculiarities of the ruminants, e.g. the pressure in the rumen (Desmecht et al, 1992b) and the eructed gases (Rollin et al, 1990).

5. CONCLUSIONS

Pulmonary function testing in domestic animals is useful not only for making an accurate diagnosis but especially for assessing the functional status of the respiratory system, for evaluating the functional effect of a treatment and for elucidating the relationships between altered function and structure. Accurate data are available only when specific technical and methodological requirements are met.

REFERENCES

ABRAHAM W.M., WATSON H.,SCHNEIDER A., KING M., YERGER L., SACKNER M.A. Noninvasive ventilatory monitoring by respiratory inductive plethysmography in conscious sheep. *J. Appl. Physiol.: Respirat. Environ. Exercise Physiol.* 1981, 51, 1657-1661.

AMIS T.C., JONES H.A., RHODES C.G., HEATHER J.D., HUGHES J.M.B. Regional distribution of pulmonary ventilation and perfusion in the conscious dog. *Am. J. Vet. Res.* 1982, 43, 1972-1977.

AMIS T.C., PASCOE J.R., HORNOF W. Topographic distribution of pulmonary ventilation and perfusion in the horse. *Am. J. Vet. Res.* 1984, 45, 1597-1601.

AMIS T.C., KURPERSHOEK C. Tidal breathing flow-volume loop analysis for clinical assessment of airway obstruction in conscious dogs. *Am. J. Vet. Res.* 1986, 47, 1002-1006.

AMORY H., ART T., DESMECHT D., ROLLIN F., LEKEUX P. Respiratory-induced variability of pulmonary arterial pressure measurements in cattle. *Vet. Res. Commun.* 1990, 14, 227-233.

ARCHER R.M., LINDSAY W.A., DUNCAN I.D. A comparison of techniques to enhance the evaluation of equine laryngeal function. *Equine Vet. J.* 1991, 23, 104-107.

ART T., LEKEUX P. A critical assessment of pulmonary function testing in exercising ponies. *Vet. Res. Commun.* 1988a, 12, 25-39.

ART T., LEKEUX P. Respiratory airflow patterns in ponies at rest and during exercise. *Can. J. Vet. Res.* 1988b, 52, 299-303.

ART T., LEKEUX P. Pulmonary mechanics during treadmill exercise in race ponies. *Vet. Res. Commun.* 1988c, 12, 245-258.

ART T., SERTEYN D., LEKEUX P. Effect of exercise on the partitioning of equine respiratory resistance. *Equine Vet. J.* 1988, 20, 268-273.

ART T, LEKEUX P, GUSTIN P, DESMECHT D., AMORY H., PAIVA M. Inertance of the respiratory system in ponies. *J. Appl. Physiol.* 1989, 67, 534-540.

ART T., ANDERSON L., WOAKES A.J., ROBERTS C., BUTLER P.J., SNOW D.H., LEKEUX P. Mechanics of breathing during strenuous exercise in thoroughbred horses. *Respir. Physiol.* 1990a, 82, 279-294.

ART T., DESMECHT D., AMORY H., LEKEUX P. Synchronization of locomotion and respiration in trotting ponies. *J. Vet. Med. A* 1990b, 37, 95-103.

ART T., DESMECHT D., AMORY H., LEKEUX P. Lobeline-induced hyperpnea in equids. Comparison with rebreathing bag and exercise. *J. Vet. Med. A* 1991, 38, 148-152.

ATTENBURROW D.P., FLACK F.C., HÖRNICKE H., MEIXNER R., POLLMAN U. Respiratory airflow and sound intensity. In : *Equine Exercise Physiology*, Snow, D.H., Persson, S.G.B., Rose, R.J. (Eds), Granta Editions, Cambridge, 1983, pp 23-26.

ATTENBURROW D.P., FLACK F.C., PORTERGILL M.J. Impedance plethysmography. *Equine Vet. J.* 1990a, 22, 114-117.

ATTENBURROW D.P., FLACK F.C., PORTERGILL M.J. The relationship between peak expiratory sound intensity and peak expiratory flow rate in the thoroughbred horse during exercise. *Equine Vet. J.* 1990b, Suppl 9, 43-46.

BAKIMA M., GUSTIN P., LEKEUX P., LOMBA F. Mechanics of breathing in goats. *Res. Vet. Sci.* 1988, 45, 332-336.

BAYLY W.M., GRANT B.D., MODRANSKY P.D. Arterial blood gas tensions during exercise in a horse with laryngeal hemiplegia, before and after corrective surgery. *Res. Vet. Sci.* 1984, 36, 256-258.

BAYLY W.M., SCHULZ D.A., HODGSON D.R., GOLLNICK P.D. Ventilatory responses of the horse to exercise: effect of gas collection systems. *J. Appl. Physiol.* 1987, 63, 1210-1217.

BEAVER W.L., WASSERMAN K., WHIPP B.J. On-line computer analysis and breath-by-breath graphical display of exercise function. *J. Appl. Physiol.* 1973, 34, 128-132.

BEECH J. Technique of tracheobronchial aspiration in the horse. *Equine Vet. J.* 1981, 13, 136-137.

BERTONE J.J., TRAUB-DARGATZ J.L., TROTTER G.W. Bilateral hypoplasia of the soft palate and aryepiglottic entrapment in a horse. *J. Am. Vet. Med. Assoc.* 1986, 188, 727-729.

BISGARD G.E., FORSTER H.V., MESINA J., SARAZIN R.G. Role of the carotid body in hypernea of moderate exercise in goats. *J. Appl. Physiol.* 1982, 52, 1216-1222.

CHAPMAN R.W., SANTIAGO T.V., ELDEMAN N.H. Effects of graded reduction of brain blood flow on ventilation in unanesthetized goats. *J. Appl. Physiol.* 1979, 47, 104-111.

CLARK W.T., JONES B.R., CLARK J. Dynamic pulmonary compliance as a measurement of lung function in dogs. *Vet. Rec.* 1977, 101, 494-499.

CLERBAUX T., SERTEYN D., WILLEMS E., BRASSEUR L. Détermination de la courbe de dissociation standard de l'oxyhémoglobine du cheval et influence, sur cette courbe, de la température, du pH et du diphosphoglycérate. *Can. J. Vet. Res.* 1986, 50, 188-192.

CLERCX C. Scintigraphical analyses of pulmonary function in dogs. PhD Thesis, Utrecht, The Netherlands, 1988.

CLERCX C., GUSTIN P., HENROTEAUX M., LANDSER F.J., VAN DE WOESTIJNE K.P. Measurements of total respiratory impedance in dogs during nasal obstruction by the forced oscillation method. In Proceedings : 8th Veterinary Respiratory Symposium, Liege, 1989, P53.

CLERCX C., GUSTIN P., LANDSER F.J. Measurement of the total respiratory impedance using the forced oscillation technique in dogs with respiratory diseases. In Proceedings : 5th IVENTA Meeting, Vienne, October 1991, p13.

CLERCX C., DUFOUR P., GUSTIN P. Development of a bronchoreactivity test in dogs. In Proceedings : 6th IVENTA Meeting, Rome, September 1992, p6.

CLOSE R., REINHOLD P., LEKEUX P. A non invasive method to estimate pulmonary compliance in calves. In Proceedings : 11th Comparative Respiratory Society Meeting, Urbana (USA), September 1992, p3.

COHEN C.A., ZAGELBAUM G., GROSS D., ROUSSOS CH., MACKLEM P.T. Clinical manifestations of inspiratory muscle fatigue. *Am. J. Med.* 1982, 73, 308-316.

COLLIE D.D.S., WATT N.J., WARREN P.M., BEGARA I., LUJAN L. Lung function and structure in sheep with maedi-visna. In Proceedings : 11th Comparative Respiratory Society Meeting, Urbana (USA), September 1992, p17.

COOK W.R. Specifications for speed in the racehorse : the Airflow Factors, The Russell Meerdink Company Ltd, Menasha, Wi, 1989.

COOK W.R. An electro-diagnostic test for the objective grading of recurrent laryngeal neuropathy in the horse. In Proceedings : 7th annual convention of the American Association of the Equine Practitioners, 1991, 275-296.

COOMBS S.L., WEBBON P.M. Observations on tracheal mucociliary clearance in horses. *Tierärztl. Prax.* 1987, suppl 2, 5-7.

DEEGEN E., KLEIN H.-K. Interpleural pressure measurement and bronchial spasmolysis tests in the horse performed with a transportable oesophageal pressure measuring instrument. *Pferdeheilkunde 3* 1987, 4, 213-221.

DERKSEN F.J., ROBINSON N.E. Esophageal and intrapleural pressures in the healthy

conscious pony. *Am. J. Vet. Res.* 1980, 41, 1756-1761.
DERKSEN F.J., SCOTT J.S., MILLER D.C., SLOCOMBE R.F., ROBINSON N.E. Bronchoalveolar lavage in ponies with recurrent airway obstruction (heaves). *Am. Rev. Respir. Dis.* 1985a, 132, 1066-1070.
DERKSEN F.J., ROBINSON N.E., ARMSTRONG P.J., STICK J.A., SLOCOMBE R.F. Airway reactivity in ponies with recurrent airway obstruction (heaves). *J. Appl. Physiol.* 1985b, 58, 598-604.
DERKSEN F.J., STICK J.A., SCOTT E.A., ROBINSON N.E., SLOCOMBE R.F. Effect of laryngeal hemiplegia and laryngoplasty on upper airway flow mechanics in exercising horses. *Am. J. Vet. Res.* 1986, 47, 16-20.
DESMECHT D., LINDEN A., AMORY H., LEKEUX P. Impaired diaphragmatic function in the pneumonic calf. In Proceedings : 10th Comparative Respiratory Society Meeting, East Lansing, (USA.), September 1991, p3.
DESMECHT D., ROLLIN F., LEKEUX P. Transdiaphragmatic pressure measurement in cattle: technical data. *Res. Vet. Sci.* 1992a, 53, 148-153.
DESMECHT D., LINDEN A., LEKEUX P. Features of pulmonary ventilation, mechanics and gas transport during rumenal distention in cattle. In Proceedings : 11th Comparative Respiratory Society Meeting, Urbana (USA), September 1992b, p6.
DE WAAL A., LITTLEJOHN A., POTGIETER G.M., VAN DER BERG J., MINNAAR P.I., SMITH A. An apparatus for collecting blood samples by radiotelemetry from horses during exercise. *Vet. Res. Commun.* 1986, 10, 65-72.
DIXON P.M. Pulmonary artery pressures in normal horses and in horses affected with chronic obstructive pulmonary disease. *Equine Vet. J.* 1978, 10, 195-198.
DOUCET M.Y., VRINS A.A., FORD-HUTCHINSON A.W. Histamine inhalation challenge in normal horses and in horses with small airway disease. *Can. J. Vet. Res.* 1991, 55, 285-293.
ESAU S.A., BELLEMARE F., GRASSINO A., PERMUTT S., ROUSSOS C., PARDY R.L. Changes in relaxation rate with diaphragmatic fatigue in humans. *J. Appl. Physiol.* 1983, 54, 1353-1360.
EVANS D.L., ROSE R.J. Maximum oxygen uptake in racehorses: changes with training state and prediction from submaximal cardiorespiratory measurements. In : *Equine Exercise Physiology 2*, Gillespie, J.R., Robinson, N.E., (Eds), ICEEP Publications, Davis, California, 1987, pp 52-67.
EVANS A.G., PARADIS M.R., O'CALLAGHAN M. Intradermal testing of horses with chronic obstructive pulmonary disease and recurrent urticaria. *Am. J. Vet. Res.* 1992, 53, 203-208.
FUNKQUIST B., HOLM K., KARLSSON A., KVART C., MOLANDER C., OBEL N. Studies on the intratracheal pressure in the exercising horse. *J. Vet. Med. A* 1988, 35, 424-441.
GALLIVAN G.J., McDONELL W.N. An evaluation of the multiple-breath nitrogen washout as a pulmonary function test in cattle. *Can. J. Vet. Res.* 1989, 53, 133-142.
GALLIVAN G.J., VIEL L., McDONELL W.N. An evaluation of the multiple-breath nitrogen washout as a pulmonary function test in horses. *Can. J. Vet. Res.* 1990, 54, 99-105.
GILLESPIE J.R., TYLER W.S., EBERLY V.E. Pulmonary ventilation and resistance in emphysematous and control horses. *J. Appl. Physiol.* 1966, 21, 416-422.
GILLESPIE J.R., TYLER W.S. Chronic alveolar emphysema in the horse. *Adv. Vet. Sci. Comp. Med.* 1969, 13, 59-65.
GROBET L. Mesure de la résistance pulmonaire chez des animaux domestiques par la technique de l'interrupteur du débit aérien. MS thesis, Université de Liège, Liège, Belgium, 1989.

GUSTIN P., LOMBA F., BAKIMA M., LEKEUX P., VAN DE WOESTIJNE K.P. Partitioning of pulmonary resistance in calves. *J. Appl. Physiol.* 1987, 62, 1826-1831.

GUSTIN P., CLERCK C., LOMBA F., LEKEUX P. The topographical distribution of the inhalation-to-perfusion ratio in double-muscled and Friesian calves. *Vet. Res. Commun.* 1988a, 12, 401-405.

GUSTIN P., DHEM A.R., LEKEUX P., LOMBA F., LANDSER F.J., VAN DE WOESTIJNE K.P. Cardio-pulmonary function values in double-muscled cattle during muscular exercise. *Vet. Res. Commun.* 1988b, 12, 407-416.

GUSTIN P., DHEM A.R., LOMBA F., LEKEUX P., LANDSER F.J., VAN DE WOESTIJNE K.P. Measurement of total respiratory impedance in calves by the forced oscillation technique. *J. Appl. Physiol.* 1988c, 64, 1786-1791.

GUSTIN P., DE GROOTE A., DHEM A.J., LOMBA F., LEKEUX P. A comparison of PO_2, PCO_2, pH and bicarbonate in blood from the carotid and coccygeal arteries of calves. *Vet. Res. Commun.* 1988d, 12, 343-346.

HANNON J.P., BOSSONE C.A., WADE C.E. Normal physiological values for conscious pigs used in biomedical research. *Lab. Anim. Sci.* 1990, 10, 293-298.

HEDENSTIERNA G., NYMAN G., KVART C., FUNKQUIST B. Ventilation-perfusion relationships in the standing horse: an inert gas elimination study. *Equine Vet. J.* 1987, 19, 514-519.

KELMAN G.R., NUNN J.F. Nomograms for correction of blood PO_2, PCO_2, pH, and base excess for time and temperature. *J. Appl. Physiol.* 1966, 21, 1484-1490.

KING L.G., HENDRICKS J.C. Total thoracic compliance measurements: a practical, safe, non-invasive measure of pulmonary function in dogs. In Proceedings : 9th Veterinary Respiratory Symposium (abstract 41.6), Orlando (USA), 1990.

KIORPES A.L., BISGARD G.E., MANOHAR M. Pulmonary function values in healthy Holstein Friesian calves. *Am. J. Vet. Res.* 1978, 39, 773-778.

KLEIN H.-J., DEEGEN E. Histamine inhalation provocation test: method to identify nonspecific airway reactivity in equids. *Am. J. Vet. Res.* 1986, 47, 1796-1800.

KOTERBA A.M., KOSCH P.C., BEECH J., WHITLOCK T. Breathing strategy of the adult horse (*Equus caballus*) at rest. *J. Appl. Physiol.* 1988, 64, 337-346.

LAWSON G.H.K., McPHERSON E.A., MURPHY J.R., NICHOLSON J.M., WOODING P., BREEZE R.G., PIRIE H.M. The presence of precipitating antibodies in the sera of horses with chronic obstructive pulmonary disease (COPD). *Equine Vet. J.* 1979, 11, 172-176.

LEKEUX P., HAJER R., BREUKINK H.J. Pulmonary function testing in calves : technical data. *Am. J. Vet. Res.* 1984a, 45, 342-345.

LEKEUX P., HAJER R., BREUKINK H.J. Elastic properties of the oesophageal wall in the dynamic measurement of intrathoracic pressure in cattle. *Res. Vet. Sci.* 1984b, 37, 366-367.

LEKEUX P., HAJER R., BREUKINK H.J. Intrathoracic pressure measurement in cattle: standardized procedure. *Can. J. Comp. Med.* 1984c, 48, 420-421.

LEKEUX P., HAJER R., BREUKINK H.J. Upper airway resistance in healthy Friesian cattle. *Res. Vet. Sci.* 1985, 38, 77-79.

LEKEUX P., ART T., CLERCX C., GUSTIN P. Influence of inertance on measurements of the mechanical properties of the bovine respiratory system. *Vet. Res. Commun.* 1988a, 12, 61-66.

LEKEUX P., ART T., AMORY H. The effect of common bovine respiratory diseases on tidal breathing flow-volume loops. *Vet. Res. Commun.* 1988b, 12, 463-473.

LE NINIVIN A., CLOSE R., ART T., LEKEUX P. Pulmonary function testing in horses by the monofrequency forced oscillation method: a preliminary study. In Proceedings : 10th Comparative Respiratory Society Meeting, East Lansing, (USA), Sept. 1991, p9.

LENS E., POSTIAUX G., CHAPELLE P. Noctural asthma monotoring by automated spectral analysis of respiratory sounds. Abstract. *Clin. Resp. Physiol.* 1987, 23, p423.

LINDFORD R.L., O'BRIEN T.R., WHEAT J.D., MEAGHER D.M. Radiographic assessment of epiglottic length and pharyngeal and laryngeal diameters in the Thouroughbred. *Am. J. Vet. Res.* 1983, 44, 1660-1666.

LITTLEJOHN A., BOWLES F. Studies on the physiopathology of chronic obstructive pulmonary disease in the horse : 5. Blood gas and acid-base values during exercise. *Onderstespoort J. Vet. Res.* 1981, 48, 239-249.

MANOHAR M. Furosemide attenuates the exercise-induced rise in pulmonary artery wedge pressure in horses. *The Physiologist* 1992, 35, 231.

McKIERNAN B.C., DYE J.A., ROZANSKI E.A., JONES S.D., HAYES B. Lung resistance and dynamic compliance in normal cats. In Proceedings : 8th Veterinary Respiratory Symposium, Liege, 1989, p24.

McKIERNAN B.C. Pulmonary function testing in dogs and cats: techniques for clinical use. In Proceedings : 10th Veterinary Respiratory Symposium, East Lansing (USA), 1991, 14-22.

McPHERSON E.A., LAWSON G.H.K., MURPHY J.R., NICHOLSON J., BREEZE R.G., PIRIE H.M. Chronic obstructive pulmonary disease (COPD) in horses : aetiological studies : responses to intradermal and inhalation antigenic challenge. *Equine Vet. J.* 1979, 11, 159-166.

MEAD J., WHITTENBERGER J.L. Evaluation of airway interruption as a method for measuring airflow resistance. *J. Appl. Physiol.* 1954, 6, 408-416.

MESSINA J.E., BISGARD G.E., ROBINSON G.M. Pulmonary function changes in goats given 3-methylindole orally. *Am. J. Vet. Res.* 1984, 45, 1526-1531.

MITCHELL B., WILLIAMS J.T. Normal blood-gas values in lamb during neonatal development and in adult sheep. *Res. Vet. Sci.* 1975, 19, 335-336.

MOORE M.P., ANDREWS F., REED S.M., GRANT B.D. Electromyographic evaluation of horses with laryngeal hemiplegia. *Equine Vet. Sci.* 1988, 8, 424-427.

MORRIS E.A., SEEHERMAN H.J. Evaluation of upper respiratory tract function during strenuous exercise in racehorses. *J. Am. Vet. Med. Assoc.* 1990, 196, 431-438.

MUIR W.W., MOORE C.A., HAMLIN R.L. Ventilatory alterations in normal horses in response to changes in inspired oxygen and carbon dioxide. *Am. J. Vet. Res.* 1975, 36, 155-159.

MUYLLE E., VAN DEN HENDE C., OYAERT W. Nitrogen clearance in horses as a respiratory function test. *J. Vet. Med. A* 1972, 19, 310-317.

MUYLLE E., NUYTTEN J., DEPREZ P., VAN DEN HENDE C., OYAERT W. Pulmonary driving pressure as a pulmonary function test in horses. *Equine Vet. Sci.* 1982, **4**, 57-59.

NELSON R.G., HAMPE D.W. Measurement of tracheal mucus transport rate in the horse. *Am. J. Vet. Res.* 1983, 44, 1165-1166.

O'CALLAGHAN M.W., GOULDEN B.E. Radiographic changes in the lungs of horses with exercise-induced epistaxis. *N. Z. Vet. J.* 1982, 30, 117-118.

O'CALLAGHAN M.W., HORNOF W.J., FISHER P.E., PASCOE J.R. Exercise-induced pulmonary haemorrhage in the horses: results of a detailed clinical, post-mortem and imaging study. VII. Ventilation/perfusion scintigraphy in horses with EIPH. *Equine Vet. J.* 1987, 19, 423-427.

PERSSON S.G.B., ESSEN B., LINDHOLM A. Oxygen uptake, red-cell volume and pulse work relationship in different states of training in horses. In Proceedings : 5th Meeting of the Academy of the Society of Large Animal in Veterinary Medicine, University of Glasgow, 1980, 34-43.

POWERS S.K., DODD S., FREEMAN J., AYERS G.D., SAMSON H., McKNIGHT T. Accuracy of pulse oximetry to estimate HbO_2 fraction of total Hb during exercise. *J. Appl. Physiol.* 1989, 67, 300-304.

REINHOLD P., CLOSE R., LEKEUX P. Validation of the monofrequency forced oscillation technique for pulmonary function investigation in calves : an in vitro and in vivo study. *Res. Vet. Sci.* 1992, 53, 165-171.

ROBINSON N.E., DERKSEN F.J., SLOCOMBE R.F. Determination of the site of airway obstruction using gases of differing density. In : *Equine Exercise Physiology*, Snow, D.H., Persson, S.G.B., Rose, R.J., (Eds), Granta Editions, Cambridge, 1983, pp 71-75.

ROLLIN F., DESMECHT D., GENICOT B., LINDEN A., LEKEUX P. Effect of inhalation of the eructed gases on the breathing pattern in cattle. In Proceedings : 9th Comparative Respiratory Society Meeting, Orlando (USA), 1990, p21(4).

ROSE R.J., HODGSON D.R., KELSO T.B., McCUTCHEON L.J., REID T.-A., BAYLY W.M., GOLLNICK P.D. Maximum O_2 uptake, O_2 debt and deficit, and muscle metabolites in Thoroughbred horses. *J. Appl. Physiol.* 1988, 64, 781-788.

SAUDER R.A., McNICOL K.J., STENCEKO A.A. Effect of age on lung mechanics and airways reactivity in lambs. *J. Appl. Physiol.* 1986, 61, 2074-2080.

SEEHERMAN H.J., MORRIS E.A. Methodology and repeatability of a standardised treadmill exercise test for clinical evaluation of fitness in horses. *Equine Vet. J.* 1990, suppl 9, 20-25.

SLOCOMBE R.F., ROBINSON N.E., DERKSEN F.J. Effect of vagotomy on respiratory mechanics and gas exchange in the neonatal calf. *Am. J. Vet. Res.* 1982, 43, 1168-1171.

SLOCOMBE R.F., DERKSEN F.J., ROBINSON N.E. Interactions of cold stress and *Pasteurella haemolytica* in the pathogenesis of pneumonic pasteurellosis in calves: changes in pulmonary function. *Am. J. Vet. Res.* 1984, 45, 1764-1770.

SLOCOMBE R., BROCK K., COVELLI G., BAYLY W. Effect of treadmill exercise on intrapleural, transdiaphragmatic and intraabdominal pressures in standardbred horses. In : *Equine Exercise Physiology 3*, Persson, S.G.B., Lindholm, A., Jeffcott, L.B., (Eds), ICEEP Publications, Davis, California, 1991, pp 83-91.

SMITH M.M., GOURLEY I.A., KURPERSHOEK C., AMIS T.C. Evaluation of a modified castellated laryngofissure for alleviation of upper airway obstruction in dogs with laryngeal paralysis. *J. Am. Vet. Med. Assoc.* 1986, 188, 1279-1283.

SPÖRRI H., LEEMAN W. Zur Untersuchung der Lungenmechanik bei Grosstieren (Research on lung mechanics in large animals). *Schw. Arch. Teirh.* 1964, 106, 699-714.

SWEENEY C.R. Tracheal mucus transport rate in healthy horses. *Am. J. Vet. Res.* 1989, 50, 2135-2137.

TURGUT K., SASSE H.H.L. Influence of clenbuterol on mucociliary transport in healthy horses and horses with chronic obstructive pulmonary disease. *Vet. Rec.* 1989, 125, 526-530.

VERHOEFF J., CRUIJSEN A.L.M., KREMER W.D.J. Mismatching of ventilation and perfusion in calves with natural bovine respiratory syncytial virus infection. *Vet. Rec.* 1988, 123, 131-134.

VIEL L. Structural-functional correlations of the lung in horses with small airway disease. PhD Thesis, University of Guelph, Guelph, Canada, 1983.

WAGNER P.D., GILLESPIE J.R., LANDGREN G.L., FEDDE M.R., JONES B.W., DEBOWES R.M., PIESCHL R.L, ERICKSON H.H. Mechanism of exercise-induced hypoxemia in horses. *J. Appl. Physiol.* 1989, 66, 1227-1233.

WILLIAMS J.W., PASCOE J.R., MEAGHER D.M., HORNOF W.J. Effects of left recurrent laryngeal neurectomy, prosthetic laryngoplasty, and subtotal arytenoidectomy on upper airway pressure during maximal exertion. *Vet. Surg.* 1990, 19, 136-141.

WILLOUGHBY R.A., McDONELL W.N. Pulmonary function testing in horses. *Vet. Clin. North Am. Large Anim. Pract.* 1979, 1, 171-196.

WILLOUGHBY R.A., ECKER G.L., McKEE S.L., RIDDOLLS L.J. Use of scintigraphy for the determination of mucociliary clearance rates in normal, sedated, diseased and exercised horses. *Can. J. Vet. Res.* 1991, 55, 315-320.

WOAKES A.J., BUTLER P.J., SNOW D.H. The measurement of respiratory airflow in exercising horses. In : *Equine Exercise Physiology 2*, Gillespie, J.R., Robinson, N.E. (Eds), ICEEP Publication, Davis, California, 1987, 194-205.

YOUNG S.S., HALL L.W. A rapid, non-invasive method for measuring total respiratory impedance in the horse. *Equine Vet. J.* 1989, 21, 99-105.

CHAPTER III

STRUCTURE-FUNCTION RELATIONSHIPS OF THE RESPIRATORY SYSTEM IN DOMESTIC ANIMALS

P. Lekeux[1] and T. Art[2]

[1] Laboratory for Functional Investigation
[2] Equine Sport Medicine Unit
Faculty of Veterinary Medicine
University of Liege

SUMMARY

This paper analyses some structure/function relationships of the respiratory system in domestic animals and their potential consequences on pulmonary capacity, performance, dysfunction and injury.

KEY WORDS

Respiratory system - Pulmonary function - Functional morphology.

1. INTRODUCTION

The function and the morphology of an organ are highly influenced by each other. At the long term, in view of the allometric and adaptative variations, the design of all the components making up a system is supposed to be matched to functional demand (Taylor and Weibel, 1981). This hypothesis of "symmorphosis" was shown to be fulfilled for all the links of the oxygen chain, except the pulmonary gas exchanger (Taylor and Weibel, 1991) which shows a redundant capacity in some species, the wild animals for example, or an insufficient capacity in some others, i.e. some domestic animals intensively selected for high performance or production (Lekeux, 1992). The lack of symmorphosis at the level of the respiratory system could be partly explained by an insufficient "structural plasticity" of the pulmonary gas exchange surface in response to chronically modified functional demand. For instance, training at a sufficient intensity and duration is able to increase the cardiac stroke volume by improving the cardiac design (Evans and Rose, 1988). This is not the case for the respiratory system where training has little morphogenetic effect on the lung structures (Art et al, 1992), although it might be somewhat effective at the level of ventilatory muscles.

On the opposite, at the short term point of view, the structure/function relationships are very important in the respiratory system. The external respiration induces important structural changes, mainly during exercise- or disease-induced hyperpnea. The effect of structural peculiarities on the function on the one hand, and the effect on the structures of pressure gradients generated by intense functioning on the other hand are so important both in physiological and pathological conditions that these mutual relationships highly influence the efficiency and integrity of the respiratory system.

This paper will analyse some examples of structure/function relationship at different levels of the respiratory system.

2. UPPER AIRWAYS

The main function of the airways is to lead air from the nose to the gas exchanging regions of the lung during inspiration, and in the opposite direction during expiration. Therefore, any change in their structure which modifies their permeability to airflow has also a direct impact on the pulmonary function.

2.1. Nostrils

Nostrils are large and mobile, especially in the equine species. Their particular structure allows their expansion during inspiration. Indeed, some muscles are able to flare the nostrils and to compress the nasal diverticulum in horses. This mechanism is particularly spectacular and of great benefit during exercise-induced hyperventilation. This can be disturbed for example by injury of the facial nerve which provides the motor efferents to the nostrils.

2.2. Nasal cavities

Because of their large turbinates and important vascularisation, the nasal cavities provide a large surface area for heat and water exchanges, but they also provide a large source of airflow resistance. Both sympathetic and parasympathetic fibers are distributed to the nasal cavities. Their stimulation may respectively constrict and dilate the vascular sinuses, which can induce a decrease and an increase of the nasal resistance. On the other hand, factors inducing an increase of the resistance of the nasal cavities (i.e. injuries due to nasal intubation or nasal septum defect) will have deleterious effects mainly during hyperpnea.

Hemorrhages resulting from upper airway endoscopy or the use of a naso-esophageal tube are frequently due to injuries of veins in the nasal septum and ventral concha.

2.3. Pharynx

The soft palate divides the pharynx into the nasopharynx and the oropharynx. Numerous lymphoid follicles are present in the mucous membrane of the dorsal and lateral walls of the nasopharynx and of the dorsal surface of the soft palate. The size of these follicles is particularly large in young horses and usually regresses in mature horses. Pharyngeal lymphoid hyperplasia appears to reflect the immature and hyperreactive condition of the submucosal lymphoid tissue present throughout the pharynx (Burrell, 1985). The clinical significance of this condition and its effect on the performance capability of the horse is still controversial. It appears to have little effect on upper airways function (Williams et al, 1990) and on the race results (Burrell, 1985), and it does not seem to impair gas exchange during exercise unless the lesions are extremely severe (Bayly et al, 1984a). However, in some horses severe pharyngitis may induce abnormal inspiratory noises during exercise. The endoscopic examination of horses suffering from this problem shows that, when the nares are obstructed, the pharyngeal walls tend to collapse easier than in healthy horses. The same horses re-examined after strenuous exercise show a further hypertrophy, and even hyperemia, of the lymphoid follicles. It can therefore be hypothetized that horses suffering from pharyngitis have an abnormally high pharyngeal resistance because, on the one hand, the pharyngeal lumen is reduced by the hypertrophied follicles and, on the other hand, a dynamic collapse of the pharyngeal walls increases further the resistance to airflow.

The stimulation of pharyngeal irritant receptors by mediators released by the lymphoid follicles could also result in reflex bronchoconstriction (Robinson, 1979).

The natural tendency of the soft structures of the nasopharynx to collapse during inspiration is limited by tensor muscle contraction.

The equine guttural pouches are diverticula of the auditory tubes which communicate with the pharynx via a slit-like opening. This structure is also present in some wild animals such as tapir and daman. The function of the guttural pouches is still unknown. They do not seem to influence directly the passage of air through the upper airways. However, these pouches are adjacent to various important structures such as blood vessels (i.e. internal and external carotid arteries), cranial nerves (i.e. vagus, cervical sympathetic trunk, glossopharyngeal nerve, hypoglossal nerve, accessory nerve) and retropharyngeal lymph nodes. Any abnormality, even subclinical, of the guttural pouches is susceptible to damage these structures and consequently to induce some dysfunction. For example, a lesion of the glossopharyngeal nerve and the vagus may induce a paralysis and dorsal displacement of the soft palate.

From a functional point of view, the most important structural peculiarity of the equine upper airways is the intrapharyngeal ostium, which is an opening in the soft palate bounded caudo-dorsally by the palatopharyngeal wall, laterally by the pillars of the soft palate and rostrally by the visible border of the soft palate. The laryngeal structures, i.e. the corniculate cartilages and the epiglottis, articulate with the ostium like a button in a button hole (Cook, 1989), forming an airtight seal when the horse breathes (Fig. 3-1.). This peculiar arrangement explains why the horse is a compulsory nasal breather, in contrast with the other domestic animals. Indeed, because of this anatomical characteristic, the equine species, unlike other animals and man, is not able to switch from nasal to oro-nasal breathing when the nasal resistance to airflow becomes too high, namely during exercise- or disease-induced hyperventilation.

Therefore, in horses, the displacement of the caudal border of the soft palate to a position above the epiglottis, called dorsal displacement of the soft palate, is not physiological, except when it occurs during swallowing, coughing or whinnying. In all other conditions, this dorsal displacement is abnormal in this species and will induce dyspnea especially during strenuous exercise. It induces a narrowing of the upper airways and causes flapping of the soft palate, sometimes inducing a dramatic asphyxia in racing horses.

The caudal margin of the intrapharyngeal ostium may also be rostrally displaced onto the corniculate processes of the arytenoid cartilages. In this position, it obstructs the laryngeal aperture and, presumably inhibiting abduction of the arytenoid cartilages, it thus increases the resistance to airflow.

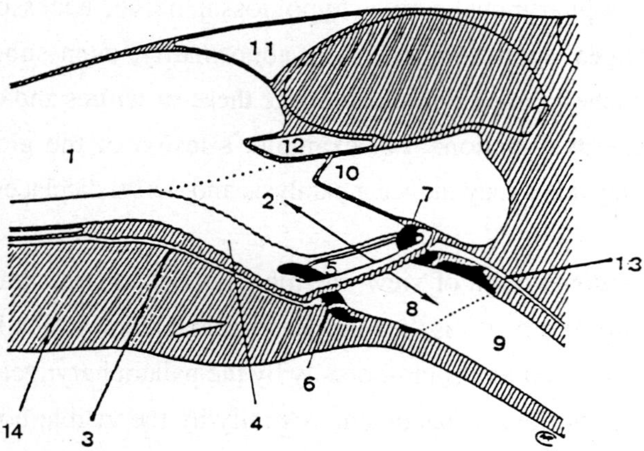

Fig. 3-1. Lateral view of the equine upper airways during normal breathing. 1 : Nasal cavity; 2 : Naso-pharynx; 3 : Oro-pharynx; 4 : Soft palate; 5 : Intrapharyngeal ostium ("button hole"); 6 : Epiglottis; 7 : Corniculate cartilage; 8 : Larynx; 9 : Trachea; 10 : Guttural pouch; 11 : Frontal sinus; 12 : Sphenopalatine sinus; 13 : Esophagus; 14 : Tongue (Cook, 1989).

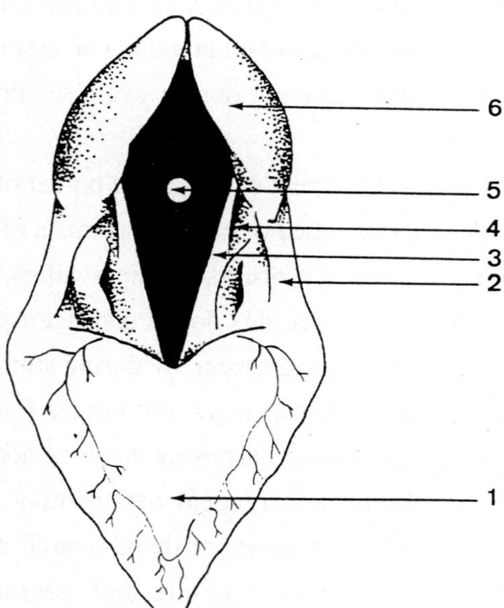

Fig. 3-2. Front view of the equine larynx. 1 : Epiglottis; 2 : Ary-epiglottic fold; 3 : Vocal cord; 4 : Laryngeal ventricle; 5 : Glottis; 6 : Corniculate cartilage.

2.4. Larynx

The structural and functional peculiarities of the larynx make this structure a potential bottleneck in the upper airways. The rostral parts of the laryngeal cartilages constitute the aditus laryngis. This pharyngeal opening is formed dorsally by the corniculate cartilages, laterally by the vocal folds and ventrally by the epiglottis (Fig. 3-2.). The aditus laryngis can vary from a tight seal, i.e. full adduction of the laryngeal structures during swallowing in order to protect the lower airways from ingesta, to a maximal opening, i.e. full abduction of these structures during hyperventilation in order to increase the permeability to high airflow. This full opening is completed by a dilation of the larynx due to contraction of intrinsic muscles which compress the laryngeal ventricles in the horse.

Some animals, like double-muscled cattle, show a proportionally narrow opening of their larynx, which is confirmed by a proportionally higher laryngeal resistance to airflow (Gustin et al, 1987) when compared to conventional cattle (Lekeux et al, 1985). The functional consequence of this structural peculiarity is an increase of the air velocity and therefore of the density of airborne contaminants at this level, which results in a higher frequency of laryngeal injuries in these animals (Lekeux and Art, 1987).

Any impairment of laryngeal dilation due to structural factors such as rostral displacement of the palato-pharyngeal arch in the horse or necrotic laryngitis in cattle, or functional factors such as laryngeal hemiparesis in the horse or laryngeal paralysis in the dog, will be responsible for an inadequate lung ventilation, mainly during hyperpnea, and will generally induce abnormal respiratory noises related to the increased airflow resistance (Venker van Haagen et al, 1978; Bayly et al, 1984b; Derksen et al, 1986; Lekeux and Art, 1987).

2.5. Trachea

The trachea is a long flexible tube formed of cartilaginous rings. Dorsally, these rings are open and completed by the dorsal tracheal membrane

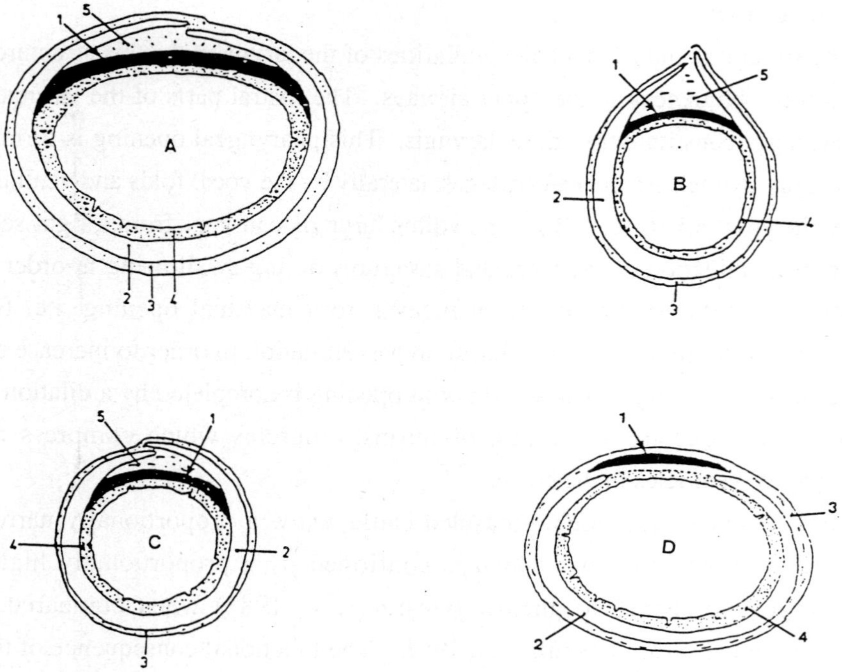

Fig. 3-3. Cross-sectional view of the cervical trachea in horse (A), cattle (B), pig (C) and dog (D). 1 : Tracheal muscle; 2 : Cartilage; 3 : Adventitia; 4 : Mucosa; 5 : Connective tissue (Collin, 1976).

(Fig. 3-3.). The latter contains smooth muscle fibers which are innervated by the autonomic nervous system.

In the horse, the free ends of the tracheal rings overlap in the cervical but not in the thoracic part of the trachea (Hare, 1975). The cross section of the equine trachea is almost circular proximally and distally (transverse diameter : 5.5 cm; sagittal diameter : 5 cm), but half-way the trachea, the lumen is more flattened dorsoventrally (transverse diameter : 7 cm; sagittal diameter : 5 cm). Routine endoscopic evaluations of the lower airways of horses examined for exercise intolerance gave evidence that sometimes there is a sharp lateral narrowing of the intra-thoracic trachea, just before the tracheal bifurcation into

both principal bronchi.
Tracheal smooth muscles take place in the dorsal tracheal membrane. They are innervated by the autonomic nervous system.
Despite its cartilaginous structure, the extrathoracic trachea is quite compliant and is susceptible to collapse by high transmural pressure occurring during forced inspiration (Art and Lekeux, 1991a). However, its compliance is significantly decreased by smooth muscle contraction (due for instance to exercise-induced adrenal discharge) and by tracheal distension (due for instance to exercise-induced head and neck stretching). Moreover, the resistance to collapse is also dependent on the shape of tracheal cross-section. From this point of view, not all animals seem to be equal. Indeed, the ratio between the transverse and sagittal diameters varies, in horses for instance, from 0.9 (i.e. circular shape) to 2 (i.e. elliptic shape) with a mean value of 1.4 (Fig. 3-4.) (Art and Lekeux, 1991b). The more ellipsoid the trachea, the more compressible it is. Therefore, horses with a transverse to sagittal diameters ratio higher than 1.5 are disadvantaged and more susceptible to present an exercise intolerance due to insuffisant lung ventilation. The size and age of the horse do not influence the compliance of the trachea (Art and Lekeux, 1991b).
This airway collapse is a good illustration of the fact that an inappropriate structure/function relationship can lead to a vicious circle. Indeed, a narrowing of the upper airways increases the resistance to airflow, which results in highly negative intratracheal pressure during inspiration. The resulting compressing transmural pressure induces some tracheal collapse which further increases the resistance to airflow.
The tracheal collapse is not limited to the equine species and is related in all species to both structural factors, i.e. design and compliance of the cartilaginous rings, and functional factors, i.e. compressing transmural pressure during respiration.
The length and dead space of the trachea affect also the respiratory mechanics at the level of the lung ventilation, influencing the inertial pressures necessary to accelerate the tracheal gases (Art et al, 1989). From a comparative point of

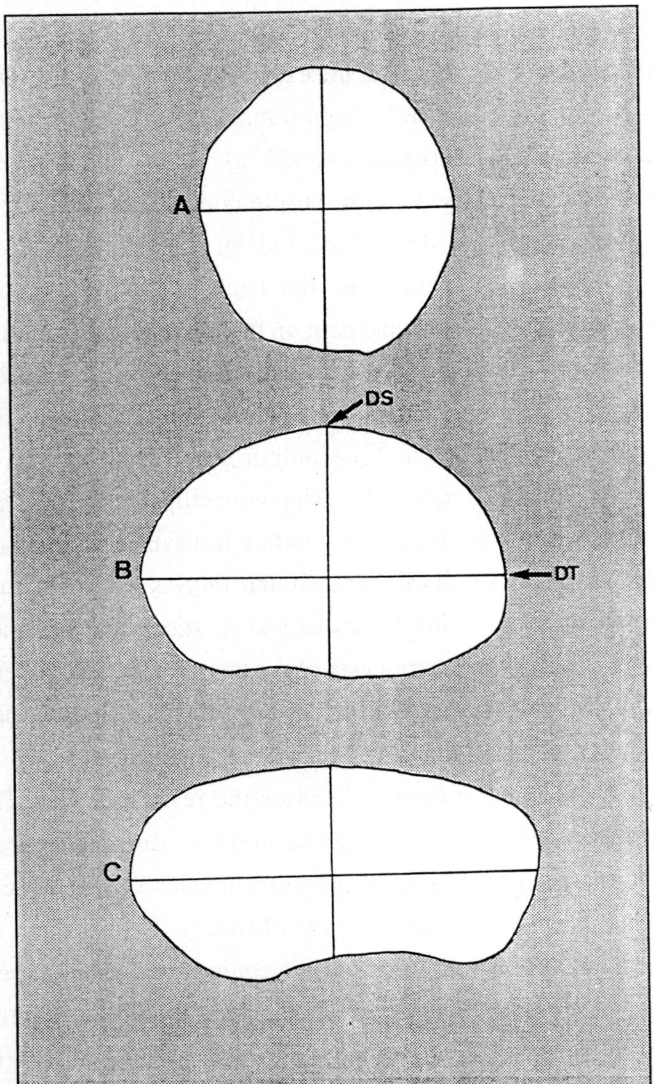

Fig. 3-4. Cross-sectional shapes of equine trachea with transverse (DT) to sagittal (DS) diameter ratios of 0.920 (A), 1.472 (B) and 2.175 (C), respectively (Art et al, 1991b).

view, the trumpeter swan presents an extreme example of tracheal elongation, which is useful for the phonation in this species (Banko, 1960).

3. LOWER AIRWAYS

After the bifurcation of the trachea into the right and left principal bronchi, the bronchial tree ramifies many times to the periphery of the lung through the primary bronchi, the segmental bronchi, the bronchioles and the terminal bronchioles.

These intrathoracic conducting airways are also susceptible to collapse when the transmural pressures exerced on their wall are compressing. This is particularly true at the level of the small airways which do not have cartilaginous support. However, in contrast with extrathoracic airways where the partial dynamic collapse occurs only during inspiration, the collapse of small airways occurs only during forced expiration, i.e. when the extraluminal pressure is more positive than the intraluminal pressure.

With airway generation, the individual diameter and length of the airways decrease but the total cross-sectional area increases. Therefore, the small airways are not a bottleneck in the healthy animal and represent only a small part of the total resistance to airflow.

4. LUNG TISSUES

The lungs of domestic animals may be subdivided into three types based upon their subgross anatomy (McLaughlin et al, 1961).

Type 1 lungs, i.e. in cattle, sheep and pig, show well developed lobulation with secondary lobules distinctly separated by complete fascial sheaths. Their pleural covering is thick and respiratory bronchioles are rare.

Type 2 lungs, i.e. in dog, cat and monkey, are not subdivided into secondary lobules. Their pulmonary pleura is thin and respiratory bronchioles are well developed.

Type 3 lungs, i.e. in horse and pony, have incomplete connective tissue septa between secondary lobules. Their pleural covering is thick and their

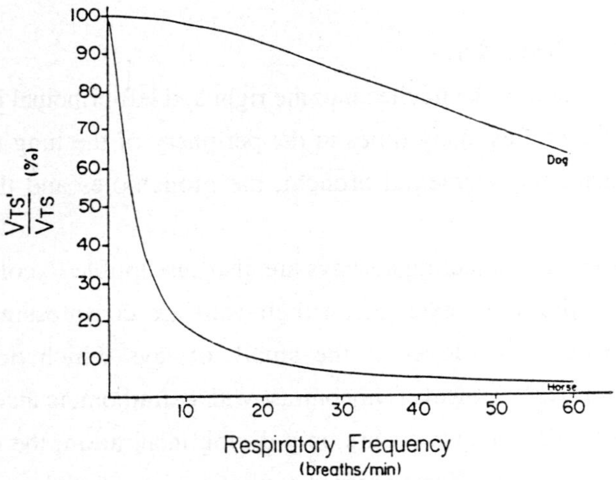

Fig. 3-5. Efficiency of the collateral ventilation as a function of respiratory rate in 2 species. VTS : Volume ventilated via the usual pathways; VTS' : Volume ventilated via the collateral pathways (Robinson ans Sorenson, 1978).

respiratory bronchioles are poorly developed.

Movement of air between adjacent regions of lung through pathways other than the tracheobronchial tree is called collateral ventilation, i.e. the transfer of air via accessory pathways like interalveolar pores of Kohn, canals of Lambert and communicating respiratory bronchioles and alveolar ducts described by Martin.

This collateral ventilation may partially compensate the ventilation in areas with obstruction of the small airways. Collateral ventilation is inexistant in type 1 lungs, important in type 2 lungs and intermediate in type 3 lungs (Robinson, 1982). Indeed, in horses these accessory pathways present a high resistance to airflow and are only able to provide a maximum of 16 % of the required respiratory volume, which is a very little proportion compared to the

96 % recorded in the canine lung (Fig. 3-5.) (Robinson and Sorenson, 1978). These percentages of course decrease with any increase in respiratory frequency (Robinson, 1982). Therefore these pathways are probably of high value for the small animal pulmonary function and of limited value for the equine pulmonary function, except maybe for the prevention of atelectasis in horses suffering from airway obstruction.

On the other hand, the high anatomical compartmentalization of the bovine and porcine lungs may be considered as a disadvantage during obstructive diseases, because it impedes any collateral ventilation (Lekeux et al, 1984), or as an advantage during infectious diseases, because it helps to contain the infectious process (Veit and Farrell, 1978).

Another important aspect of the structure/function relationships in the lung is the mechanical interaction between adjacent regions of the lung parenchyma and between the thorax and the lung. This is called interdependence (Menkes and Traystman, 1977). This mechanism is responsible for lobar differences in direct and collateral ventilation. This could partly explain why the incidence of atelectasis and pneumonia is greater in cranial, middle and accessory pulmonary lobes than in caudal lobes (Robinson, 1982) and why atelectasis is more frequent in animals with high thoracic compliance, such as neonates (Fisher and Wood, 1980).

5. LUNG VASCULARIZATION

The lung receives blood from two circulations (Table 3-1.).

The *pulmonary circulation* receives the total cardiac output from the right heart. The branches of the pulmonary trunk carry venous blood to the lung, accompany the bronchi and form rich capillary plexuses on the walls of the alveoli.

Vasoconstriction of the small pulmonary arteries may be induced by hypoxia. The intensity of this hypoxic vasoconstriction varies from species to species and is correlated with the thickness of the medial smooth muscle layer of these arteries (Tucker et al, 1975).

Table 3-1. Comparison between pulmonary and bronchial circulation.

	Pulmonary	Bronchial
Aims	gas exchange venous blood filtration blood reservoir	nutrition of airways, vessels and visceral pleura thermoregulation
Structure	right ventricle ↓ pulmonary artery ↓ pulmonary arterioles ↓ pulmonary capillaries ↓ pulmonary veins ←	left ventricle ↓ bronchial and bronchoesophageal arteries ↓ peribronchial plexus subepithelial plexus pleural, vascular and ganglia pl. ↓ azygos veins
Blood flow	± 99 % of the right ventricle	± 2 % of the left ventricle
Capillary flow	pulsatile	constant

Cattle and pigs, which present the greatest response to hypoxia, have the thickest muscular layer. Dogs and cats, which fail to develop pulmonary hypertension, have the thinnest muscular layer. Horses and goats show an intermediate response (Robinson, 1982).

This hypoxic vasoconstriction may be considered as an advantage when it contributes to improve the ventilation/perfusion adequation, by matching the local blood flow to the local ventilation (Marshall et al, 1981). On the other hand, during chronic hypoxia, an excessive vasoconstriction induces pulmonary hypertension which can lead to right heart insufficiency in some species (Will et al, 1975).

The *bronchial circulation*, a branch of the systemic circulation, carries arterial blood for the nutrition of the lung structures. It originates from two arteries : (1) the broncho-esophageal artery, supplying the airways and interlobular septa of most of the lung, and (2) the right apical bronchial artery, supplying the airways of the right apical lobe. Bronchial arteries form a circulatory plexus in the connective tissues along the airways. Branches from this plexus penetrate the bronchial walls to form a sub-epithelial vascular plexus, the role of which is probably to ensure some heat dissipation. The bronchial circulation is drained by either the azygos or the pulmonary veins.

Pulmonary and bronchial circulations anastomose at the level of the terminal bronchioles. Most of these anastomoses occur at the level of the capillaries and veins rather than at the level of the arteries (Magno and Fishman, 1982; McLaughlin, 1983).

These anastomoses are frequent in the horse lungs and may be a potential etiological factor for exercise-induced pulmonary hemorrhage, which occurs in 75 % of the racing thoroughbreds (Raphel, 1982). Indeed, micropathological examination of exercise-induced pulmonary hemorrhage lesions shows extensive proliferations of bronchial blood vessels and greatly increased numbers of anastomoses between the bronchial and pulmonary circulations. The extent of the anastomic flow depends on the relative pressure in the bronchial and pulmonary vasculature and on the alveolar pressure (Modell et al, 1981). The increase of the pressure gradient between the bronchial and the pulmonary arteries could perhaps favour bronchial blood flow from the first into the second group of vessels.

6. RIB CAGE

The differences in size, shape and position of the abdomen in relation to the lungs, as well as the high rigidity of the thorax are probably advantageous for the locomotion and for the stabilization of the relaxation volume of the respiratory system during postural changes in the equine species (Leith and Gillespie, 1971). On the other hand, the high thoracic compliance of the neonates in general and the newborn calf in particular is partly responsible for the low functional residual capacity and the high sensitivity to atelectasis of these animals (Slocombe et al, 1982).

7. RESPIRATORY MUSCLES AND THEIR INNERVATION

The diaphragm is the main inspiratory muscle. It is a domed musculotendinous sheet separating the abdomen and the thorax. Its insertion to the rib cage is put forward in production animals, such as cattle and pig, when compared to athletic species, such as horse and dog. This influences directly the specific volume of the thoracic cavity.

The *phrenic nerve*, which innervates the diaphragm, comes from the cervical cord and lies on both sites of the heart. In horses suffering from electrolytes imbalance (after prolonged sudation, diarrhea, ...) the phrenic nerve may become hyperexcitable, and, sometimes, a diaphragmatic flutter may be observed, i.e. diaphragmatic contraction in phase with cardiac depolarization.

The laryngeal muscles are innervated by *the recurrent nerves*. The recurrent nerve is one of the longest nerves of the body. The left laryngeal nerve originates from the brain, travels down the neck into the chest as a part of the vagus. At the level of the heart, the recurrent nerve branches off the 10th cranial nerve and become an individual nerve, which has to travel all the way back up the neck before it finally reaches the larynx. The high incidence of left laryngeal hemiplegia in the horse has been related to neural injuries due to the specific course of the left recurrent laryngeal nerve. However, this theory is challenged by the occurrence of right hemiplegia in this species.

8. ABDOMINAL PISTON

When a coupling exists between locomotion and respiration in athletic animals, it seems that the "abdominal piston" acts in synergy with the respiratory pump (Fig. 3-6.) (Art et al, 1990). Therefore, this strategy probably reduces the cost of breathing. During gallop, there is a compulsory linkage between step and respiratory rates (Bramble and Carrier, 1983; Attenburrow 1982; 1983; Young et al, 1992). This is probably due to a mechanical linkage : the role of the visceral content acting as a piston, the flexion of the back and the loading of the thorax by the forelimbs has been put forward to explain the mechanical advantages of this synchronisation

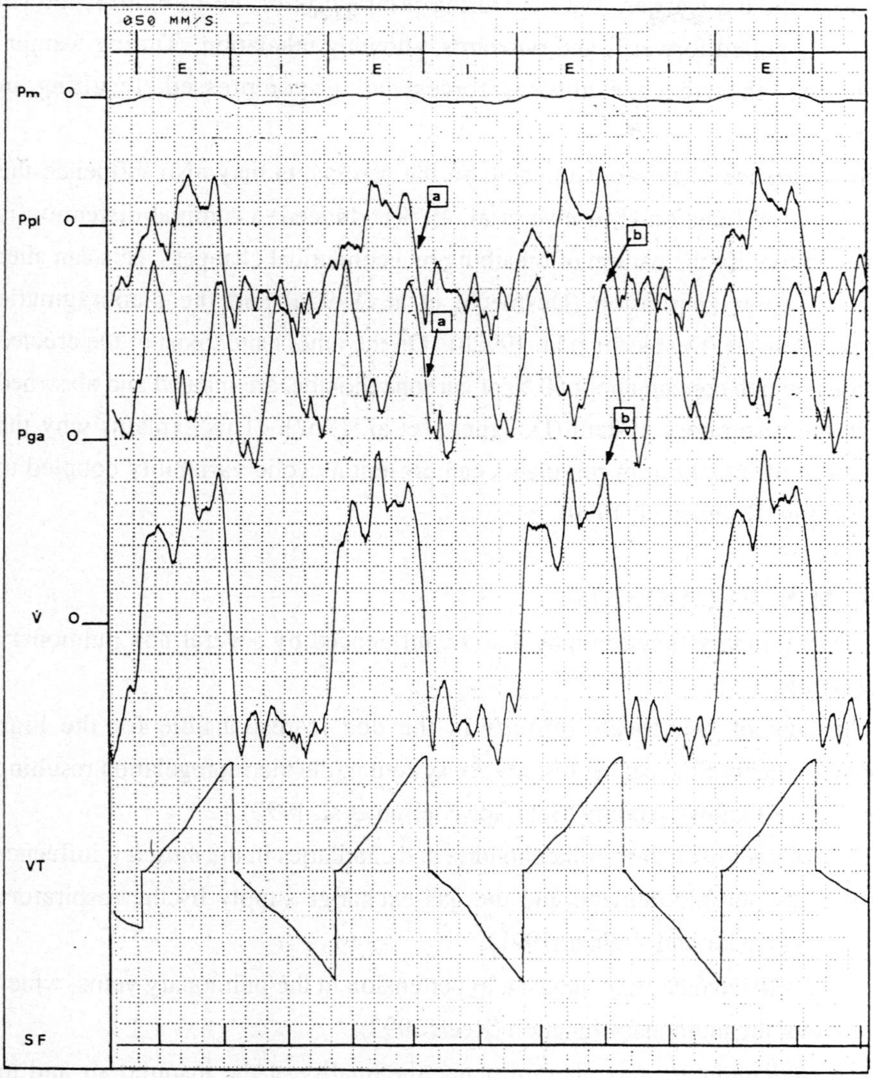

Fig. 3-6. Simultaneous recording of mask pressure (Pm), pleural pressure (Ppl), gastric pressure (Pga), respiratory airflow ($\dot{V}$), tidal volume (VT) and step frequency (SF) in a pony during the first minute of trot (3.5 $m.s^{-1}$). SF was retraced from the original recordings. The SF/Respiratory frequency ratio was 2/1; Ppl and Pga decreased simultaneously during the first part of inspiration (point a) and expiratory peaks $\dot{V}$ were simultaneous with Pga peaks (point b); I : Inspiration; E : Expiration (Art et al, 1990).

(Bramble and Carrier, 1983). During protraction of the forelimbs, the rib cage is pulled forwards and outwards, allowing inhalation. During weight-bearing, the rib cage absorbs forces and is compressed, resulting in exhalation.

The presence of the forestomachs in the ruminants may also influence the pulmonary function (Musewe et al, 1979). Indeed, a ruminal distention is able to modify the pattern of breathing by geometrical changes. This can alter the alveolar ventilation (Desmecht et al, 1992a) and the diaphragmatic performances (Desmecht et al, 1992b). On the other hand, most of the eructed gases, which contain about 50 % of carbone dioxide, are inhaled and absorbed via the respiratory system (Dougherty et al, 1962). This explains why the pattern of breathing in ruminants can present a cyclic variability coupled to belching (Rollin et al, 1990).

9. MISCELLANEOUS

The pulmonary function may also be influenced by several non pulmonary structures.

The lack of skin *sweat glands* in the dog is responsible for the high involvement of the canine respiratory system in the thermoregulation resulting in the well known panting (Schmidt-Nielsen et al, 1970).

The volumes of both the mitochondria and capillaries in the *muscles* influence the body aerobic demand and the gas exchange supply by the respiratory system (Taylor and Weibel, 1991).

A left *heart defect* may induce a hypertension in the pulmonary veins, which can alter the pulmonary function (Reef, 1992).

The *environment* may also influence the quality of the inspired air and its effects on the mechanics of breathing, the mucociliar clearance and the pulmonary hemodynamics (Rom and Crystal, 1991).

10. CONCLUSIONS

Analysis of structure/function relationships is essential for understanding the functioning of the respiratory system. These interactions are complex and their effects may be weak or strong, uni- or multilateral, short- or long-term, and positive or negative.

In any case, these structure/function relationships are responsible for the capacity and performance of the pulmonary function in physiological conditions and for the type and severity of both pulmonary dysfunctions and injuries in pathological conditions.

REFERENCES

ART T., LEKEUX P., GUSTIN P., DESMECHT D., AMORY H., PAIVA M. Inertance of the respiratory system in ponies. *J. Appl. Physiol.* 1989, 67, 534-540.

ART T., DESMECHT D., AMORY H., LEKEUX P. Synchronization of locomotion and respiration in trotting ponies. *J. Vet. Med. A* 1990, 37, 95-103.

ART T., LEKEUX P. Mechanical properties of the isolated equine trachea. *Res. Vet. Sci.* 1991a, 51, 55-60.

ART T., LEKEUX P. The effect of shape, age, and extension on the compliance of equine tracheal segment. *Vet. Res. Commun.* 1991b, 15, 135-146.

ART T., VOTION D., Mc ENTEE K., AMORY H., LINDEN A., CLOSE R., LEROY P., LEKEUX P. Influence of training on ventilatory and cardio-respiratory parameters measured during a standardised exercise in thoroughbred horses. In Proceedings : 11th Comparative Respiratory Society Meeting, Urbana (USA), September 1992, p1.

ATTENBURROW D.P. Time relationship between the respiratory cycle and limb cycle in the horse. *Equine Vet. J.* 1982, 14, 69-72.

ATTENBURROW D.P. Respiration and locomotion. In : *Equine Exercise Physiology*, Snow, D.H., Persson, S.G.B., Rose, R.J. (Eds), Granta Editions, Cambridge, 1983, pp 17-22.

BANKO W.E. The trupeter swan. North American Fauna, n° 63, Washington D.C. U.S. Dept of the Interior, Fish and Wildlife Service, 1960.

BAYLY W.M., GRANT B.D., BREEZE R.G. Arterial blood gas tensions and acid base balance during exercise in horses with pharyngeal lymphoid hyperplasia. *Equine Vet. J.* 1984a, 16, 435-438.

BAYLY W.M., GRANT B.D., MODRANSKY P.D. Arterial blood gas tensions during exercise in a horse with laryngeal hemiplegia, before and after corrective surgery. *Res. Vet. Sci.* 1984b, 36, 256-258.

BRAMBLE D.M., CARRIER D.R. Running and breathing in mammals. *Science* 1983, 219, 251-256.

BURRELL M.H. Endoscopic and virological observations on respiratory disease in a group of young thoroughbred horses in training. *Equine Vet. J.* 1985, 17, 99-103.

COLLIN B. Atlas d'Anatomie. Ed. Université de Liège, Liège, Belgium, 1976.

COOK W.R. Specifications for speed in the racehorse : the Airflow Factors, The Russell Meerdink Company Ltd, Menasha, Wi, 1989.

DERKSEN F.J., SCOTT E.A., STICK J.A., ROBINSON N.E., SLOCOMBE R.F. Effect of laryngeal hemiplegia and laryngoplasty on upper airway flow mechanics in exercising horses. *Am. J. Vet. Res.* 1986, 47, 16-20.

DESMECHT D., LINDEN A., LEKEUX P. Features of pulmonary ventilation, mechanics and gas transport during ruminal distention in cattle. In Proceedings : 11th Comparative Respiratory Society Meeting, Urbana (USA), September 1992a, p6.

DESMECHT D., LINDEN A., LEKEUX P. Alteration in the electromechanical coupling of the diaphragm is associated with ruminal tympanism in cattle. In Proceedings : 11th Comparative Respiratory Society Meeting, Urbana (USA), September 1992b, p3.

DOUGHERTY R.W., STEWART W.E., NOLD M.M., LINDAHL I.L., MULLENAX C.H., LEEK B.F. Pulmonary absorption of eructated gas in ruminants. *Am. J. Vet. Res.* 1962, 23, 205-212.

EVANS D.L., ROSE R.J. Cardiovascular and respiratory responses to submaximal exercise training in the thoroughbred horse. *Pflügers Arch.* 1988, 411, 316-321.

FISHER C.J., WOOD L.D.H. Effect of lobar acid injury on pulmonary perfusion and gas exchange in dogs. *J. Appl. Physiol. : Respirat. Environ. Exercise Physiol.* 1980, 49, 150-156.

GUSTIN P., BAKIMA M., LEKEUX P., LOMBA F., VAN DE WOESTIJNE K.P. Partitioning of upper airway resistance in Friesian and double-muscled calves. *Respir. Physiol.* 1987, 69, 299-306.

HARE W.C.D. Equine respiratory system. In : *Sisson and Grossman's The Anatomy of the Domestic Animals,* 5th edn, Volume 1, Getty, R. (Ed.), W.B. Saunders Company, Philadelphia, 1975, pp 498-523.

LEITH D.E., GILLESPIE J.R. Respiratory mechanics of normal horses and one with chronic obstructive lung disease. *Fed. Proc.* 1971, 30, 551.

LEKEUX P., HAJER R., BREUKINK H.J. Effect of somatic growth on pulmonary function values in healthy Friesian cattle. *Am. J. Vet. Res.* 1984, 45, 2003-2007.

LEKEUX P., HAJER R., BREUKINK H.J. Upper airway resistance in healthy Friesian cattle. *Res. Vet. Sci.* 1985, 38, 77-79.

LEKEUX P., ART T. Functional changes induced by necrotic laryngitis in double-muscled calves. *Vet. Rec.* 1987, 121, 353-355.

LEKEUX P. La fonction respiratoire en tant que facteur potentiellement limitant de la santé, des productions et des performances animales. *Ann. Méd. Vét.* 1992, 136, 560-564.

MAGNO M.G., FISHMAN A.P. Origin, distribution and blood flow of bronchial circulation in anesthetized sheep. *J. Appl. Physiol.* 1982, 53, 272-279.

MARSHALL B.E., MARSHALL C., BENUMOF J., SAIDMAN L. Hypoxic pulmonary vasoconstriction in dogs: effects of lung segment size and oxygen tension. *J. Appl. Physiol.* 1981, 51, 1543-1551.

McLAUGHLIN R.F., TYLER W.S., CANADA R.O. A study of subgross pulmonary anatomy in various mammals. *Am. J. Anat.* 1961, 108, 149-165.

McLAUGHLIN R.F. Jr. Bronchial artery distribution in various mammals and in humans. *Am. Rev. Respir. Dis.* 1983, 128, S57-S58.

MENKES H., TRAYSTMAN R.J. State of the art: collateral ventilation. *Am. J. Vet. Res.* 1977, 116, 287-309.

MODELL H.E., BECK K., BUTLER J. Functional aspects of canine bronchial-pulmonary vascular communications. *J. Appl. Physiol.* 1981, 50, 1045-1051.

MUSEWE V.O., GILLESPIE J.R., BERRY J.D. Influence of ruminal insufflation on pulmonary function and diaphragmatic electromyography in cattle. *Am. J. Vet. Res.* 1979, 40, 26-31.

RAPHEL C.F. Endoscopic findings in the upper respiratory tract of 479 horses. *J. Am. Vet. Med. Assoc.* 1982, 181, 470-473.

REEF V.B. Cardiovascular problems associated with poor performance. In : *Current Therapy in Equine Medicine 3*, section 9, *Cardiovascular Disease*, Robinson, N.E. (Ed.), Saunders Company, Philadelphia, 1992, pp 381-383.

ROBINSON N.E., SORENSON P.R. Collateral flow resistance and time constant in dog and horse lungs. *J. Appl. Physiol.* 1978, 44, 63-68.

ROBINSON N.E. Functional abnormalities caused by upper airway obstruction and heaves: their relationship to the etiology of epistaxis. *Vet. Clin. North Am. Large Anim. Pract.* 1979, 1, 17-34.

ROBINSON N.E. Some functional consequences of species differences in lung anatomy. *Adv. Vet. Sci. Comp. Med.* 1982, 26, 1-33.

ROLLIN F., DESMECHT D., GENICOT B., LINDEN A., LEKEUX P. Effect of inhalation of the eructed gases on the breathing pattern in cattle. *The Physiologist* 1990, 33, p44.

ROM W.N., CRYSTAL R.G. Consequences of chronic inorganic dust exposure. In : *The Lung Scientific Foundations*, volume 2, Crystal, R.G., West, J.B. (Eds), Raven Press, New York, 1991, pp 1885-1897.

SCHMIDT-NIELSEN K., BRETZ W.L., TAYLOR C.R. Panting in dogs: unidirectional air flow over evaporative surfaces. *Science* 1970, 169, 1102-1104.

SLOCOMBE R.F., ROBINSON N.E., DERKSEN F.J. Effect of vagotomy on respiratory mechanics and gas exchange in the neonatal calf. *Am. J. Vet. Res.* 1982, 43, 1168-1171.

TAYLOR C.R., WEIBEL E.R. Design of the mammalian respiratory system. I. Problem and strategy. *Respir. Physiol.* 1981, 44, 1-10.

TAYLOR C.R., WEIBEL E.R. Learning from comparative physiology. In : *The Lung Scientific Foundations*, volume 2, Crystal, R.G., West, J.B. (Eds), Raven Press, New York, 1991, pp 1595-1607.

TUCKER A., McMURTRY I.F., REEVES J.T., ALEXANDER A.F., WILL D.H., GROVER R.F. Lung vascular smooth muscle as a determinant of pulmonary hypertension at high altitude. *Am. J. Physiol.* 1975, 228, 762-767.

VEIT H.P., FARRELL R.L. The anatomy and physiology of the bovine respiratory system relating to pulmonary disease. *Cornell Vet.* 1978, 68, 555-581.

VENKER-VAN HAAGEN A.J., HARTMAN W., GOEDEBUURE S.A. Spontaneous laryngeal paralysis in young Bouviers. *J. Am. An. Hosp. Ass.* 1978, 14, 714-721.

WILL D.H., HICKS J.L., CARD C.S., REEVES J.T., ALEXANDER A.F. Correlation of acute with chronic hypoxic pulmonary hypertension in cattle. *J. Appl. Physiol.* 1975, 38, 495-498.

WILLIAMS J.W., MEAGHER D.M., PASCOE J.R., HORNOF W.J. Upper airway function during maximal exercise in horses with obstructive upper airway lesions. Effect of surgical treatment. *Vet. Surg.* 1990, 19, 142-147.

YOUNG I.S., WARREN R.D., ALTRINGHAM J.D. Some properties of the mammalian locomotory and respiratory systems in relation to body mass. *J. exp. Biol.* 1992, 164, 283-294.

CHAPTER IV

MECHANICS OF BREATHING IN RESTING AND EXERCISING ANIMALS

P. Lekeux[1] and T. Art[2]

[1] Laboratory for Functional Investigation
[2] Equine Sport Medicine Unit
Faculty of Veterinary Medicine
University of Liege

SUMMARY

This review paper describes the principles and applications of the mechanics of breathing in domestic animals, taking into account the effects of species, breed, age and exercise.

KEY WORDS

Respiratory system - Pulmonary function - Mechanics of breathing

1. INTRODUCTION

The respiratory system consists of the lungs which act as a gas exchanger, and of the chest wall which acts as a pump. This last property was recognized much earlier than the first one. Indeed, the role of the diaphragm and the other ventilatory muscles in breathing was described by Erasistratus (300 B.C.) and Galen (150), respectively. Later, Leonardo da Vinci (1500) concluded that the lungs expand like bellows. Many other scientists like Rohrer, who formulated quantitative respiratory mechanics, and Fenn, who elaborated pressure/volume relationship, contributed to the understanding of the mechanics of breathing.

Volume changes of the respiratory apparatus imply work performed on the respiratory system, mainly expanding or compressing the gas in the lungs, and displacing it in and out of the airways. The driving forces exerted by the respiratory muscles are opposed mainly by static forces (elastic, gravitational and surface) and dynamic flow resistive forces (viscous and turbulent resistance of the gases and viscous resistance of the tissues). The inertial forces (i.e. the pressure necessary to accelerate the airflow), are negligible at rest but are of importance in hyperventilating large animals.

Therefore, at each time of the respiratory cycle, the change in pleural pressure (ΔPpl) equals the sum of the elastic (Pel), resistive (Pr) and inertial (Pin) pressure changes. ΔPpl is determined by the change in lung volume (ΔV_T), lung compliance (C), airflow ($\dot{V}$), respiratory resistance (R), volume acceleration ($\ddot{V}$) and inertance (I) of the respiratory system :

$$\Delta Ppl = Pel + Pr + Pin = \Delta V_T/C + R\dot{V} + I\ddot{V}$$

The mechanics of breathing study the relationship between the pressures exerted by the respiratory system and the resulting changes in volume and airflow.

2. THE RESPIRATORY PUMP

The functioning of this pump is based on several structures, i.e. the rib cage and the intercostal and accessory muscles, the diaphragm and the abdomen and its muscles.

Inspiration is most of the time an active event based mainly on the contraction of the diaphragm. The other inspiratory muscles play a minor role during quiet breathing.
Expiration is most of the time a passive event based on the elastic recoil of the lung and chest wall. When expiration becomes active, the main expiratory muscles are those of the abdominal wall.

3. PLEURAL PRESSURE CHANGES

Because the visceral and parietal pleurae are maintained in close apposition, the lung and the thorax interact mechanically. The work performed by the ventilatory muscles induces changes in the pressure of the intrapleural space, which in turn causes the pressure in the alveoli to rise and fall. The resulting pressure gradient between the atmosphere and the alveoli causes air to flow through the airways.
There is a vertical pressure gradient throughout the thorax : pleural pressure is more subatmospheric in the dorsal than in the ventral regions. Furthermore, the changes in the pleural pressure during respiration are greatest in the middle and in the bottom, and less in the top of the thorax. This results in preferential ventilation of the ventral regions of the lungs in dog (Banchero et al, 1966), horse (Derksen and Robinson, 1980) and cattle (Lekeux et al, 1984a). On the other hand, some pressure gradient along the craniocaudal dimensions has also been described, which could be explained by non uniform ventilation of the lung.

4. ELASTIC PROPERTIES OF THE LUNG

The lung has an inherent elasticity due to the tissue elasticity (the normal lung is an elastic structure that contains a network of elastin and collagen fibres) and the surface tension forces. The latter are lowered by the pulmonary surfactant, a complex material composed of 80 % lipids and 20 % proteins. The surfactant maintains alveolar stability and prevents pulmonary atelectasis.

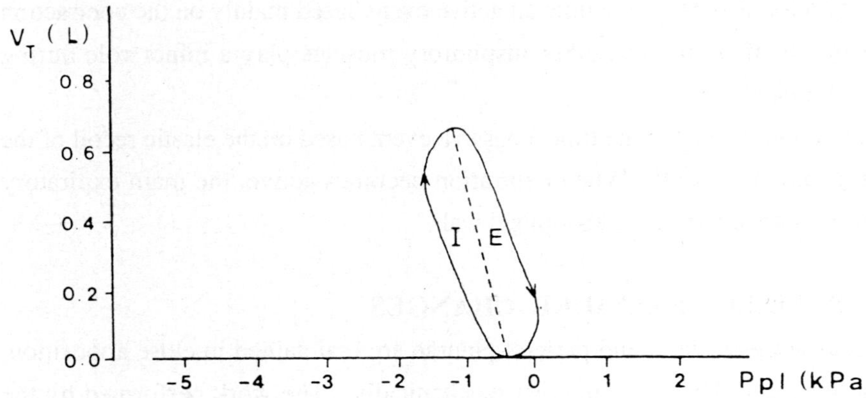

Fig. 4-1. Pressure/volume loop recorded during tidal breathing. The dashed line represents the mechanical work of breathing. V_T : Tidal volume; Ppl : Intrapleural pressure.

The elastic properties of the lung are well documented by the pressure/volume relation curve constructed by plotting the different driving pressures necessary to inflate the lung up to a given level, versus the lung inflation. These static pressure/volume curves require the measurement of transpulmonary pressure during stepwise inflation of the lung, which is only possible in intubated anesthetized animals (Robinson et al, 1972; Gallivan et al, 1989b). Decreased static compliance may be due to fibrosis, lung consolidation or edema. Increased static compliance may occur with age or emphysema (Robinson and Gillespie, 1973).

The relationship established during spontaneous tidal breathing represents the dynamic compliance of the lung, i.e. the volume change (tidal volume) per unit of pleural pressure change (ΔPpl) measured at two points of zero flow (start and end of inspiration) (Fig. 4-1.). Although the dynamic compliance depends on the intrinsic properties of the lung, it is also influenced by dynamic factors such as lung inflation and respiratory frequency. Dynamic compliance increases with lung inflation and may decrease with increasing respiratory frequency. The latter is especially true in lungs presenting a certain degree of sub-obstruction of the lower airways. Therefore, dynamic compliance measurement is used as an index of not only lung elasticity but also of ventilatory asynchronism.

5. ELASTIC PROPERTIES OF THE CHEST WALL

The chest wall and the lungs work in concert but they have different elastic properties. The pressure applied to the chest wall is the difference between pleural and atmospheric pressures and can be used for measuring the chest wall pressure/volume curves.

The compliance of the thorax varies with species and age. It is much higher in a newborn small animal than in an adult large one (Leith and Gillespie, 1971). This has consequences on the pattern of breathing, the lung capacities and the sensitivity to atelectasis.

6. PULMONARY RESISTANCE

The total pulmonary resistance quantifies the permeability of the airways to the airflow. It can be calculated as the pleural pressure change per unit of flow change measured between two points of equal lung volume during inspiration and expiration (50 % for instance).

Both the frictional resistance between the air molecules and the walls of the airways and the viscous drag of the tissues interfere with the respiratory flow. The resistance (R) to airflow passing through a tube is determined by the radius (r) and the length (L) of the tube, as well as by the physical properties of the gas breathed (μ), according to the following formula :

$$R = (8\,\mu\,L)/\,r^4$$

This formula points out the critical importance of the airway radius : if the radius is divided by two, the resistance increases 16 times.

During quiet nasal breathing, about 50 % of the total pulmonary resistance is opposed by the nose passage, 30 % by the remaining upper airways and 20 % by the intrathoracic airways (Lekeux et al, 1985; Gustin et al, 1987; Art et al, 1988d). This means that about 80 % of the total pulmonary resistance is due to the extra-thoracic airways

A major factor affecting the diameter of the tracheobronchial tree, and consequently its influence on airflow, is smooth muscle contraction or relaxation. When irritant materials such as dust are inhaled, the tracheobronchial irritant receptors are stimulated, resulting in a bronchoconstriction. The afferent pathway of this reflex is elicited by the parasympathetic system. Furtheron, any factor which impairs the mucociliar clearance will also decrease the permeability of the airways. For example, keeping the heads of healthy horses raised for a long time during transportation may impair the physiological upper airway clearance and interfere the permeability of the airways (Racklyeft and Love, 1990).

A noncholinergic excitatory system, with tachykinins as transmitter and activated by axon reflexes from airway receptors, may also cause bronchoconstriction (Barnes, 1989).

Relaxation of the tracheobronchial smooth muscle occurs following stimulation of β_2-adrenergic receptors by circulating cathecolamines. The nonadrenergic noncholinergic inhibitory nervous system is also a bronchodilator system. Its efferent fibres are located in the vagus and its neurotransmitter(s) in the airways could be nitric oxide (Kannan and Johnson, 1992).

7. PULMONARY INERTANCE

Inertial forces are those forces that are necessary to accelerate or decelerate the air in the respiratory airways. Pulmonary inertance can be calculated as the ratio of the pressure gradient due to inertia to the simultaneous volume acceleration. In human beings, the inertance of the respiratory system is negligible. Consequently, the pressures necessary to induce accelerations and decelerations of the air in the airways (inertial pressures) may be neglected, even during intense exercise. On the contrary, the inertial pressures can be rather high in hyperventilating large animals (Lekeux et al, 1988; Art et al, 1989).

8. MECHANICAL WORK OF BREATHING

A classical approach for the assessment of the mechanical work of breathing is based on the measurement of the area of the pressure/volume loops (Fig. 4-1.). Although it is well known that the total work of breathing is underestimated by this method, the latter gives a good estimation of the dynamic components of the work of breathing, i.e. the energetical cost necessary to overcome the non-elastic forces in the lungs.

9. EFFECT OF THE SPECIES ON THE MECHANICS OF BREATHING

9.1. Pattern of breathing

The equine species differs from the other domestic animals as regards its breathing strategy (Art and Lekeux, 1988a; Koterba et al, 1988; Gallivan et al, 1989a). Unlike man, horses at rest breath around, rather than from, the relaxed volume of the respiratory system (i.e. the equilibrium position where the tendency of the lung to recoil inward is equal to the tendency of the chest wall to passively recoil outward) (Koterba et al, 1988). Inversely to the other species, the second part of exhalation is active in the horse, and consequently the very first part of inhalation is passive. The physiological reason for this strategy is still unknown, but it has been hypothetized that it could minimize the work of breathing. Indeed, the equine chest wall is very stiff in comparison to other species (Leith and Gillespie, 1971). This implies that the work done to overcome this stiffness during inspiration (named the elastic work) will be proportionally higher. Breathing around, rather than from, the relaxed respiratory volume implies that the energy stored during the latter active part of expiration will be restored during the first passive part of inhalation. Thus, the abdominal muscles, by performing positive work during expiration, share the total work of breathing with the inspiratory muscles.

A direct consequence of this specific breathing strategy, is that the pattern of the respiratory airflow is bi- or polyphasic in horses (Art and Lekeux, 1988a; Koterba et al, 1988; Gallivan et al, 1989a).

Table 4-1. Specific values of the mechanics of breathing in several species.

Value	Unit	Beef Cattle	Dairy Cattle	Horse	Goat	Small Animals
sCdyn	$L.kPa.L.kg^{-1}$	2.3	2.4	4.3	5.0	3.3
sR_L	kPa	8.5	7.0	3.6	5.0	1.6
$s\dot{W}vis$	kPa	0.74	0.47	0.40	0.40	0.22

s : Specific value independent of the body size and weight. Cdyn : Dynamic lung compliance; R_L : Total pulmonary resistance; $\dot{W}vis$: Minute work of breathing.

9.2. Compulsory nasal breathing

Another species peculiaritiy is the occurrence of a compulsory nasal breathing in horses. This is not the case in other domestic animals. This peculiarity has little impact in resting quiet conditions, but may become a serious disadvantage during hyperpnea or during nasal obstruction. Indeed, about 50 % of total pulmonary resistance is due to nasal resistance (Art et al, 1988d). When the latter is too high, horses, unlike other species, are not able to switch from nasal to oronasal breathing.

9.3. Lung compartmentalization

Bovine and porcine lungs show a well developed lobulation with the secondary lobules distincly separated from each others by complete fascial sheaths and covered by a thick pleura (Robinson, 1982). This high level of compartmentalization is partly responsible for the low specific lung compliance in these species (2.4 versus 3.3 L/kPa.kg in other mammals) (Lekeux et al, 1984b) and for their high lung tissue resistance to airflow (80 versus 30 % of peripheral resistance in other mammals) (Gustin et al, 1987) (Table 4-1.).

10. EFFECT OF THE BREED ON THE MECHANICS OF BREATHING

10.1. Hypermuscled animals

Compared to conventional cattle, the double-muscled animals show a higher specific total pulmonary resistance (8.5 versus 7 kPa) and a higher ratio of upper airway to lower airway resistance (76 versus 62 %) (Fig. 4-2.) (Gustin et al, 1987; 1988). They also show a higher specific mechanical work of breathing (0.74 versus 0.47 kPa) (Gustin et al, 1988). Therefore the energetical cost of breathing in these animals represents a greater part of the total energetical cost of their body metabolism, even in physiological conditions (Table 4-2.).

Double-muscled cattle show also a lower specific dynamic lung compliance (2.2 versus 2.4 L/kPa.kg in conventional cattle). This could be explained by their relatively greater ventilatory asynchronism due to their higher respiratory rate (Gustin et al, 1988).

10.2. Sleep-disordered breathing

Some dog breeds, like the English bulldog, have anatomically narrowed upper airways. This could explain why they suffer from sleep-disorders breathing (Hendricks et al, 1991). They compensate this by a hyperactivity in upper airway muscles in order to maintain patency of the airways (Hendricks et al, 1992).

11. EFFECT OF AGE ON THE MECHANICS OF BREATHING

11.1. Effect of somatic growth

Mechanical data are highly influenced by the somatic growth (Table 4-2.). Dynamic lung compliance and total pulmonary resistance show a positive linear and a negative exponential relation with the independent variables of the somatic growth, respectively (Fig. 4-3.) (Lekeux et al, 1984b). Therefore, the growth of the airway and the alveolar structure seems to be non-isotropic in large animals, similarly as it has been postulated in man (Gaultier, 1980).

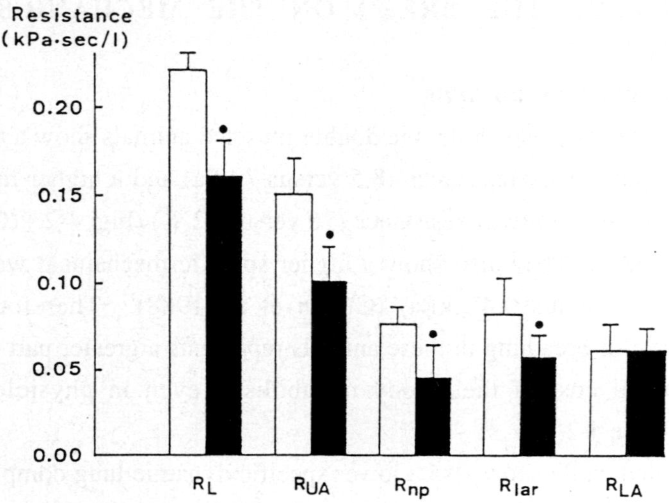

Fig. 4-2. Partitioning of total pulmonary resistance (R_L) in double-muscled (□) and conventional cattle (■). UA : Upper airway; np : Nasopharynx; lar : Larynx; LA : Lower airway (Gustin et al, 1987).

Table 4-2. Predicted values of the mechanics of breathing in healthy dairy and beef cattle.

Value	Unit	Dairy cattle		Beef cattle	
		a	b	a	b
Pplmin	kPa (-)	0.83	0.09	0.65	0.14
Pplmax	kPa (-)	0.33	0.11	0.99	-0.21
maxΔPpl	kPa	0.43	0.10	0.28	0.22
Cdyn	L.kPa^{-1}	0.05	0.82	0.03	0.87
R_L	kPa.sec.L^{-1}	2.68	-0.59	3.31	-0.57
Wvis	J	0.002	1.1	0.004	1.06
$\dot{W}$vis	J.min^{-1}	0.24	0.83	0.19	0.97

Allometric equations, i.e. $x = a.y^b$ where x is the pulmonary value and y is the body weight. Pplmin : Peak intrapleural pressure during inspiration; Pplmax : Peak intrapleural pressure during expiration; maxΔPpl : Maximum change in intrapleural pressure; Cdyn : Dynamic lung compliance; R_L : Total pulmonary resistance; Wvis : Viscous work of breathing; $\dot{W}$vis : Minute work of breathing.

On the other hand, the specific values of the mechanics of breathing differ significantly before and after one year of age (Lekeux et al, 1984b). This suggests that the functional maturity of the respiratory system is not reached before one year of age in the bovine species. This is much later than the occurrence of the functional maturity of their forestomachs. In contrast, the functional maturity and the optimal capacity of the caprine respiratory system occur at three month of age, which is approximately at the same time as the occurrence of mature ruminal function (Bakima et al, 1988). This might be one of the reasons for the highly frequent and severe respiratory disorders observed in cattle between three months and one year of age. This is not the case in goats.

The somatic growth has also a significant effect on the collateral ventilation which is absent in all neonates and present in some adult mammals (Macklem, 1971). Indeed, in dogs, the number of interalveolar pores of Kohn increases until one year of age (Martin, 1963). This phenomenon influences the homogeneity of the lung ventilation and therefore its mechanical properties.

11.2. Effect of aging

Studies on the effect of aging on the animal lung are sparse and difficult to analyse. Indeed, the observed changes may occur with age or because of age, i.e. due to pathological or environmental factors. However, it seems that the loss of elastic recoil (Robinson and Gillespie, 1973; Knudson et al, 1977) and the increase in closing volume (Anthonisen et al, 1970) are a normal consequence of aging.

12. EFFECT OF EXERCISE ON THE MECHANICS OF BREATHING

The hyperventilation generated during exercise has important effects on the mechanics of breathing. This has been mainly studied in horses (Table 4-3.).

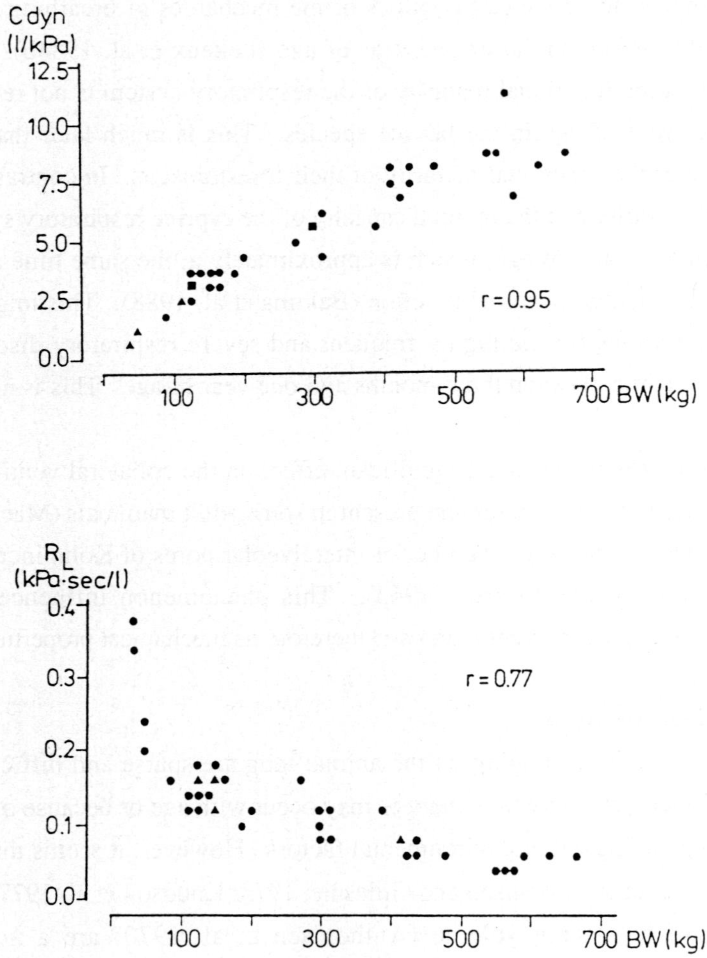

Fig. 4-3. Effect of somatic growth on bovine lung dynamic compliance (Cdyn) and total pulmonary resistance (R_L) (Lekeux et al, 1984b).

12.1. Effect of exercise on the total pulmonary resistance

While exercise does not modify significantly the relative contribution of the different parts of the respiratory tract to the total pulmonary resistance, it induces a substantial increase in resistance (Fig. 4-4.) (Art et al, 1988c; 1990a).

Table 4-3. Mean values of the mechanics of breathing in healthy adult thoroughbred horses (mean body weight : 470 kg).

Value	Unit	Rest	Slow Trot	Fast Gallop
Pplmin	kPa	-0.78	-1.78	-4.85
Pplmax	kPa	-0.34	0.55	3.62
maxΔPpl	kPa	0.44	2.33	8.47
P_{in}	kPa	0.02	1.16	4.26
$\Delta P_{\dot{V}=0}$	kPa	0.24	-0.90	-3.88
Cdyn	$L.kPa^{-1}$	23	-6.8	-3.4
R_L	$Pa.sec.L^{-1}$	25	30	57
R_{UA}	$Pa.min.L^{-1}$	20	23	46
R_{LA}	$Pa.min.L^{-1}$	5	7	11
Wvis	J	1.4	14	82
$\dot{W}vis$	$J.min^{-1}$	17	1274	9922
$\dot{W}vis/\dot{V}e$	$J.L^{-1}$	0.22	2.2	6.2
$\dot{W}vis/\dot{V}O_2$	$J.L^{-1}$	7.7	106	148

Pplmin : Peak intrapleural pressure recorded during inspiration; Pplmax : Peak intrapleural pressure recorded during expiration; maxΔPpl : Maximum change in intrapleural pressure; Pin : Inertial pressure; $\Delta P_{\dot{V}=0}$: Intrapleural pressure gradient between the 2 points of zero flow; Cdyn : Dynamic lung compliance; R_L : Total pulmonary resistance; R_{UA} : Upper airways resistance; R_{LA} : Lower airways resistance; Wvis : Viscous work of breathing; $\dot{W}vis$: Minute work of breathing; $\dot{W}vis/\dot{V}e$: Work of breathing per ventilated litre; $\dot{W}vis/\dot{V}O_2$: Work of breathing per litre of oxygen uptake.

During exercise, physiological adjustments such as dilatation of the external nares, full abduction of the larynx and bronchodilation, tend to facilitate the increase of flow and to decrease the resistance by enlarging the cross-sectional area of the airways and therefore the airways radius. However, despite these exercise-induced adaptations, heavy exercise induces a more than two fold increase in the total pulmonary resistance. Actually, the total pulmonary resistance is the result of two kinds of opposed factors : decreasing resistance due to physiological changes and increasing resistance due to physical effects

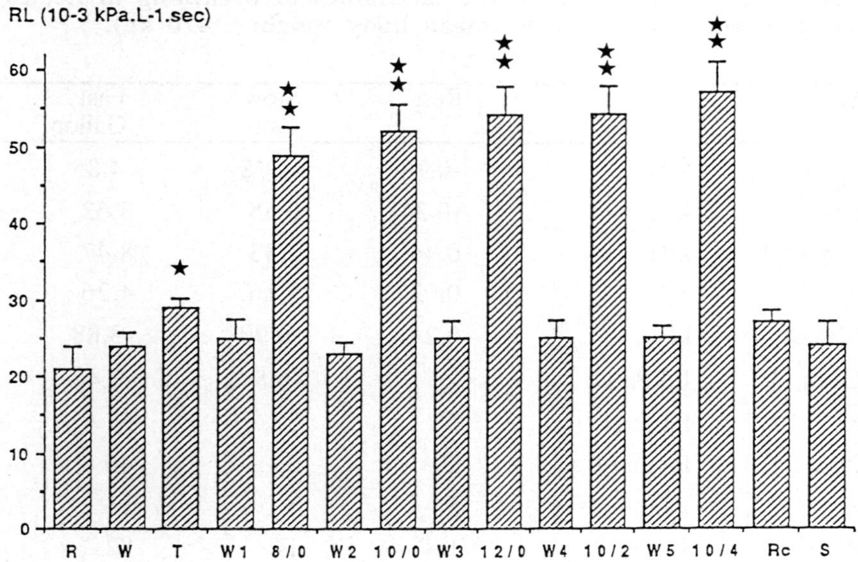

Fig. 4-4. Total pulmonary resistance (R_L) in horses performing exercise of increasing intensity. R : Rest; W : Walk; T : Trot; 8/0, 10/0, 12/0 : Gallops at 8, 10 and 12 $m.sec^{-1}$ at incline 0°; 10/2 and 10/4 : Gallops at 10 $m.sec^{-1}$ at incline 2 and 4°; Rc : Recovery; S : Stop. * : Different from rest value with $P < 0.05$; ** : $P < 0.001$ (Art et al, 1990a).

(mainly frictions, turbulences, inhomogeneous distribution of the resistance among airways and alveoli, and changes of the cross-sectional area of the airways induced by compressing transmural pressures) tending to increase it. When the horse walks or trots slowly, both factors cancel each other and the resistance remain unchanged. On the contrary, during heavy exercise the physical factors depending on flow amplitude and increasing the total pulmonary resistance, predominate largely over the physiological ones and the resistance increases. Lastly during recovery, while the ventilatory parameters return progressively to their base-line, the physiological factors overcome and the resistance may be less than during quiet breathing at rest (Art et al, 1988c). Several factors may explain the exercise-induced increase in resistance.

The importance of frictions and turbulences in the increase of the total pulmonary resistance has been demonstrated by experiments in which exercising horses were breathing a helium-oxygen mixture. This mixture has a lesser density than air and therefore minimizes turbulences and frictions. During exercise, there was a significant increase in minute ventilation due to an increase in respiratory frequency, as well as a 50 % decrease of total pulmonary resistance and mechanical work of breathing (Art et al, 1991).
The study of the inspiratory and expiratory components of the resistance values in trotting horses have shown that, during inspiration, the extra-thoracic airways account for more than 90 % of the total pulmonary resistance, while during expiration the intra-thoracic airways are responsible for more than 50 % of the pulmonary resistance (Art et al, 1988d). This observation could be explained by the fact that, during exercise, a dynamic partial collapse may occur in the airways when the pressure surrounding the airways exceeds the pressure within the lumen of the airways (Gillespie, 1974). When horses inhale, sub-atmospheric pressures in the extra-thoracic airways may be as low as minus 5 kPa while the pressure in the surrounding tissues remains atmospheric. During expiration, the intra-thoracic pressure become greater than the pressure prevailing inside some of the intra-thoracic airways. Submitted to compressive pressures, these structures tend to collapse, consequently increasing their resistance to airflow. Because of their bony support, the nasal cavities are less subjected to compression than less well supported structures such as the nares, pharynx, trachea and bronchi.
If this collapse already occurs in healthy horses, one may expect that this phenomenon dramatically aggravates in horses suffering from airways obstruction, a condition accompanied by substantial transmural pressures during exercise (Funkquist et al, 1988).
It has been shown that both the extra- and intra-thoracic parts of the trachea are sufficiently compliant to decrease their cross sectional area when submitted to high but nevertheless physiological compressive transmural pressures (Art and Lekeux, 1991a; 1991b). Moreover, the shape of the cross sectional area

influences significantly the tendency of the trachea to collapse : tracheae with a circular shape of the cross sectional area are less compressible than tracheae with a more ellipsoidal shape (Art and Lekeux, 1991b). This is particularly important in view of the variability observed in this shape among individual horses, some horses being probably more susceptible than others to dynamic tracheal collapse. In other words, during intense exercise, when high level of ventilation are reached, horses having an ellipsoidal trachea may be disadvantaged when compared to those having a more circular trachea.

Lastly, the extension of the trachea decreases its collapsibility (Art and Lekeux, 1991b). This means that hyperextension stiffens the trachea, decreases its resistance to airflow and consequently increases the maximal airflow through this trachea. This could explain why horses extend their neck during maximal exercise : as well as providing maximum patency of the nasopharyngeal airways, the cervical extension and the consequent longitudinal extension of the trachea decrease the tracheal compliance and minimize the phenomenon of dynamic collapse.

12.2. Effect of exercise on the pulmonary inertance

Tracheal length in mammals is designed by the physiological and anatomical peculiarities of each species (Leith, 1982). Horses are grass-eating animals and have proportionally longer legs and longer necks than other domestic grass-eating species. They also have a deep thorax. The anatomical consequence of this feature is that they also have a proportionally longer trachea than other species. Therefore, the tracheal diameter is matched with the dominant constraints such as tracheal resistance, inertance (which is proportional to the tracheal length and inversely related with the tracheal radius), flow limitation, dead space and minimum work of breathing (Leith, 1982) : a larger diameter would be advantageous for low pulmonary resistance and inertance but disadvantageous for the anatomical dead space.

During quiet breathing, respiratory frequency is about 14 cycles/min, tidal volume about 5.5 L, the total pressure change to which the lungs are subjected about 0.44 kPa and the pressure associated to volume acceleration about 0.02 kPa (Art et al, 1989). During fast gallop, respiratory frequency increases up to 121 cycles/min, tidal volume up to 13.2 L; the maximal pressure change reaches values of 8.5 kPa and total volume acceleration more than 3000 L/sec^2. The pressure required to produce these accelerations is then 4.3 kPa or 50 % of the total pressure change. Therefore, it appears that these inertial pressures become of great importance in the exercising horse. They may even be a limiting or at least a constraining factor to any further increase of ventilation (Art et al, 1989).

12.3. Effect of exercise on the pulmonary dynamic compliance

The great importance of the respiratory inertial factors in running horses explains why the dynamic compliance become negative when measured during exercise (Art and Lekeux, 1988b; Art et al, 1991). Classically, the dynamic compliance is measured at points of zero flow and is defined by the equation :

$$Cdyn = V_T/(\Delta Pel - 4\ \Pi^2.f^2.V_T.I).$$

In this formula, ΔPel is the elastic pressure change and the term $4\ \Pi^2.f^2.V_T.I$ indicates the inertial pressure changes. As the latter is generally considered as negligible the equation is simplified as follows :

$$Cdyn = V_T/\Delta Pel$$

In exercising horses, $4\ \Pi^2.f^2.V_T.I$ increases and its absolute value may become equal to or greater than ΔPel. This explains why, in these specific conditions, Cdyn is either overestimated, infinite or negative.

12.4. Effect of exercise on the mechanical work of breathing

It has been shown that the work per respiratory cycle, the work per liter of air ventilated and the work per minute are dramatically increased during exercise (Fig. 4-5.) (Art and Lekeux, 1989). For example, the power output (i.e. the work of breathing per minute) increases 475 times from rest to strenuous gallop (Table 4-3.) (Art et al, 1990a).

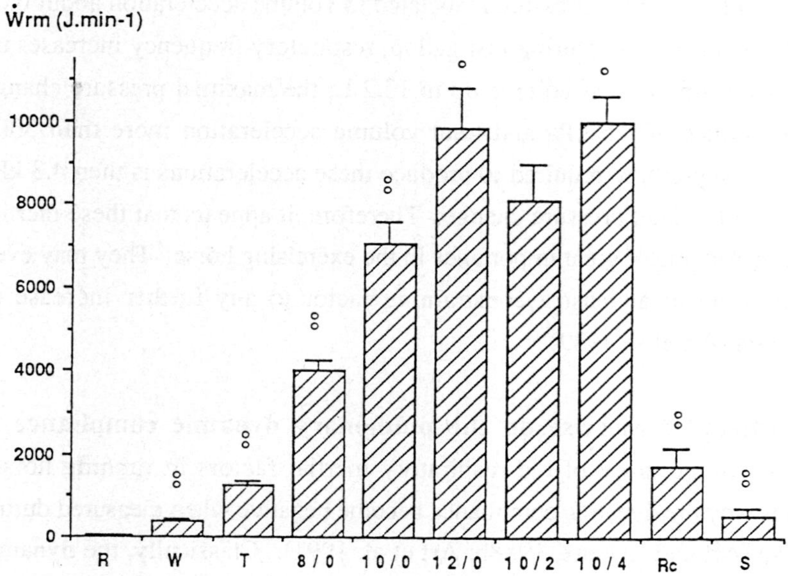

Fig. 4-5. Minute work of breathing (Ẇrm) from horses performing exercise of increasing intensity. R : Rest; W : Walk; T : Trot; 8/0, 10/0, 12/0 : Gallops at 8, 10 and 12 $m.sec^{-1}$ at incline 0°; 10/2 and 10/4 : Gallops at 10 $m.sec^{-1}$ at incline 2 and 4°; Rc : Recovery; S : Stop. ° : Different from the preceding value with $P < 0.05$; °° : $P < 0.01$ (10/0 was taken as the preceding value of 10/2) (Art et al, 1990a).

The relationship between the mechanical work of breathing per minute and the minute volume in running horses is curvilinear with an upwards concavity. The curve is of ever-increasing slope, implying that the mechanical cost of breathing for any additional unit of air ventilated becomes greater with any increase of ventilation (Art and Lekeux, 1989; Art et al, 1990a).

The sharp increase of the work of breathing associated with the exercise-induced hyperventilation is explained by the increase of resistive, elastic and inertial work. The increase of the resistive work is related with the increase of the total pulmonary resistance (Art and Lekeux 1989; Art et al, 1990a). The latter factor itself results from the compulsory nasal breathing (Art and Lekeux, 1988c), which is associated with frictions and turbulences (Art et al,

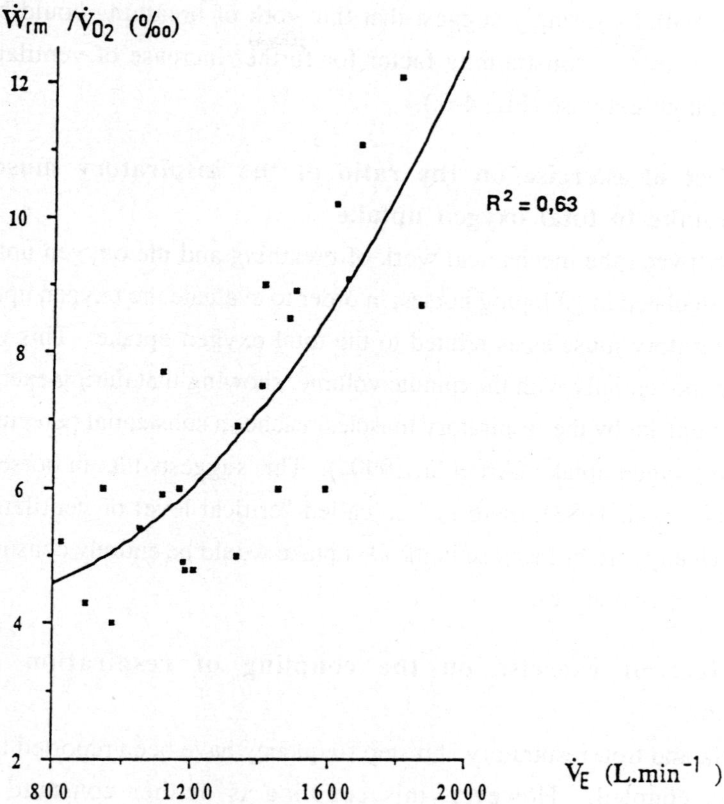

Fig. 4-6. Relationship between the ratio of minute work of breathing to oxygen consumption ($\dot{W}rm.\ \dot{V}O_2^{-1}$) and the minute volume ($\dot{V}e$) for horses galloping on a treadmill. $\dot{W}rm$ is given in per thousand of $\dot{V}O_2$; R^2 : Coefficient of determination (Art et al, 1990a).

1991) and dynamic partial collapse of the airways (Art and Lekeux, 1991a). The three fold increase of the breathed volume probably increases highly the elastic work (Art and Lekeux, 1989) namely because of the chest wall stiffness. Lastly, the length of the airways and the magnitude of flow accelerations during exercise result in a non-negligible importance of the inertial work (Art et al, 1989).

These observations strongly suggest that the work of breathing could be a limiting or at least a constraining factor for further increase of ventilation during strenuous exercise (Fig. 4-6.).

12.5. Effect of exercise on the ratio of the inspiratory muscles oxygen uptake to total oxygen uptake

The ratio between the mechanical work of breathing and the oxygen uptake has been calculated in galloping horses, in order to evaluate the oxygen uptake by the respiratory muscles as related to the total oxygen uptake. This ratio increases exponentially with the minute volume, showing that during exercise the oxygen uptake by the respiratory muscles reaches a substantial percentage of the total oxygen uptake (Art et al, 1990a). This suggests that in horses as in man (Bye et al, 1983), there is a so called "critical level of ventilation" above which any further increase in the O_2 uptake would be entirely consumed by the respiratory muscles.

12.6. Effect of exercise on the coupling of respiration and locomotion

At the walk and trot, respiratory and step frequency have been reported to be sometimes coupled. However, this coupling is neither constant, nor compulsory (Karlsen and Brejtsen, 1965; Art et al, 1990b). When the coupling exists, it seems that the "abdominal piston" acts in synergy with the respiratory pump (Art et al, 1990b), inducing probably a reduction in the cost of breathing.

Once the horse gallops, there is a compulsory linkage between step and respiratory rates (Attenburrow, 1982; 1983; Bramble and Carrier, 1983; Young et al, 1992). The mechanisms underlying this coupling are not well understood. It is probably due to a mechanical linkage : the role of the viscera acting as a piston, the flexion of the back and the loading of the thorax by the forelimbs may profit mechanically from this synchronisation (Bramble and Carrier, 1983). During protraction of the forelimbs, the rib cage is pulled forwards and outwards, allowing inhalation. During weight-bearing, the rib cage absorbs forces and is compressed, resulting in exhalation. Experimental evidence shows that, in galloping horses, breathing is assisted more by back flexion rather than by the visceral piston mechanism (Young et al, 1992).

It must be emphasized that this coupling is not absolute in healthy horses. Indeed, some galloping horses, both on the track and on the treadmill, show sporadically a "big breath" which run on two or three strides. The reason of this remains to be investigated but these horses seem to run better after this hyperinflation of the lungs.

12.7. Effect of exercise on the recruitment of respiratory muscles

The diaphragm and the external intercostal muscles are the main inspiratory muscles in mammals. However, in horses, the serratus ventralis muscle has the most important role in assisting the inspiratory effort of the diaphragm, both at rest (Hall et al, 1991) and during exercise (Manohar, 1991). On the other hand, the transversal abdominal muscle is the principal auxillary muscle actively involved in expiration. Lastly, the intercostal muscles are also activated during the second part of inspiration and expiration (Hall et al, 1991).

The study of the recruitment of respiratory muscles has been performed by electromyography in healthy resting horses (Koterba et al, 1988; Hall et al, 1991) and in ponies during hypoxia (Brice at al, 1990). Until now, this measurement has not been reported in exercising horses. However, during exercise, the activity of both inspiratory and expiratory muscles increases and the metabolic needs of the muscles become substantial. The increase in blood flow in the activated tissues may be related to the increase in the metabolic needs. Therefore, the activity of the ventilatory muscles in ponies has been indirectly estimated by the increase in the perfusion of the muscles (Manohar, 1990a; 1990b; 1991). The ventilatory muscles comprise 5.5 % of the total body weight and receive 10 % and ± 15 % of the cardiac output at rest and at maximal exercise, respectively. The increase in blood flow in these muscles is accompanied by a precipitous decrease in their vascular resistance (Manohar, 1990a; 1991).

During exercise, the blood flow in the costal part of the diaphragm exceeds the blood flow of all other inspiratory or expiratory muscles : it increases over 20-folds in maximally exercised ponies. During maximal exercise, diaphragmatic blood flow reaches its upper limit (Manohar, 1987) and adenosine infusion, which causes a marked vasodilatation in the pony's diaphragm at rest, fails to elicit any further vasodilation, indicating that the vasodilator capacity is completely utilized (Manohar, 1986). This suggests a potential limiting factor of the ventilatory machinery during heavy exercise.

13. CONCLUSIONS

Mechanics of breathing are an essential factor of the pulmonary efficiency in all species and even a limiting factor in some of them such as large domestic animals. Therefore, the mechanical peculiarities may explain many differences in lung function between species. On the other hand, any mechanical impairment, even moderate, is susceptible to decrease the pulmonary efficiency, which can lead to a poor performance syndrome and sometimes to lung damages.

REFERENCES

ANTHONISEN N.R., DANSON J., ROBERTSON P.C. Airway closure as a function of age. *Respir. Physiol.* 1970, 8, 58-65.

ART T., LEKEUX P. Effect of environmental temperature and relative humidity on breathing pattern and heart rate in ponies during and after standardised exercise. *Vet. Rec.* 1988a, 123, 295-299.

ART T., LEKEUX P. Respiratory airflow patterns in ponies at rest and during exercise. *Can. J. Vet. Res.* 1988b, 52, 299-303.

ART T, LEKEUX P. Pulmonary mechanics during treadmill exercise in race ponies. *Vet. Res. Commun.* 1988c, 12, 245-258

ART T., SERTEYN D., LEKEUX P. Effect of exercise on the partitioning of equine respiratory resistance. *Equine Vet. J.* 1988d, 20, 268-273.

ART T, LEKEUX P. Work of breathing in exercising ponies. *Res. Vet. Sci.* 1989, 46, 49-53.

ART T., LEKEUX P., GUSTIN P., DESMECHT D., AMORY H., PAIVA M. Inertance

of the respiratory system in ponies. *J. Appl. Physiol.* 1989, 67, 534-540.
ART T., ANDERSON L., WOAKES A.J., ROBERTS C., BUTLER P.J., SNOW D.H., LEKEUX P. Mechanics of breathing during strenuous exercise in thoroughbred horses. *Respir. Physiol.* 1990a, 82, 279-294.
ART T, DESMECHT D, AMORY H, LEKEUX P. Synchronization of locomotion and respiration in trotting ponies. *J. Vet. Med. A* 1990b, 37, 95-103.
ART T, LEKEUX P. Mechanical properties of the isolated equine trachea. *Res. Vet. Sci.* 1991a, 51, 55-60.
ART T, LEKEUX P. The effect of shape, age, and extension on the compliance of equine tracheal segment. *Vet. Res. Commun.* 1991b, 15, 135-146.
ART T., DESMECHT D., AMORY H., LEKEUX P. Heliox-induced changes in the breathing mechanics of ponies during exercise. In : *Equine Exercise Physiology 3*, Persson, S.G.B., Lindholm, A., Jeffcott, L.B. (Eds), ICEEP Publications, Davis, California, 1991, pp 47-53.
ATTENBURROW D.P. Time relationship between the respiratory cycle and limb cycle in the horse. *Equine Vet. J.* 1982, 14, 69-72.
ATTENBURROW D.P. Respiration and locomotion. In : *Equine Exercise Physiology*, Snow, D.H., Persson, S.G.B., Rose, R.J. (Eds), Granta Editions, Cambridge, 1983, pp 17-22.
BANCHERO N., RUTISHAUSER W.J., TSAKIRIS A.G., WOOD E.H. Respiratory changes in pleural pressures at different sites and body positions. *J. Appl. Physiol.* 1966, 22, 1075-1080.
BAKIMA M., GUSTIN P., LEKEUX P., LOMBA F. Mechanics of breathing in goats. *Res. Vet. Sci.* 1988, 45, 332-336.
BARNES P.J. Airway neuropeptides: roles in fine tuning and in disease. *NIPS* 1989, 4, 116-120.
BRAMBLE DM, CARRIER D.R. Running and breathing in mammals. *Science* 1983, 219, 251-256.
BRICE A.G., FORSTER H.V., PAN L.G., LOWRY T.F., MURPHY C.L. Respiratory muscle electromyogram responses to acute hypoxia in awake ponies. *J. Appl. Physiol.* 1990, 68, 1024-1032.
BYE P.T.P., FARKAS G.A., ROUSSOS Ch. Respiratory factors limiting exercise. *Ann. Rev. Physiol.* 1983, 45, 439-451.
DERKSEN F.J., ROBINSON N.E. Esophageal and intrapleural pressures in the healthy conscious pony. *Am. J. Vet. Res.* 1980, 41, 1756-1761.
FUNKQUIST B., HOLM K., KARLSSON A., KVART C., MOLANDER G., OBEL N. Studies on the intratracheal pressure in the exercising horse. *J. Vet. Med. A* 1988, 35, 424-441.
GALLIVAN G.J., McDONELL W.N., FORREST J.B. Comparative pulmonary mechanics in the horse and the cow. *Res. Vet. Sci.* 1989a, 46, 322-330.
GALLIVAN G.J., McDONELL W.N., FORREST J.B. Comparative ventilation and gas exchange in the horse and the cow. *Res. Vet. Sci.* 1989b, 46, 331-336.
GAULTIER C. Développement postnatal de la fonction pulmonaire chez l'enfant. Thesis, University of Paris-Sud UER Kremlin-Bicètre, 1980.
GILLESPIE J.R. The role of the respiratory system during exertion. *Jl S. Afr. vet. Ass.* 1974, 45, 305-309.
GUSTIN P., BAKIMA M., LEKEUX P., LOMBA F., VAN DE WOESTIJNE K.P. Partitioning of upper airway resistance in Friesian and double-muscled calves. *Respir. Physiol.* 1987, 69, 299-306.
GUSTIN P., BAKIMA M., LEKEUX P., LOMBA F., VAN DE WOESTIJNE K.P. Pulmonary function values and growth in Belgian White Blue double-muscled cattle.

Res. Vet. Sci. 1988, 45, 405-410.

HALL L.W., AZIZ H.A., GROENENDYK J., KEATES H., REX M.A. Electromyography of some respiratory muscles in the horse. *Res. Vet. Sci.* 1991, 50, 328-333.

HENDRICKS J.C., KOVALSKI R.J., KLINE L.R. Phasic respiratory muscle patterns and sleep-disordered breathing during rapid eye movement sleep in bulldogs. *Am. Rev. Respir. Dis.* 1991, 144, 1112-1120.

HENDRICKS J.C., PETROF B.J., PANCKERI,K., PACK A.I. Compensatory hyperactivity of an upper airway dilator in bulldogs. *Am. Rev. Respir. Dis.* 1992, 145, A402.

KANNAN M.S., JOHNSON D.E. Nitric oxide mediates the neural nonadrenergic, noncholinergic relaxation of pig tracheal smooth muscle. *Am. J. Physiol. (Lung Cell Mol. Physiol.)* 1992, 2, L511-L514.

KARLSEN G., BREJTSEN N. Synchronisation of rythm of respiration and movement: a basis for the development of a fast trotter. (In russian,) *Konevodstvo I Konnyj Sport* 1965, 33, 22-24.

KNUDSON R.J., CLARK D.F., KENNEDY T.C., KNUDSON D.E. Effect of aging alone on mechanical properties of the normal adult human lung. *J. Appl. Physiol.* 1977, 43, 1054-1062.

KOTERBA A.M., KOSCH P.C., BEECH J., WHITLOCK T. Breathing strategy of the adult horse (*Equus caballus*) at rest. *J. Appl. Physiol.* 1988, 64, 337-346.

LEITH D.E., GILLESPIE J.R. Respiratory mechanics of normal horses and one with chronic obstructive lung disease. *Fed. Proc.* 1971, 30, 551.

LEITH D.E. Mammalian tracheal dimensions: scaling and physiology. *J. Appl. Physiol.* 1982, 55, 196-200.

LEKEUX P., HAJER R., BREUKINK H.J. Pulmonary function testing in calves: technical data. *Am. J. Vet. Res.* 1984a, 45, 342-345.

LEKEUX P., HAJER R., BREUKINK H.J. Effect of somatic growth on pulmonary function values in healthy Friesian cattle. *Am. J. Vet. Res.* 1984b, 45, 2003-2007.

LEKEUX P., HAJER R., BREUKINK H.J. Upper airway resistance in healthy Friesian cattle. *Res. Vet. Sci.* 1985, 38, 77-79.

LEKEUX P., ART T., CLERCX C., GUSTIN P. Influence of inertance on measurements of the mechanical properties of the bovine respiratory system. *Vet. Res. Commun.* 1988, 12, 61-66.

MACKLEM P.T. Airway obstruction and collateral ventilation. *Physiol. Rev.* 1971, 51, 368-436.

MANOHAR M. Vasodilator reserve in respiratory muscles during maximal exertion in ponies. *J. Appl. Physiol.* 1986, 60, 1571-1577.

MANOHAR M. Blood flow in respiratory muscles during maximal exertion in ponies with laryngeal hemiplegia. *J. Appl. Physiol.* 1987, 62, 229-237.

MANOHAR M. Inspiratory and expiratory muscle perfusion in maximally exercised ponies. *J. Appl. Physiol.* 1990a, 68, 544-548.

MANOHAR M. Diaphragmatic perfusion heterogeneity during exercise with inspiratory resistive breathing. *J. Appl. Physiol.* 1990b, 68, 2177-2181.

MANOHAR M. Respiratory muscle perfusion during strenuous exercise. In : *Equine Exercise Physiology 3*, Persson, S.G.B., Lindholm, A., Jeffcott, L.B. (Eds), ICEEP Publications, Davis, California, 1991, pp 1-8.

MARTIN H.B. The effect of aging on the alveolar pores of Kohn in the dog. *Am. Rev. Respir. Dis.* 1963, 88, 773-778.

RACKLYEFT D.J., LOVE D.N. Influence of head posture on the respiratory tract of healthy horses. *Austr. Vet. J.* 1990, 67, 402-405.

ROBINSON N.E., GILLESPIE J.R., BARRY J.D., SIMPSON A. Lung compliance, lung volume and single-breath diffusing capacity in dogs. *J. Appl. Physiol.* 1972, 33, 808-812.

ROBINSON N.E., GILLESPIE J.R. Lung volumes in aging beagle dogs. *J. Appl. Physiol.* 1973, 35, 317-321.

ROBINSON NE. Some functional consequences of species differences in lung anatomy. *Adv. Vet. Sci. Comp. Med.* 1982, 26, 1-33.

YOUNG I.S., WARREN R.D., ALTRINGHAM J.D. Some properties of the mammalian locomotory and respiratory systems in relation to body mass. *J. exp. Biol.* 1992, 164, 283-294.

CHAPTER V

GAS EXCHANGE IN RESTING AND EXERCISING ANIMALS

P. Lekeux[1] and T. Art[2]

[1] Laboratory for Functional Investigation
[2] Equine Sport Medicine Unit
Faculty of Veterinary Medicine
University of Liege

SUMMARY

This paper describes the different steps of the pulmonary and peripheral gas exchange in resting and exercising domestic animals.

KEY WORDS

Respiratory system - Pulmonary function - Gas exchange - Exercise.

1. INTRODUCTION

The oxygen uptake by the respiratory system and the oxygen transport by the blood circulation must always be matched to the oxygen consumption in the mitochondria of the tissues. This allows the aerobic breakdown of the alimentary substrates, which provides energy for the phosphorylation of ADP to ATP.

Therefore, the ability for an animal to sustain a high level of exercise depends not only on the capacity of the striated muscle cells to generate ATP aerobically, but also on the capacity and integration of the various links of the oxygen transporting chain. In most physiological conditions, the oxygen uptake by the organism is almost equal to the carbon dioxide output. The respiratory quotient, i.e. the ratio between the CO_2 output and the O_2 uptake, increases from 0.8 at rest to 1.1 during heavy exercise. This occurs mainly because of an increased utilization of carbohydrates as energetic substrate but also because of the nonmetabolic production of CO_2, for instance during the buffering of lactic acid.

The maximal oxygen uptake is the rate of oxygen consumption beyond which additional energy demand must be met by anaerobic metabolism, which results in lactic acid accumulation. The maximal oxygen uptake is about 2.3 ml/sec.kg in athletic species such as horse and dog, and is 2.5 times lower in non athletic species such as the ruminants (Weibel et al, 1987; Wagner et al, 1991). The ratio between maximal and resting oxygen consumption is at least 30 in sport horses (Rose et al, 1988) and only 10 in cattle (Kuhlmann et al, 1985).

This paper will mainly deal with the processes of pulmonary gas exchange in the horse, which is the most intensively investigated species in this field.

2. PULMONARY GAS EXCHANGE

2.1. Ventilation

2.1.1. Lung volumes

The volume of air inhaled or exhaled during a normal breath is termed tidal volume. Its value in common mammals is about 10 ml/kg of body weight (Stahl, 1967), varying from 12 ml/kg in horses to 8 ml/kg in cattle (Lekeux et al, 1984). Multiplying the tidal volume by the respiratory frequency gives the minute ventilation.

Exercise imposes a potent stress on the ventilatory pump : as speed increases, minute ventilation increases almost linearly and the minute ventilation, which averages 80 L/min in resting horses (Table 5-1.), may reach values of ± 1800 L/min during heavy exercise (Art et al, 1992). The adaptation of the minute ventilation to the gas exchange requirements can be reached by changing the tidal volume, the respiratory frequency or both parameters.

Trotting horses running at low work intensity increase their minute ventilation by a simultaneous increase in tidal volume and respiratory frequency. At high exercise intensity minute ventilation increases mainly by an increase in respiratory frequency (Art and Lekeux, 1988b). Values as high as 133 breaths/min have been reported in standardbred horses running on a treadmill (Dahl et al, 1987). Values of tidal volume of racing trotting horses are sparse: tidal volumes of about 12 L have been reported in horses trotting at 10 m/sec, with a respiratory frequency of 87 breaths/min (Gottlieb-Vedi et al, 1991).

In galloping horses, respiration and locomotion are compulsory coupled (Bramble and Carrier, 1983) : step and respiratory frequencies average 110 to 130/min, with maximum values of 148/min observed in the field (Hörnicke et al, 1983; 1987). When the horse gallops, the increase in minute ventilation with increasing speed is mainly due to the increase in tidal volume rather than in respiratory frequency. Tidal volumes between 12 and 15 L are reported in fast galloping horses (Bayly et al, 1987; Hörnicke et al, 1987; Art et al, 1990; Landgren et al, 1991). An extreme value of 29.7 L has been observed in a horse decoupling the 1:1 ratio of step to respiratory frequencies for a 2:1 ratio

Table 5-1. Mean ventilatory values in adult thoroughbred horses.

Value	Unit	Rest	Slow Trot	Fast Gallop
$\dot{V}O_2max$	%	3.3	18	100
V_T	L	5.6	6.2	13.2
V_D	L	3.4	3.5	2.6
V_A	L	2.2	2.8	10.6
V_D/V_T	%	60	57	20
f	min^{-1}	14	91	121
t_I	sec	1.9	0.34	0.25
t_E	sec	2.4	0.32	0.25
t_I/t_{TOT}	%	44	52	50
$\dot{V}_e$	$L.min^{-1}$	78	564	1598
$\dot{V}_D$	$L.min^{-1}$	47	321	320
$\dot{V}_A$	$L.min^{-1}$	31	243	1278
$\dot{V}_e/\dot{V}O_2$	$L.L^{-1}$	35	47	24
$\dot{V}_e/\dot{V}CO_2$	$L.L^{-1}$	43	51	23
mean$\dot{V}i$	$L.sec^{-1}$	2.9	19	53
mean$\dot{V}e$	$L.sec^{-1}$	2.3	20	53
$\dot{V}imax$	$L.sec^{-1}$	4.1	27	64
$\dot{V}emax$	$L.sec^{-1}$	4.2	30	79
$\ddot{V}i$	$L.sec^{-2}$	8	632	1685
$\ddot{V}e$	$L.sec^{-2}$	7	566	1595

$\dot{V}O_2max$ % : % of maximal oxygen uptake; V_T : Tidal volume; V_D : Physiological dead space; V_A : Alveolar volume; V_D/V_T : Ratio of dead space to tidal volume; f : Breathing frequency; t_I : Inspiratory time of the breathing cycle; t_E : Expiratory time; t_I/t_{TOT} : Ratio of inspiratory to total time of the breathing cycle; $\dot{V}_e$: Minute volume; $\dot{V}_D$: Dead space ventilation; $\dot{V}_A$: Alveolar ventilation; $\dot{V}e/\dot{V}O_2$: Ventilatory equivalent for oxygen uptake; $\dot{V}e/\dot{V}CO_2$: Ventilatory equivalent for carbon dioxide output; mean$\dot{V}i$: Mean inspiratory flow or inspiratory drive; mean$\dot{V}e$: Mean expiratory flow; $\dot{V}imax$: Peak inspiratory flow; $\dot{V}emax$: Peak expiratory flow; $\ddot{V}i$: Volume acceleration at the onset of inspiration; $\ddot{V}e$: Volume acceleration at the onset of expiration.

(Gillespie et al, 1991).
On the opposite, in dogs, the exercise-induced hyperventilation is mainly due to an increase in respiratory rate, with little change in tidal volume (Szlyk et al, 1981).
In cattle, the exercise-induced hyperventilation is due to an equal increase in tidal volume and respiratory rate during moderate exercise. For higher work load, increased minute ventilation is obtained by an increase in tidal volume (Kuhlmann et al, 1985). Compared to conventional cattle, double-muscled cattle show a lower tidal volume and a higher respiratory rate for an equal minute ventilation, both in resting and exercising conditions (Gustin et al, 1988a).
Only a part of the inspired volume reaches the part of the lung where gas exchange takes place : this is the alveolar ventilation. The remaining part of the minute ventilation is wasted in the regions of lung where no gas exchange occurs : this is the physiological dead space ventilation which includes the conducting airways (anatomical dead space) and the alveoli which are ventilated but not perfused (alveolar dead space). The ratio between the dead space and the tidal volume averages 50-60 % in resting horses and cattle (Gustin et al, 1988a; Gallivan et al, 1989; Lekeux et al, 1992), a percentage which is twice greater than that reported in other species such as dog (Musch et al, 1986).
For a given minute ventilation, the lower the physiological dead space ventilation, the higher the alveolar ventilation and the better the gas exchange. However, adequate gas exchange is maintained with very low tidal volume and very high respiratory frequency (600 cycles/min) (i.e. high frequency or jet ventilation). This suggests that factors like mass convection, convective dispersion and molecular diffusion may provide an adequate gas transport between the atmospheric air and the alveoli, despite a very high ratio between dead space and tidal volume (Froese and Bryan, 1981; Chang, 1984).
This ratio as well as exercise-induced changes in alveolar ventilation in horses depend on the type of exercise performed (Pollmann and Hörnicke, 1984;

Bayly et al, 1987; Pelletier et al, 1987; Rose and Evans, 1987). During mild to moderate exercise, the dead space volume does not change significantly (Pelletier et al, 1987). Therefore, an increase in tidal volume will increase the alveolar ventilation and decrease the dead space to tidal volume ratio.

If the exercise is prolonged at a constant rate, the dead space ventilation will increase by a simultaneous increase of the respiratory frequency and of the ratio between dead space and tidal volume (Pelletier et al, 1987; Rose and Evans, 1987). This adaptation reflects probably the thermoregulatory role of the respiratory system.

Lastly, during intense effort, there is a decrease of the dead space to tidal volume ratio from ± 60 % (resting value) to ± 20 % (fast galloping value) (Table 5-1.) (Rose and Evans 1987; Lekeux et al, 1992). In absolute values, the physiological dead space is reduced from 3.5 L at rest to 2.5 L during heavy exercise. The anatomical dead space averages 2.5 L at rest (Pollmann and Hörnicke, 1984) and is expected to remain unchanged during exercise. Therefore, the exercise-induced difference in the dead space (1 L) is probably due to the disappearance of the alveolar dead space (i.e. alveoli which are ventilated but not perfused). This can be induced by the recruitment of previously non-functional pulmonary capillaries (Lekeux et al, 1992).

On the opposite, the physiological dead space volume was reported to increase slightly with exercise in cattle (Kuhlmann et al, 1985). This suggests that alveolar dead space would be more important in exercising than in resting cattle.

2.1.2. Distribution of ventilation

The distribution of ventilation is not uniform throughout the lung, even in healthy animals. This results from two different facts.

The main reason is that the intrapleural pressure changes are not uniform all over the thoracic cage. Because of gravitational effects, pressure is more negative in the dorsal than in the ventral part of the lung (Derksen and Robinson, 1980; Lekeux et al, 1984). Consequently, the dorsal alveoli are

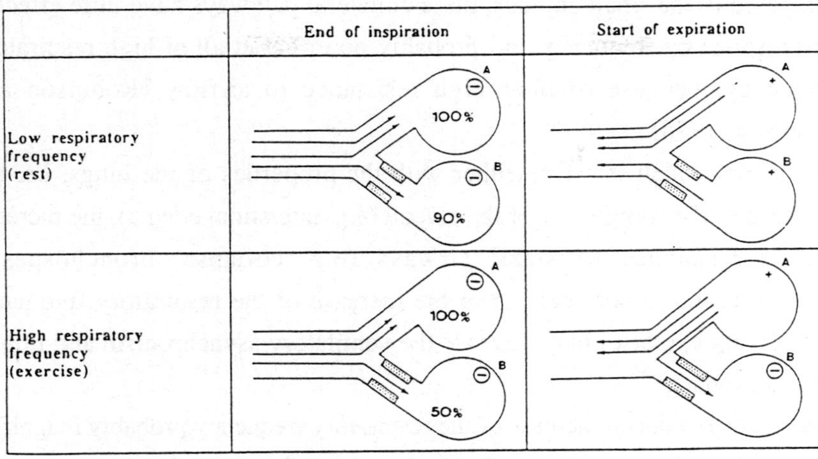

Fig. 5-1. Effect of ventilatory asynchronism on alveolar ventilation. The higher the respiratory frequency, the lower the ventilation in obstructed area.

more distended, less compliant, and receive less air during inspiration at any ventilatory rate.

A second reason may be the occurrence of some inequalities in the regional small airways resistance and/or alveoli compliance : inhaled air enters preferentially the area of the lungs with low resistive airways and high compliant alveoli. This induces a ventilatory asynchronism which is moderate in healthy animals and does not have significant effect on gas exchange at low respiratory frequency. However, in animals with important asynchronism (i.e. subclinical small airway diseases) and with a high respiratory frequency (i.e. exercising ones), this phenomenon will significantly impair gas exchange (Fig. 5-1.).

The interdependence between adjacent lung regions tends to limit the non-uniform changes in regional ventilation (Robinson and Sorenson, 1978). These mechanical interactions are the result from the intricate network of interconnecting elastic and collagenous tissue fibers of the lung.

Collateral ventilation between adjacent lung areas may also reduce the non-uniformity of the ventilation distribution. However, in the horse, when compared to the small animals, these collateral pathways have little effect at low respiratory frequency and probably no effect at all at high respiratory frequency, because of their high resistance to airflow (Robinson and Sorenson, 1978).

All factors which interfere either with the properties of the lungs, i.e. the decrease of the compliance of the alveoli (e.g. interstitial edema), the increase of the resistance of small airways (e.g. collapse, bronchospasm, hypersecretion, blood, etc ...) or the increase of the respiratory frequency (e.g. during exercise) may increase the ventilatory asynchronism and impair the gas exchange.

The exercise-induced increase of the respiratory frequency probably magnifies the regional differences in ventilation. Lung lobules with a long time constant for filling are not adequately filled up before the start of expiration. This results in ventilation/perfusion mismatching and hypoxemia. Moreover, because of the interdependence, the lobules with increased airflow resistance and/or decrease compliance are stretched and compressed by the surrounding lung parts (Mead et al, 1970). This may induce abnormal stresses on the tissues of these lobules. It has been suggested that exercise-induced pulmonary hemorrhage could be a consequence of this pulmonary overstretching (Robinson, 1979).

2.2. Pulmonary perfusion

The lungs are perfused by the pulmonary artery, which supplies the gas exchange regions. The distribution of the blood flow throughout the lung is influenced by the pressure difference between the pulmonary arteries and the pulmonary veins, by the vascular resistance and by the gravitational forces.

Blood flow to the conducting airways, interlobular septa and pleura is supplied by the bronchial artery and the filtrated fluid is drained by the lymphatic circulation.

There are some differences between the pulmonary and bronchial circulation. The pulmonary vascular resistance is very low : it is estimated at only one seventh of the resistance of the systemic circulation. Consequently, the mean pressure throughout these vessels is much lower than in the systemic circulation (26 mmHg versus 124 mmHg). While the vascular resistance in the systemic circulation is totally due to the pre-capillary vessels, the pulmonary vascular resistance is equally distributed between the pre- and the post-capillary vessels. Because of the peculiar distribution and of the low value of the pulmonary vascular resistance, the pressure in the pulmonary capillaries remains pulsatile.

During strenuous exercise, pulmonary blood flow increases up to eight times in horses (Thomas and Fregin 1981; Thomas et al, 1983; Thornton et al, 1983), ponies (Parks and Manohar, 1983) and dogs (Vancitters and Frabklin, 1969; Pendergast et al, 1985). A marked pulmonary hypertension is a feature of exercising horses and ponies : the mean pulmonary arterial pressure raises about 3 times, from 28 mmHg at rest to about 84 mmHg at fast gallop (Table 5-2.) with maximal reported values of 100 mmHg (Goetz and Manohar, 1986; Evans and Rose, 1988a,b,c; Wagner et al, 1989; Erickson et al, 1990; 1992). The pulmonary right-to-left shunt of the cardiac output is approximately 1 % at rest, i.e. perfusion through non-ventilated areas. It may decrease to 0.4 % during heavy exercise in horses (Wagner et al, 1989).

2.3. Ventilation/perfusion ratio

Gas exchanges ultimately depend on the optimization of the ventilation/perfusion ratio : efficient gas exchange occurs in the lung regions where this ratio is 0.8 to 1.0.

Most lung regions have a ventilation/perfusion ratio of 0.8. However there are lung regions that are excessively perfused (ratio < 0.8) or ventilated (ratio > 0.8). When ventilation is impaired (e.g. by subtotal obstruction of the airways), the ventilation/perfusion ratio decreases. In extreme cases of total obstruction of the airways, the ventilation/perfusion ratio is 0 : this corresponds to a right-to-left shunt. If perfusion is inadequate because of pulmonary vasoconstriction or hypotension, the ventilation/perfusion ratio

Table 5-2. Pulmonary hemodynamic values in adult thoroughbred horses.

Value	Unit	Rest	Slow Trot	Fast Gallop
HR	min^{-1}	35	103	210
SV	L	1.05	1.12	1.36
$\dot{Q}$	$L.min^{-1}$	37	115	285
PaPs	mmHg	37	78	152
PaPd	mmHg	22	39	50
PaPm	mmHg	28	52	82
Pw	mmHg	16	30	49
P(aP-w)	mmHg	12	22	33
PVR	$mmHg.min.L^{-1}$	0.32	0.19	0.11
T°a	°C	37.5	38.1	41.3
$\dot{V}O_2/HR$	L/beat	0.06	0.12	0.32
$\dot{V}A/\dot{Q}$	$L.L^{-1}$	0.84	2.11	4.48

HR : Heart rate; SV : Stroke volume; $\dot{Q}$: Cardiac output; PaPs : Systolic pulmonary artery pressure; PaPd : Diastolic pulmonary artery pressure; PaPm : Mean pulmonary artery pressure; Pw : Pulmonary artery wedge pressure; P(aP-w) : Pulmonary driving pressure; PVR : Pulmonary vascular resistance; T°a : Arterial blood temperature; $\dot{V}O_2/HR$: Oxygen pulse; $\dot{V}A/\dot{Q}$: Global ventilation perfusion ratio.

will increase. In extreme cases of non-perfusion, e.g. due to lung emboli, the ventilation/perfusion ratio becomes infinite.

In the quiet resting horse, the ventilation/perfusion ratio is not influenced by the gravitation, suggesting that the gradient in lung ventilation is matched by the gradient in lung perfusion (Amis et al, 1984).

In the heavily exercising horse, there is only a very mild mismatch of the ventilation/perfusion relationship. This mismatch accounts for 25 % of the increase of the alveolo-arterial difference in oxygen partial pressure (Wagner et al, 1989).

The physiological characteristics of the ventilation/perfusion ratio in horses

contrast with those of human beings. In the latter, the ventilation/perfusion ratio is not uniform at rest and a true mismatching occurs during exercise.
In subjects suffering from airway diseases, exercise will enhance ventilation/perfusion mismatching, mainly by the impairment of ventilation. This is particularly true as regards the equine species in which the collateral ventilation has little effect in compensating the non-permeability of small airways (Robinson and Sorenson, 1978). Therefore, the pulmonary lobules with a longer filling time constant will have an inadequate ventilation/perfusion ratio resulting in hypoxemia and sometimes hypercapnia.

2.4. Pulmonary diffusion

2.4.1. Composition of the respiratory gases

The ambient O_2 partial pressure, i.e. the relative contribution of the O_2 pressure to the total pressure of the ambient gas mixture, is about 20.93 % of the atmospheric pressure (760 mmHg at sea level). CO_2 partial pressure in ambient air is negligible (0.03 %).
After passing through the nasal cavities and the upper airways, inhaled air is saturated with H_2O. At normal body temperature, the partial pressure of the water vapor represents about 6.1 % of the total pressure, or 47 mmHg. Therefore the other gases account for a pressure of only 713 mmHg (i.e. 760 mmHg - 47 mmHg). The actual O_2 pressure in the trachea decreases therefore from 159 mmHg to 149 mmHg.
The alveolar air is quite different from the inspired air, because CO_2 is continuously expelled in the alveoli and O_2 is removed from the alveoli. Alveolar air composition is not constant because it is subjected to the cyclic variations of the respiratory phase (alveolar partial pressure in O_2 increases during inspiration and decreases during expiration). The mean values of alveolar air composition are : 14.5 % of O_2, 5.5 % of CO_2 and 79 % of nitrogen. However, after expiration, the air remaining in the lungs is mixed with the air of the next inspiration, whereby the variation of alveolar gas composition is damped (Fig. 5-2.).

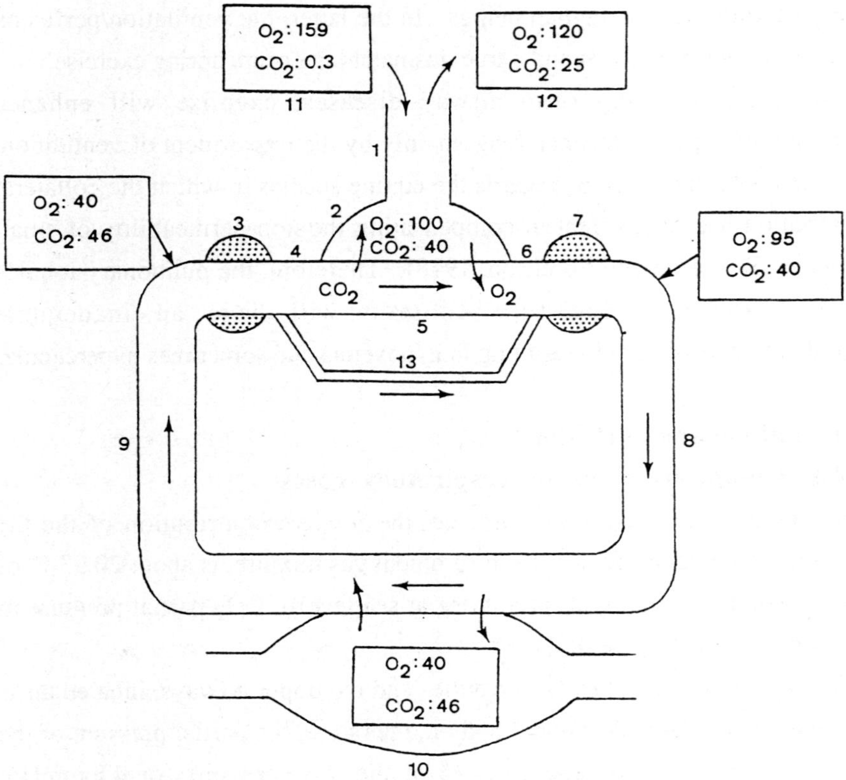

Fig. 5-2. O_2 and CO_2 partial pressures (mmHg) in relation to ventilation, perfusion and diffusion processes. 1 : Airways; 2 : Alveoli; 3 : Right heart; 4 : Pulmonary artery; 5 : Pulmonary capillaries; 6 : Pulmonary veins; 7 : Left heart; 8 : Arteries; 9 : Veins; 10 : Locomotor muscles; 11 : Inspired air; 12 : Expired air; 13 : Blood shunt.

2.4.2. Alveolar diffusion

Alveolar diffusion is a passive process whereby O_2 passes from the alveoli to the capillary blood and CO_2 passes in the opposite direction. As indicated by the following formula, the rate of diffusion (v) is influenced by the pressure gradient between the gases in the alveoli (PA) and the gases in the capillaries (Pcap), by the physical properties of the gases (D = diffusion coefficient), by the alveolar surface area available (A) and by the thickness of the alveolar-capillary barrier (X).

$$v = [D \times A \times (PA\text{-}Pcap)] / X$$

The alveolo-arterial pressure gradient is not constant : on the one hand, it decreases progressively as the blood passes through the alveolar capillaries, and on the other hand, it varies according to the time of the respiratory cycle. The maximal pressure gradients encountered are about 60 mmHg and 6 mmHg as regards O_2 and CO_2, respectively. The coefficient of diffusion of O_2 in horse averages 0.45 L/min/mmHg (Hare, 1975). The diffusion coefficient of CO_2 is 25 times higher than that of O_2.

The horse, along with other habitually active cursorial animals, appears to have an appropriately enlarged alveolar-capillary surface area, when compared to sedentary animals (Weibel, 1979). Moreover, during exercise, this area is enlarged by the recruitment of unperfused vessels induced by the increase in pulmonary arterial pressure and maybe by some mediators.

At rest and at moderate exercise levels, no measurable limitation of diffusion is observed in the healthy horse. The alveolar-arterial difference in O_2 tension averages 4 mmHg. On the opposite, during heavy but not necessarily maximal exercise (from 60 % of VO_2max), arterial hypoxemia and hemoglobin desaturation occur in horses (Fig. 5-3.) (Bayly et al, 1983b; Thornton et al, 1983; Art et al, 1990). Simultaneously, the alveolar-arterial difference in O_2 tension increases and may reach values as high as 30 mmHg (Lekeux et al, 1992).

Hypoxemia is primarily related to one, or to the combination of two or more of the following factors : (1) a decrease in the O_2 partial pressure in the inspired air, (2) right to left vascular shunts, (3) a ventilation/perfusion mismatching, (4) a diffusion impairment and (5) an alveolar hypoventilation.

The first factor can of course be eliminated when horses exercise in normal environmental conditions.

The right-to-left shunts and the matching of ventilation and perfusion have been shown to be accessory factors in the occurrence of hypoxemia during exercise (Wagner et al, 1989). A mild inequality of the ventilation/perfusion

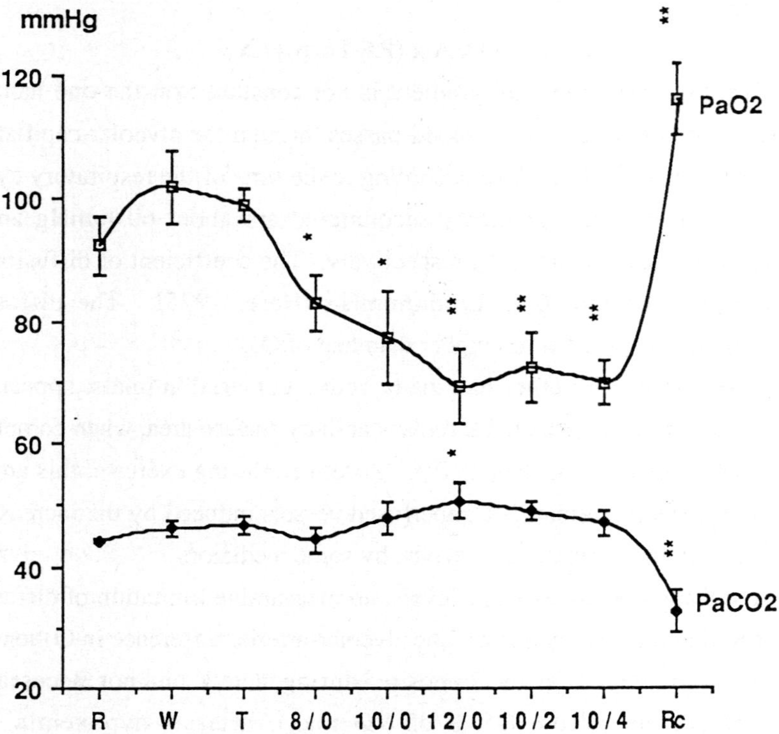

Fig. 5-3. Effect of velocity and incline on arterial blood gas values in thoroughbred horses. R : Rest; W : Walk; T : Trot; 8/0 : Gallop at 8 m/sec with 0° incline; Rc : Recovery. * : Significantly different from rest value with $P \leq 0.05$; ** : $P \leq 0.01$.

ratio accounts for 25 % of the widening of the alveolar-arterial O_2 tension difference. Alveolar-capillary diffusion desequilibrium is responsible for the remaining 75 % of this widening. Actually, during heavy exercise, different and opposite factors may influence the diffusion capacity.

On the one hand, the capillary transit time is strongly shortened and so is the time for O_2 equilibration. This will impair the diffusion.

On the other hand, there are adjustments which will improve the diffusion.

Firstly, mixed venous O_2 pressures as low as 16 mmHg have been reported

during fast gallop (Bayly et al, 1989). Because the alveolar O_2 pressure remains rather steady, the pressure gradient between the capillary blood and the alveolar air is increased, improving the O_2 extraction and diffusion.
Secondly, a large percentage of alveoli which are not perfused at rest, becomes functional, because of the exercise-induced increase in blood flow. This results in an increase of the exchanging alveolar surface. Furtheron, a vasodilation of the pulmonary capillaries and thus an increase of the capillary blood volume occur. In man, the capillary blood volume increases about 3 times above its resting value with an only 4- to 5-fold increase in pulmonary blood flow (Dempsey, 1986). In horses, the blood flow increases 8 times. Therefore, the capillary blood volume expands presumably more than 3 times. Lastly, the increase in the packed cell volume promotes the O_2 diffusion by increasing the hemoglobin concentration.
The fact that the equine species shows evidence of diffusion limitation during heavy exercise (Wagner et al, 1989) suggests that the physiological adjustments improving the pulmonary diffusion are overcome by the short capillary blood transit time. However, other athletic species have a short transit time during exercise (0.29 sec in the dog, 0.35 sec in the pony and 0.5 sec in man) but none of these demonstrate diffusion limitation during exercise (Parks and Manohar, 1984). Therefore, it may be hypothetized that these species are able to compensate their short capillary transit time by other physiological adaptations, which seem to be absent in horses.

2.5. Blood gas transport

2.5.1. Oxygen

The O_2 partial pressure in air or in liquids represents the relative pressure exerted by O_2 when mixed with other gases. The hemoglobin saturation in O_2 represents the percentage of the total hemoglobin binding sites occupied by O_2. The O_2 content represents the total amount of O_2 in the blood : a small amount of O_2 is dissolved in the plasma while the largest part is bound to hemoglobin.

2.5.1.1. O_2 dissolved in plasma

Once O_2 passes through the alveolar-capillary barrier, it either dissolves in the plasma or combines with hemoglobin. At rest, complete equilibration between alveolar and capillary O_2 tensions occurs before the blood leaves the capillary. Oxygen has a low solubility in the plasma : only 0.3 ml of O_2 will be dissolved in 100 ml of plasma, when alveolar partial pressure in O_2 is ± 100 mmHg. However, this O_2 dissolved in the plasma determines the arterial partial pressure in O_2 and therefore plays an important role in both O_2 diffusion and O_2 blood transport.

Resting values of arterial blood gases show little differences between species and breeds, except the difference between immature dairy and hypermuscled cattle (Table 5-3.).

During exercise, most species show physiological values of arterial blood gas partial pressures. Indeed, exercising dogs (Flandrois et al, 1971; Musch et al, 1986), cattle (Kuhlmann et al, 1985) and ponies (Pan et al, 1983) are normoxemic and normocapnic. On the opposite, high intensity and short term exercise induces hypoxemia (down to 60 mmHg) and hypercapnia (up to 55 mmHg) in both race horses, i.e. thouroughbreds (Bayly et al, 1983b; Art et al, 1990) and trotters (Thornton et al, 1983), and in double-muscled cattle (Gustin et al, 1988a).

2.5.1.2. O_2 bound to hemoglobin

Each molecule of hemoglobin can bind 4 molecules of O_2, forming the oxyhemoglobin complex. Beyond its capital role in O_2 transport, hemoglobin provides a sink for O_2 and therefore contributes to maintain an adequate pressure gradient during the alveolo-capillary diffusion. Each gram of hemoglobin is able to bind 1.36-1.39 ml of O_2 .

The blood hemoglobin concentration is largely increase (plus 50 %) during exercise in athletic species such as horses (Persson, 1967) and dogs (Ilkiw et al, 1989; Rose and Bloomberg, 1989) but not (plus 10 %) in non athletic species such as cattle (Kuhlmann et al, 1985; Gustin et al, 1988a).

Table 5-3. Predicted values of ventilation and arterial blood gas values in healthy dairy and beef cattle.

Value	Unit	Dairy cattle a	Dairy cattle b	Beef cattle a	Beef cattle b
V_T	L	0.009	1.00	0.009	0.95
$\dot{V}_e$	$L.min^{-1}$	0.99	0.74	0.48	0.86
Ti/T_{tot}		0.58	-0.04	0.42	0.01
mean$\dot{V}$i	$L.sec^{-1}$	0.03	0.78	0.02	0.84
mean$\dot{V}$e	$L.sec^{-1}$	0.04	0.70	0.01	0.87
$\dot{V}$imax	$L.sec^{-1}$	0.03	0.80	0.03	0.78
$\dot{V}$emax	$L.sec^{-1}$	0.04	0.77	0.02	0.87
PaO_2	kPa	8.64	0.09	8.51	0.07
$PaCO_2$	kPa	6.96	-0.04	9.66	-0.11

The data listed are allometric equations, i.e. $x = a.y^b$ in which x is the pulmonary value and y is the body weight. V_T : Tidal volume; $\dot{V}_e$: Minute volume; Ti/T_{tot} : Ratio of inspiratory to total time of the breathing cycle; mean$\dot{V}$i : Mean inspiratory flow or inspiratory drive; mean$\dot{V}$e : Mean expiratory flow; $\dot{V}$imax : Peak inspiratory flow; $\dot{V}$emax : Peak expiratory flow; PaO_2 : Arterial oxygen partial pressure; $PaCO_2$: Arterial carbon dioxide partial pressure.

2.5.1.3. Oxygen content of blood

The O_2 content of blood is mainly determined by the hemoglobin concentration and its saturation in O_2. When hemoglobin is satured in O_2, 100 ml of blood carries ± 20 ml of O_2, in addition to the 0.3 ml of O_2 dissolved per 100 ml of plasma.

The saturation of hemoglobin depends on the arterial O_2 partial pressure which depends in turn on the amount of O_2 dissolved in the plasma (Fig. 5-4.). At partial pressure in O_2 higher than 70 mmHg, the oxyhemoglobin curve is almost flat and hemoglobin saturation is nearly 100 %. Any increase in O_2 partial pressure has little influence because only few (3-5 %) of the

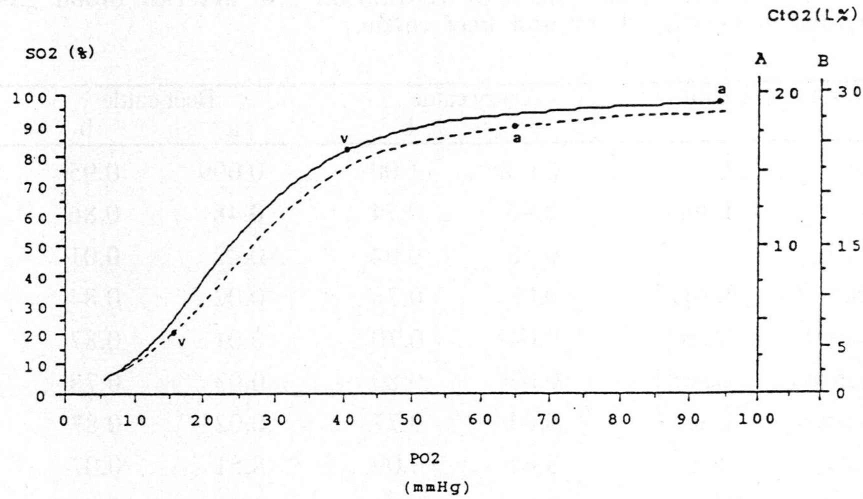

Fig. 5-4. Oxyhemoglobin dissociation curve in resting (solid line) and heavily exercising (dashed line) horses. PO_2 : Partial pressure for O_2; SO_2 : Percent saturation of hemoglobin (Hb) for O_2; CtO_2 : O_2 content at rest (A) (Hb : 140 g/L) and during exercise (B) (Hb : 220 g/L); A : Arterialized blood; B : Mixed venous blood.

oxygen binding sites of hemoglobin are still available. When partial pressure in O_2 becomes lower than 60 mmHg, the oxyhemoglobin saturation curve shows a sharp decreasing slope. Such partial pressure is encountered in the tissues which have a mean partial pressure in O_2 of ± 40 mmHg. In this condition, blood loses ± 25 % of its O_2 at the profit of the tissues. When the metabolism is high, i.e. during exercise, the tissue partial pressure in O_2 is even lower and more O_2 will be released. Lastly, blood temperature, pH, partial pressure in CO_2 and intracellular concentration of certain organic phosphates induce a right-sided shift of the curve, promoting a better O_2 release at the level of the metabolizing tissues.

The oxyhemoglobin dissociation curve in horses is slighlty different from the classical curve reported for human beings. The affinity of the equine hemoglobin for O_2 is higher than in man but less influenced by changes in temperature (Clerbaux et al, 1986). On the other hand, the bovine oxyhemoglobin dissociation curve is shifted to the left and less influenced by temperature, pH and 2-3 diphosphoglycerate than in man (Gustin et al, 1988b).

When the number of erythrocytes and consequently the hemoglobin concentration is reduced, for instance during anemia, the O_2 content of blood is reduced, despite normal arterial O_2 partial pressure and hemoglobin saturation. On the contrary, when the packed cell volume increases, for instance during exercise in horses and dogs, the O_2 content increases, even if the arterial O_2 partial pressure is reduced (Table 5-4.). The increase in the packed cell volume and the consequent increase in hemoglobin due to splenic contraction is an adaptation to exercise specific to the athletic species, providing almost 50 % more binding sites for O_2 during exercise in horses (Persson, 1967) and dogs (Longhurst et al, 1986). In the horse, this could represent a compensatory adjustment to the fall in arterial O_2 partial pressure and the hemoglobin desaturation, which is observed during heavy exercise. However, a too large increase in packed cell volume may interfere with the microcirculation, because it increases the blood viscosity (Boucher et al, 1981).

2.5.2. Carbon dioxide

CO_2 is produced during metabolic processes in the tissues and it diffuses from the cells into the capillary blood. In resting conditions, when the blood leaves the tissues, partial pressure in CO_2 has increased from 40 to 46 mmHg. Approximately 5 % of the CO_2 is dissolved in the plasma : this fraction determines the partial pressure in CO_2. The remaining CO_2 is transported in two chemical combinations, i.e. bicarbonate carbamino-compounds. Most of the CO_2 combines reversibly with H_2O, forming carbonic acid, which then dissociates into bicarbonate and hydrogen ion :

$$H_2O + CO_2 \longleftrightarrow H_2CO_3 \longleftrightarrow HCO_3^- + H^+$$

Sixty to 80 % of the CO_2 is transported as HCO_3^-. The reaction may take

Table 5-4. Gas exchange values in adult thoroughbred horses.

Value	Unit	Rest	Slow Trot	Fast Gallop
$\dot{V}O_2$	$L.min^{-1}$	2.2	12	67
$\dot{V}CO_2$	$L.min^{-1}$	1.8	11	69
RQ	-	0.82	0.92	1.03
PvO_2	mmHg	39	30	16
$PvCO_2$	mmHg	47	50	96
HCO_3^-	$mmol.L^{-1}$	28.8	27.5	23.0
PaO_2	mmHg	95	99	69
$PaCO_2$	mmHg	45	43	50
$[A\text{-}a]DO_2$	mmHg	4	4	29
pHa	-	7.39	7.40	7.26
PCV	%	38	44	58
Hb	g/L	140	160	220
SaO_2	%	97	97	90
CaO_2	L%	20	22	28
CvO_2	L%	14	11	5
$C(a\text{-}v)O_2$	L%	6	11	23
PAO_2	mmHg	99	103	98
$PACO_2$	mmHg	44	42	49
$F_{me}O_2$	%	16.2	17.7	14.3
$F_{me}CO_2$	%	2.6	2.5	5.4
Fet O_2	%	14.0	14.5	13.9
Fet CO_2	%	6.3	6.0	7.0

$\dot{V}O_2$: Oxygen uptake; $\dot{V}CO_2$: Carbon dioxide output; RQ : Respiratory quotient; PvO_2 : Venous oxygen partial pressure; $PvCO_2$: Venous carbon dioxide partial pressure; PaO_2 : Arterial oxygen partial pressure; $PaCO_2$: Arterial carbon dioxide partial pressure; HCO_3^- : Bicarbonate content; $[A\text{-}a]DO_2$: Alveolar-arterial oxygen gradient; pHa : Arterial pH; PCV : Packed cell volume; Hb : Blood hemoglobin concentration; SaO_2 : Percent saturation of hemoglobin with oxygen; $CaCO_2$: Arterial oxygen content; CvO_2 : Venous oxygen content; $C(a\text{-}v)O_2$: Arterio-venous oxygen content gradient; PAO_2 : Alveolar oxygen partial pressure; $PACO_2$: Alveolar carbon dioxide partial pressure; $F_{me}O_2$: Mixed expired oxygen fraction; $F_{me}CO_2$: Mixed expired carbon dioxid fraction; Fet O_2 : End-tidal oxygen fraction; Fet CO_2 : End-tidal carbon dioxide fraction.

place in the plasma, but occurs mainly in the erythrocytes. The presence of carbonic anhydrase accelerates this process several hundred times. Actually, the first step of this reaction reaches equilibrium before the blood leaves the capillaries. The reverse reaction, i.e. the formation of CO_2, occurs when the blood reaches the lungs.

The formation of carbamino compounds (15-20 % of the total CO_2 blood content), by coupling the CO_2 to the -NH groups of proteins (mainly hemoglobin) is the last form of CO_2 transport.

At high exercise intensities, i.e. 100 % of VO_2max, the large muscular mass produces very high amounts of CO_2 and the lung seems unable to eliminate this CO_2. The development of a relative CO_2 retention observed in healthy running horses is unique among domestic animals (Table 5-4.) (Bayly et al, 1989; Art et al, 1990). On the opposite, dogs (Szlyk et al, 1981) and ponies (Parks and Manohar, 1984) develop a compensatory hyperventilation during heavy exercise which increases the alveolar partial pressure in O_2 but also decreases the arterial partial pressure in CO_2 (down to 30 mmHg). Obviously, in exercising horses, there is a lack of truly compensatory hyperpnea contributing to the development of exercise-induced hypercapnia (Bayly et al, 1989; Lekeux et al, 1992).

3. PERIPHERAL GAS EXCHANGE

Peripheral gas exchanges are mainly influenced by the capillary density and blood hemoglobin concentration, by the mitochondria volume and by the diffusion from the capillaries to the mitochondria. These data have been reviewed elsewhere (Taylor and Weibel, 1991).

4. GAS EXCHANGE DURING POST-EXERCISE RECOVERY

After exercise, all physiological parameters return progressively to their resting values, the speed of this return being dependent on both the intensity and the duration of the exercise performed, the state of fitness of the horse and the bioclimatological conditions.

The excess of O_2 uptake after the exercise is mainly used for resynthesis of the phosphocreatin in the exercised muscles, for the catabolism or anabolism of blood lactate, and for the restoration of hormonal reserves (Rose et al, 1988). This excess of the O_2 uptake is associated with an elevated minute volume which is mainly due to an increase in respiratory frequency (Art and Lekeux, 1988a). Obviously, 5 minutes after exercise, the horses hyperventilate, as assessed by the high ventilatory equivalent for O_2, i.e. minute ventilation per L of oxygen uptake. Despite a high dead space to tidal volume ratio, this hyperventilation results in an alveolar hyperventilation and a consequent hyperoxia and hypocapnia (Fig. 5-3.) (Art et al, 1990). Furtheron, the end-tidal expired gases have high O_2 levels (17.2 % versus 14 % at rest) and a low CO_2 concentration (4.5 % versus 6.3 % at rest) .
Several assumptions may be put forwards to explain this post-effort hyperventilation. When the animal stops, limb motion does not longer influence the respiratory control and other factors such as acidosis or lactacidosis could become major respiratory stimulants. The resulting alveolar hyperventilation induces a respiratory alkalosis which could be advantageous to compensate for the metabolic acidosis.
The pulmonary resistance after exercise becomes significantly lower once the ventilatory parameters return near their resting values : this means that the physiological adjustments like bronchodilation or dilation of the larynx are no longer overcome by the physical phenomenons which tend to increase pulmonary resistance (Art and Lekeux, 1988c).
The post-effort hyperventilation, mainly based on an increase of the respiratory frequency, plays a major role in the body thermoregulation. This is not only true in dogs (Schmidt-Nielsen et al, 1970) which are highly dependent on the panting for their thermoregulation, but also in other species. It has been shown that ponies recovering from treadmill exercise tests in hot and humid conditions have a significantly higher respiratory frequency than ponies recovering from the same tests in dry and cold conditions (Art and Lekeux, 1988a). This observation should be hold in mind when horses,

performing endurance races in hot and humid conditions, are examined at the "vet-gate". Indeed, the respiratory frequency in these conditions is a poor indicator of the actual ventilatory demand of the horse (Rose et al, 1983).

5. EFFECT OF TRAINING ON GAS EXCHANGE

The effects of training in the equine species have received increasing attention during the last decades. The use of standardized treadmill tests has largely contributed to the improvements of the knowledge in this field. However, differences in the experimental observations have been found. They show that physiological adjustments to training may differ according to various parameters such as the age of the athlete, the previous stage, history, intensity and duration of training, etc ... Indeed, during training, the multiple steps of the oxygen chain are stimulated and adapted, but each of them respondes to training with different delays : the oxydative machinery of the muscles develops faster than the neovascularization in the muscles; the hemoglobin concentration increases only in the early stage of training; the cardiac output increases only after several weeks of training. They also depend on the breed and discipline, as well as on the training programmes (treadmill or field, duration and intensity). Furthermore, the kind of test used to point out the effects of training also influences the observations : short or prolonged exercise; standardized mild, moderate, submaximal heavy effort or maximal exercise up to fatigue are used for this purpose. However, despite the many problems related to the study of training effects, some information is now available.

Without doubt, training improves rapidly and significantly the maximal oxygen consumption (Fig. 5-5.) (Evans and Rose, 1987; 1988a; Knight et al, 1991; Art et al, 1992). The cardio-vascular mechanisms underlying the improvement of the O_2 uptake with training have already been studied, but the ventilatory mechanisms have been investigated much less so far. The improvement of the O_2 uptake with training is related to an increase in cardiac output (Bayly et al, 1983a) and/or in O_2 extraction. Actually, the results

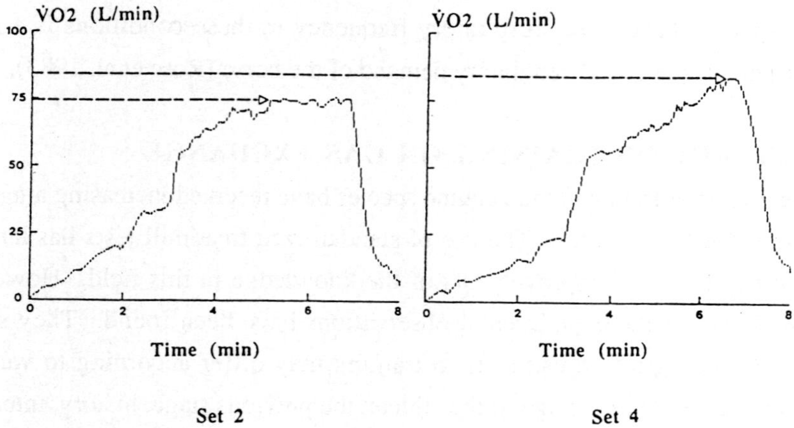

Fig. 5-5. Oxygen consumption ($\dot{V}O_2$) during standardized treadmill exercise before (Set 2) and after (Set 4) a 6-week period of training (Art et al, 1992).

concerning the effects of training on the arterio-venous difference in O_2 content are rather conflicting : this parameter is reported to be unchanged during submaximal exercise (Bayly et al, 1983a; Thornton et al, 1983), and increased during maximal exercise (Knight et al, 1991) or decreased during maximal exercise (Evans and Rose, 1988a). The discrepancy between these investigations can largely be explained by the difference in intensity and duration of the training programs applied and the standardised exercise tests used. For example, the decrease of arterio-venous difference in O_2 content with training during maximal exercise was simultaneous with a sharp increase of the cardiac output. The latter shortens the transit time of the blood in the tissues and consequently reduces the time for adequate diffusion (Evans and Rose, 1988a). On the other hand, no changes in the cardiac output were found in the study reporting an increase in arterio-venous difference in O_2 content (Knight et al, 1991).

Training does not seem to modify the exercise-induced alterations of blood gas tensions during and after heavy exercise (Thornton et al, 1983; Evans and Rose 1988a; Butler et al, 1991), nor the pulmonary arterial pressure and the pulmonary blood flow velocity during a mild standardized exercise (Erickson et al, 1987).

Although all the systems involved in exercise physiology, i.e. bones, tendons, muscles, cardio-vascular system, can be efficiently improved by training, there are only limited adaptations to training in the ventilatory capacity. The significant increase of the O_2 uptake induced by training is not accompanied by an equivalent increase in the minute volume. The ventilatory rate is unchanged during a maximal exercise test up to fatigue (Evans and Rose, 1988a) or is slighty lower during a standardised exercise test (Art et al, 1992) after a period of training. This results in a significant decrease of the ventilatory equivalent (minute volume to O_2 uptake ratio), obvious even in the early stage of training (Art et al, 1992). The mechanisms underlying this training adjustment are still unclear.

In human athletes, the improvement of the ventilatory equivalent for O_2 is explained by a training-induced reduction in respiratory frequency and an increase in tidal volume. The time available for gas exchange at the level of the alveoli is thus increased by training, and this induces a better alveolar O_2 extraction : the mean expired O_2 concentration is about 18 % in untrained men and 14 % in well trained athletes (Jirka and Adamus, 1965; Fringer and Stull, 1974).

In equine athletes, the decrease of the ventilatory equivalent after training is also associated with an improvement of the alveolar O_2 extraction (Art et al, 1992). However, in contrast with man, the reason for this improvement seems not to be a change in the pattern of breathing but probably an increase of the affinity of hemoglobin for O_2. This could be explained by a training-induced left-sided shift of the oxyhemoglobin curve resulting from a lower exercise-induced acidosis and hyperthermia (Art et al, 1992).

Whatever the reason may be, the decrease in the ventilatory equivalent means that horses breath less air to ensure a given O_2 uptake. Theoretically, this could imply that (1) the relative energetic cost of ventilation is reduced, (2) the fatigue of the respiratory muscles is delayed, and/or (3) the reduction of the O_2 uptake by the muscles is profitable to the working locomotor muscles. However, these assumptions remain also to be proved.

6. EFFECT OF DETRAINING ON GAS EXCHANGE

After a 3-weeks period of detraining, most of the training-modified ventilatory parameters, i.e. the O_2 uptake, the ventilatory equivalent for O_2 and the minute ventilation during a standardized exercise, return to their pre-training levels (Knight et al, 1991; Art et al, 1992). This indicates that the ventilatory adaptations are transient, despite the fact that they occur rapidly when the intensity of training is sufficient.

7. CONCLUSIONS

Because the various systems for oxygen delivery can adapt their functioning to the demand, the pulmonary gas exchange requirements are met in most physiological conditions, except in race horses and double-muscled calves which become hypoxemic and hypercapnic during high intensity exercise.

REFERENCES

AMIS T.C., PASCOE J.R., HORNOF W. Topographic distribution of pulmonary ventilation and perfusion in the horse. *Am. J. Vet. Res.* 1984, 45, 1597-1601.

ART T., LEKEUX P. Effect of environmental temperature and relative humidity on breathing pattern and heart rate in ponies during and after standardised exercise. *Vet. Rec.* 1988a, 123, 295-299.

ART T., LEKEUX P. Respiratory airflow patterns in ponies at rest and during exercise. *Can. J. Vet. Res.* 1988b, 52, 299-303.

ART T., LEKEUX P. Pulmonary mechanics during treadmill exercise in race ponies. *Vet. Res. Commun.* 1988c, 12, 245-258.

ART T., ANDERSON L., WOAKES A.J., ROBERTS C., BUTLER P.J., SNOW D.H., LEKEUX P. Mechanics of breathing during strenuous exercise in thoroughbred horses. *Respir. Physiol.* 1990, 82, 279-294.

ART T., VOTION D., Mc ENTEE K., AMORY H., LINDEN A., CLOSE R., LEROY P., LEKEUX P. Influence of training on ventilatory and cardio-respiratory parameters measured during a standardised exercise in thoroughbred horses. In Proceedings : 11th

Comparative Respiratory Society Meeting, Urbana (USA), September 1992, p1.

BAYLY W.M., GABEL A.A., BARR S.A. Cardiovascular effects of submaximal aerobic training on a treadmill in standardbred horses, using a standardized exercise test. *Am. J. Vet. Res.* 1983a, 44, 544-553.

BAYLY W.M., GRANT B.D., BREEZE R.G. The effects of maximal exercise on acid-base balance and arterial blood gas tension in thoroughbred horses. In : *Equine Exercise Physiology*, Snow, D.H., Persson, S.G.B., Rose, R.J. (Eds), Granta Editions, Cambridge, 1983b, pp 400-407.

BAYLY W.M., SCHULZ D.A., HODGSON D.R., GOLLNICK P.D. Ventilatory response to exercise in horses with exercise-induced hypoxemia. In : *Equine Exercise Physiology 2*, Gillespie, J.R., Robinson, N.E. (Eds), ICEEP Publications, Davis, California, 1987, pp 172-182.

BAYLY W.M., HODGSON D.R., SCHULZ D.A., DEMPSEY J.A., GOLLNICK P.D. Exercise-induced hypercapnia in the horse. *J. Appl. Physiol.* 1989, 67, 1958-1966.

BOUCHER J.H., FERGUSON E.W., WILHELMSEM C.L., STATHAM N., Mc MEEKIN R.R. Erytrocyte alterations during endurance exercise in horses. *J. Appl. Physiol.* 1981, 51, 131-134.

BRAMBLE D.M., CARRIER D.R. Running and breathing in mammals. *Science* 1983, 219, 251-256.

BUTLER P.J., WOAKES A.J., ANDERSON L.S., SMALE K., ROBERTS C.A., SNOW D.H. The effect of cessation of training on cardiorespiratory variables during exercise. In : *Equine Exercise Physiology 3*, Persson, S.G.B., Lindholm, A., Jeffcott, L.B. (Eds), ICEEP Publications, Davis, California, 1991, pp 71-76.

CHANG H.K. Mechanisms of gas transport during ventilation by high frequency oscillation. *J. Appl. Physiol.* 1984, 56, 553-559.

CLERBAUX T., SERTEYN D., WILLEMS E., BRASSEUR L. Détermination de la courbe de dissociation standard de l'oxyhémoglobine du cheval et influence, sur cette courbe, de la température, du pH et du diphosphoglycérate. *Can. J. Vet. Res.* 1986, 50, 188-192.

DAHL L.G., GILLESPIE J.R., KALLINGS P., PERSSON S.G., THORNTON J.R. Effects of a cold environment on exercise tolerance in the horse. In : *Equine Exercise Physiology 2*, Gillespie, J.R., Robinson, N.E. (Eds), ICEEP Publications, Davis, California, 1987, pp 235-242.

DEMPSEY J.A. Is the lung built for exercise ? *Med. Sci. Sp. Ex.* 1986, 18, 143-155.

DERKSEN F.J., ROBINSON N.E. Esophageal and intrapleural pressures in the healthy conscious pony. *Am. J. Vet. Res.* 1980, 41, 1756-1761.

ERICKSON B.K., ERICKSON H.H., COFFMAN J.R. Pulmonary artery, aortic and oesophageal pressure changes during high intensity treadmill exercise in the horse: a possible relation to exercise-induced pulmonary hemorrhage. *Equine Vet. J.* 1990, suppl 9, 47-52.

ERICKSON B.K., ERICKSON H.H., COFFMAN J.R. Pulmonary artery and aortic pressure changes during high intensity treadmill exercise in the horse: effect of frusemide and phentolamine. *Equine Vet. J.* 1992, 24, 215-219.

ERICKSON H.H., SEXTON W.L., ERICKSON B.K., COFFMAN J.R. Cardiopulmonary response to exercise and detraining in the Quarter Horse. In : *Equine Exercise Physiology 2*, Gillespie, J.R., Robinson, N.E. (Eds), ICEEP Publications, Davis, California, 1987, pp 41-51.

EVANS D.L., ROSE R.J. Maximum oxygen uptake in racehorses: changes with training state and prediction from submaximal cardiorespiratory measurements. In : *Equine Exercise Physiology 2*, Gillespie, J.R., Robinson, N.E. (Eds), ICEEP Publications, Davis, California, 1987, pp 52-67.

EVANS D.L., ROSE R.J. Cardiovascular and respiratory responses to submaximal exercise training in the thoroughbred horse. *Pflügers Arch.* 1988a, 411, 316-321.

EVANS D.L., ROSE R.J. Dynamics of cardiorespiratory function in Standardbred horses during different intensities of constant-load exercise. *J. Comp. Physiol. B* 1988b, 157, 791-799.

EVANS D.L., ROSE R.J. Cardiovascular and respiratory responses in thoroughbred horses during treadmill exercise. *J. Exp. Biol.* 1988c, 134, 397-408.

FLANDROIS R., LACOUR J.R., OSMAN H. Control of breathing in the exercising dog. *Respir. Physiol.* 1971, 13, 361-371.

FRINGER M.N., STULL G.A. Changes in cardiorespiratory parameters during periods of training and detraining in young adult females. *Med. Sci. Sports* 1974, 6, 20-25.

FROESE A.B., BRYAN A.C. High frequency ventilation. *Am. Rev. Respir. Dis.* 1981, 123, 249-250.

GALLIVAN G.J., McDONELL W.N., FORREST J.B. Comparative ventilation and gas exchange in the horse and the cow. *Res. Vet. Sci.* 1989, 46, 331-336.

GILLESPIE J.R., LANDGREN G.L., LEITH D.E. 1:2 ratio of breathing to stride frequencies in a galloping horse breathing 6 % CO_2. In : *Equine Exercise Physiology 3*, Persson, S.G.B., Lindholm, A., Jeffcott, L.B. (Eds), ICEEP Publications, Davis, California, 1991, pp 66-70.

GOETZ T.E., MANOHAR M. Pressures in the right side of the heart and esophagus (pleura) in ponies during exercise before and after furosemide administration. *Am. J. Vet. Res.* 1986, 47, 270-276.

GOTTLIEB-VEDI M., ESSEN-GUSTAVSSON B., PERSSON S.G.B. Draught load and speed compared by submaximal tests on a treadmill. In : *Equine Exercise Physiology 3*, Persson, S.G.B., Lindholm, A., Jeffcott L.B. (Eds), ICEEP Publications, Davis, California, 1991, pp 92-96.

GUSTIN P., DHEM A.R., LEKEUX P., LOMBA F., VAN DE WOESTIJNE K.P. Cardio-pulmonary function values in double-muscled cattle during muscular exercise. *Vet. Res. Commun.* 1988a, 12, 407-416.

GUSTIN P., CLERBAUX TH., WILLEMS E., LEKEUX P., LOMBA F., FRANS A. Oxygen transport properties of blood in two different bovine breeds. *Comp. Biochem. Physiol.* 1988b, 89A, 553-558.

HARE W.C.D. Equine respiratory system. In : *Sisson and Grossman's The Anatomy of the Domestic Animals*, 5th edn, Volume 1, Getty, R. (Ed.), W.B. Saunders Company, Philadelphia, 1975, pp 498-523.

HÖRNICKE H., MEIXNER R., POLLMANN U. Respiration in exercising horses. In : *Equine Exercise Physiology*, Snow, D.H., Persson, S.G.B., Rose, R.J. (Eds), Granta Editions, Cambridge, 1983, pp 7-16.

HÖRNICKE H., WEBER M., SCHWEIKER W. Pulmonary ventilation in thoroughbred horses at maximum performance. In : *Equine Exercise Physiology 2*, Gillespie, J.R., Robinson, N.E. (Eds), ICEEP Publications, Davis, California, 1987, pp 216-224.

ILKIW J., DAVIS P., CHURCH D. Hematologic, biochemical, blood-gas, and acid-base values in greyhounds before and after exercise. *Am. J. Vet. Res.* 1989, 50, 583-586.

JIRKA Z., ADAMUS M. Changes of ventilation equivalents in young people in the course of 3 years training. *J. Sport Med.* 1965, 5, 1-6.

KNIGHT P.K., SINHA A.K., ROSE R.J. Effects of training intensity on maximum oxygen uptake. In : *Equine Exercise Physiology 3*, Persson, S.G.B., Lindholm, A., Jeffcott, L.B. (Eds), ICEEP Publications, Davis, California, 1991, pp 77-82.

KUHLMANN W.D., HODGSON D.S., FEDDE M.R. Respiratory, cardiovascular, and metabolic adjustments to exercise in the Hereford calf. *J. Appl. Physiol.* 1985, 58, 1273-1280.

LANDGREN G.L., GILLESPIE J.R., LEITH D.E. No ventilatory response to CO_2 in thoroughbreds galloping at 14 $m.s^{-1}$. In : *Equine Exercise Physiology 3*, Persson, S.G.B., Lindholm, A., Jeffcott, L.B. (Eds), ICEEP Publications, Davis, California, 1991, pp 59-65.

LEKEUX P., HAJER R., BREUKINK H.J. Effect of somatic growth on pulmonary function values in healthy Friesian cattle. *Am. J. Vet. Res.* 1984, 45, 2003-2007.

LEKEUX P., ART T., DESMECHT D. Effect of exercise on equine alveolar ventilation. In Proceedings : 11th Comparative Respiratory Society Meeting, Urbana (USA), September 1992, S12.

LONGHURST J.C., MUSCH T.I., ORDWAY G.A. Oxygen consumption during exercise in dogs - roles of splenic contraction and adrenergic vasoconstriction. *Am. J. Physiol.* 1986, 251, H502-H509.

MEAD J., TAKISHIMA T., LEITH D. Stress distribution in lungs: a model of pulmonary elasticity. *J. Appl. Physiol.* 1970, 28, 596-608.

MUSCH T., FRIEDMAN D., HAIDET G., STRAY-GUNDERSEN J., WALDROP T., ORDWAY G. Arterial blood gases and acid-base status of dogs during graded dynamic exercise. *J. Appl. Physiol.* 1986, 61, 1914-1919.

PAN L.G., FORSTER H.V., BISGARD G.E., KAMINSKI R.P., DORSEY S.M., BUSCH M.A. Hyperventilation in ponies at the onset of and during steady-state exercise. *J. Appl. Physiol.: Respirat. Environ. Exercise Physiol.* 1983, 54, 1394-1402.

PARKS C.M., MANOHAR M. Distribution of blood flow during moderate and strenous exercise in ponies (Equus Cabalus). *Am. J. Vet. Res.* 1983, 44, 1861-1866.

PARKS C.M., MANOHAR M. Blood-gas tensions and acid-base status in ponies during treadmill exercise. *Am. J. Vet. Res.* 1984, 45, 15-19.

PELLETIER N., BLAIS D., VRINS A., ROBINSON N.E. Effect of sub-maximal exercise and training on dead space ventilation in the horse. In : *Equine Exercise Physiology 2*, Gillespie, J.R., Robinson, N.E. (Eds), ICEEP Publications, Davis, California, 1987, pp 225-234.

PENDERGAST D.R., KRASNEY J.A., ELLIS A., McDONALD B., MARCONI C., CERRETELLI P. Cardiac output and muscle blood flow in exercising dogs. *Respir. Physiol.* 1985, 61, 317-326.

PERSSON S.G.B. On blood volume and working capacity in horses. *Acta Vet. Scand.* (suppl) 1967, 19, 1.

POLLMANN U., HÖRNICKE H. The respiratory dead space of the horse during exercise measured telemetrically. In : *Biotelemetry VI*, Sansen, W. (Ed.), Leuven, 1984, pp 129-132.

ROBINSON N.E., SORENSON P.R. Collateral flow resistance and time constant in dog and horse lungs. *J. Appl. Physiol.* 1978, 44, 63-68.

ROBINSON N.E. Functional abnormalities caused by upper airway obstruction and heaves: their relationship to the etiology of epistaxis. *Vet. Clin. North Am. Large Anim. Pract.* 1979, 1, 17-34.

ROSE R.J., ALLEN J.R., BROCK K.A., CLARK C.R., HODGSON D.R., STEWART J.H. Effects of clenbuterol hydrochloride on certain respiratory and cardiovascular parameters in horses performing treadmill exercise. *Res. Vet. Sci.* 1983, 35, 301-305.

ROSE R.J., EVANS D.L. Cardiovascular and respiratory function in the athletic horse. In : *Equine Exercise Physiology 2*, Gillespie, J.R., Robinson, N.E. (Eds), ICEEP Publications, Davis, California, 1987, pp 1-24.

ROSE R.J., HODGSON D.R., KELSO T.B., Mc CUTCHEON L.J., REID T.A., BAYLY W.M., GOLLNICK P.D. Maximum oxygen uptake, oxygen debt and deficit, and muscle metabolites in thoroughbred horses. *J. Appl. Physiol.* 1988, 64, 781-788.

ROSE R.J., BLOOMBERG M.S. Responses to sprint exercise in the greyhound: effects on haematology, serum biochemistry and muscle metabolites. *Res. Vet. Sci.* 1989, 47, 212-218.

SCHMIDT-NIELSEN K., BRETZ W.L., TAYLOR C.R. Panting in dogs: unidirectional air flow over evaporative surfaces. *Science* 1970, 169, 1102-1104.

STAHL W.R. Scaling of respiratory variables in mammals. *J. Appl. Physiol.* 1967, 22, 453-460.

SZLYK P.C., McDONALD B.W., PENDERGAST D.R., KRASNEY J.A. Control of ventilation during graded exercise in the dog. *Respir. Physiol.* 1981, 46, 345-365.

TAYLOR C.R., WEIBEL E.R. Learning from comparative physiology. In : *The Lung: Scientific Foundations*, Crystal, R.G., West, J.B. (Eds), Raven Press, New York, 1991, pp. 1595-1607.

THOMAS D.P., FREGIN G.F. Cardiorespiratory and metabolic responses to treadmill exercise in the horse. *J. Appl. Physiol.* 1981, 50, 864-868.

THOMAS D.P., FREGIN G.F., GERBER N.H., AILES N.B. Effects of training on cardiorespiratory function in the horse. *Am. J. Physiol.* 1983, 245, R160-R165.

THORNTON J.R., ESSEN-GUSTAVSSON B., LINDHOLM A. Effects of training and detraining on oxygen uptake, cardiac output, blood gas tensions, pH and lactate concentrations during and after exercise in the horse. In : *Equine Exercise Physiology*, Snow, D.H., Persson, S.G.B., Rose, R.J. (Eds), Granta Editions, Cambridge, 1983, pp 470-486.

VANCITTERS R.L., FRABKLIN D.L. Cardiovascular performance of Alaska sled dog during exercise. *Circ. Res.* 1969, 24, 33-42.

WAGNER P.D., GILLESPIE J.R., LANDGREN G.L., FEDDE M.R., JONES B.W., DEBOWES R.M., PIESCHL R.L., ERICKSON H.H. Mechanism of exercise-induced hypoxemia in horses. *J. Appl. Physiol.* 1989, 66, 1227-1233.

WAGNER P.D., HOPPELER H., SALTIN B. Determinants of maximal oxygen uptake. In : *The Lung: Scientific Foundations*, Crystal, R.G., West, J.B. (Eds), Raven Press, New York, 1991, pp. 1585-1593.

WEIBEL E.R. Oxygen demand and the size of respiratory structures in mammals. In : *Evaluation of Respiratory Processes*, Wood, S.C., Lenfant, C. (Eds), Marcel Dekker Inc, New York, 1979, pp 289-346.

WEIBEL E.R., MARQUES L.B., CONSTANTINOPOL M., DOFFEY F., GEHR P., TAYLOR C.R. Adaptive variation in the mammalian respiratory system in relation to energetic demand. VI. The pulmonary gas exchanger. *Respir. Physiol.* 1987, 69, 81-100.

CHAPTER VI

CONTROL OF BREATHING IN RESTING AND EXERCISING ANIMALS

P. Lekeux[1], F. Rollin[2], T. Art[3]

[1] Laboratory for Functional Investigation
[2] Department of Large Animals Medicine
[3] Equine Sport Medicine Unit
Faculty of Veterinary Medicine
University of Liege

SUMMARY

This paper analyses the current knowledge concerning the control of breathing in resting and exercising healthy domestic animals.

KEY WORDS

Respiratory system - Pulmonary function - Control of breathing.

1. INTRODUCTION

With the exception of the changes induced by strenuous exercise, it can be assumed that the arterial blood gases remain remarkably steady. This means that oxygen (O_2) uptake and carbon dioxide (CO_2) production are constantly matched by the alveolar ventilation. This homeostasis is under the control of a central system, which receives afferent information from peripheral and central receptors and which regulates, via motor neurons, the ventilatory muscles accordingly. The respiratory control center is located in the medulla oblongata and its activity is modulated by a variety of neural inputs. The metencephalic pons is also involved in controlling the respiratory rythm and higher centers of consciousness can intervene to modify the pattern of breathing.

2. RESPIRATORY CONTROL AT REST

2.1. The central control

Breathing is controlled by neurons located in the pons and the medulla oblongata. The respiratory center in the medulla is divided into two groups of neurons. A dorsal group is located in the ventral portion of the nucleus tractus solitarii and contains mainly inspiratory neurons. A ventral group is located near the nucleus ambiguus and nucleus retroambiguus and has both inspiratory and expiratory neurons. If the medulla is experimentally isolated from all neural inputs, the animal continues to breath rythmically. The activity of both medullar centers is modulated by two respiratory centers in the pons : (1) the apneustic center, located in the lower pons, which stimulates the inspiratory neurons of the medulla and (2) the pneumotaxic center, located in the upper pons, which switches off the inspiration.

2.2. Chemoreceptors and humoral control

Because the primary function of the lungs is the supply of O_2 and the removal of CO_2, it is clear that the ventilation must ultimately be controlled according to information on gas exchange (Fig. 6-1.).

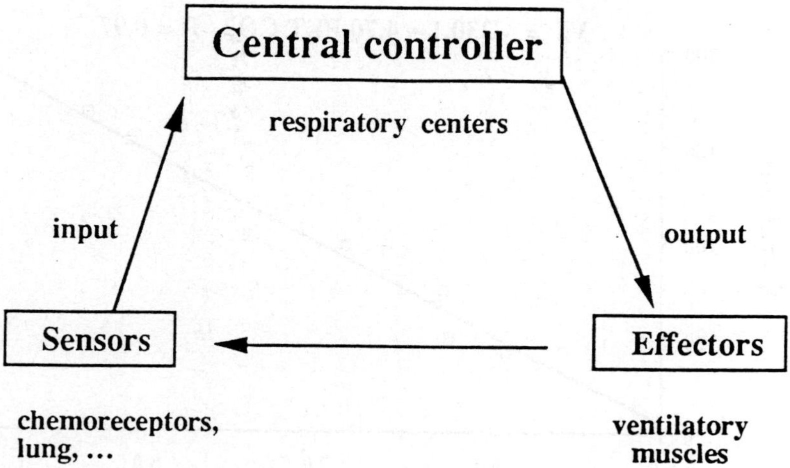

Fig. 6-1. General pathway of the control of breathing in physiological conditions.

Chemoreceptors are receptors which detect changes in arterial blood gases or chemical composition. Changes in arterial partial pressure in CO_2 and in pH are detected by both peripheral and central chemoreceptors, while changes in arterial O_2 partial pressure are detected by peripheral chemoreceptors only. At rest, lung ventilation is predominantly regulated by partial pressure in CO_2 and/or H^+ concentration. Indeed, small changes in arterial partial pressure in CO_2 and/or pH are more potent regulators of ventilation than changes in arterial O_2 partial pressure.

The *central chemoreceptor* tissue is located near the ventral aspect of the medulla obloganta. It lies in the intracerebral interstitial fluid and is separated from the blood by the brain barrier. It apparently responds to the pH changes of the interstitial tissue fluid. The latter can be induced by changes in arterial CO_2 partial pressure, giving a fast response because CO_2 diffuses freely through the blood brain barrier and induces a fast decrease of the pH of the interstitial fluid (Fig. 6-2.). It can also be induced by change in blood pH,

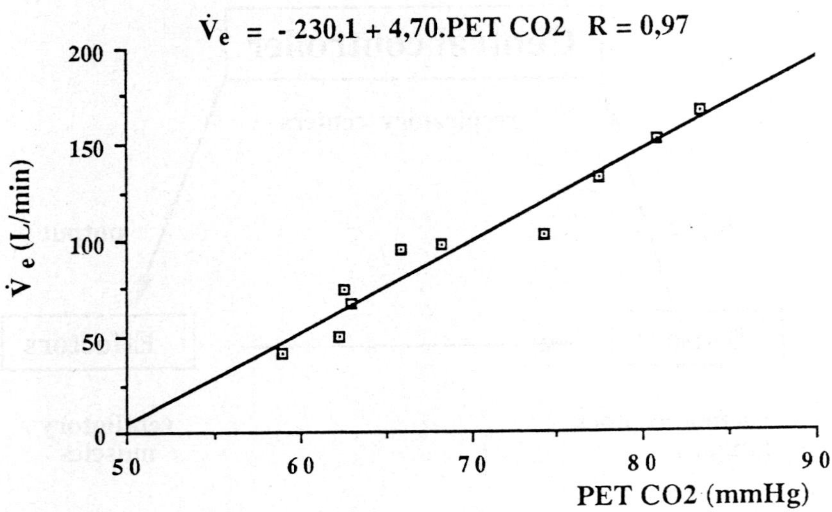

Fig. 6-2. Linear response to hyperoxic rebreathing relating ventilation ($\dot{V}_e$) to end-tidal partial pressure in CO_2 (PET CO_2) in one calf.

giving a delayed response because the brain barrier is relatively impermeable to H^+. Therefore, an acute increase of the H^+ concentration is at first detected by the peripheral receptors.

The *peripheral chemoreceptors* are located in the carotid bodies at the bifurcation of the common carotid arteries and in the aortic bodies, near the aortic arch. These chemoreceptors send afferent impulses to the respiratory control center via the vagus and the glossopharyngeal nerves. Their activity is enhanced by hypercapnia, hypoxemia and acidosis, but also by hyperthermia and by a decrease in blood pressure. While their response to CO_2 and pH is quite linear, their response to changes in arterial O_2 partial pressure is non linear : they only show enhanced activity once arterial O_2 partial pressure drops below 60 mmHg (Fig. 6-3.).

The carotid bodies are sensitive to changes in arterial O_2 partial pressure but not in oxyhemoglobin content. A decrease in arterial O_2 partial pressure also

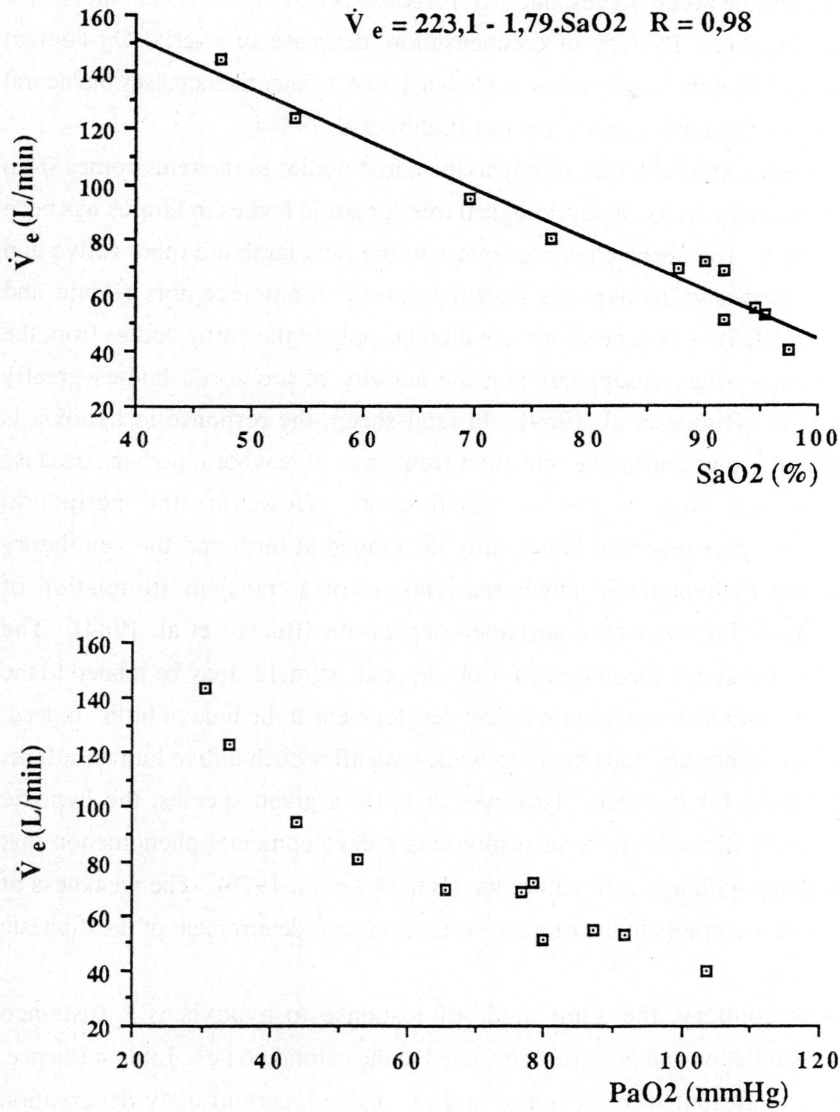

Fig. 6-3. Plotting of ventilation ($\dot{V}_e$) against O_2 saturation (SaO_2) (linear hypoxic response) and against arterial partial pressure in O_2 (PaO_2) (hyperbolic relationship) during isocapnic hypoxia in one calf.

stimulates the aortic bodies, but their response is less vigorous than that of the carotid bodies. By way of compensation, decrease in arterial O_2 content generated by either carbon monoxide inhalation or anemia increases the neural activity of the aortic chemoreceptors (Lahiri et al, 1981a).

Because the arterial blood supply to the aortic bodies in the fetus comes from the pulmonary artery, a physiological role for aortic bodies in fetuses has been suspected. The aortic chemoreceptors in the fetal lamb are more active and more responsive to hypoxia than the carotid chemoreceptors (Ponte and Purves, 1973). In the newborn, the blood supply to the aortic bodies from the pulmonary artery disappears and the activity of the aortic bodies greatly decreases (Biscoe et al, 1969). In fetal sheep, the response to hypoxia is weak but grows during the transition from fetus to newborn, perhaps because of the occlusion of the umbilical cord. However, the peripheral chemoreceptor response is not fully developed at birth and the ventilatory response to hypoxia in newborns consists of a transient stimulation of ventilation followed by a sustained depression (Bureau et al, 1984). The species difference encountered for this hypoxic stimulus may be related to the state of anatomical and physiological development at the time of birth. Indeed, newborn lambs and kids begin to walk soon after birth unlike human infants and kittens for instance. However, even in a given species, the hypoxic ventilatory diphasic mode of response is a developmental phenomenon that disappears with age and maturation (Belenky et al, 1979). The weakness of the chemoreceptors in the newborn is thus a major determinant of the diphasic response.

On the contrary, the adult mode of response to hypoxia is a sustained hyperventilation and is mainly attributed to the carotid bodies. Little influence, if any, is attributed to the aortic bodies. Indeed, carotid body denervation results in hypoventilation, hypoxemia and hypercapnia in goats, sheep, calves and ponies (Bisgard and Vogel, 1971; Bisgard et al, 1976; Forster et al, 1981; Lahiri et al, 1981b). In calves following carotid body denervation, the increase in ventilation after injection of potassium cyanide or lobeline, 2 potent stimulants of the peripheral chemoreceptors, represents only 20 % of control values. However, Bisgard et al (1980) showed in a 4-year period study that the aortic chemoreceptors become functional in a time-dependent manner after carotid body denervation in the pony. In the same way, blood gas values showed a trend toward normalization 6 months after carotid body denervation in calves. This technique allowed to demonstrate that carotid chemoreceptors are responsible for at least 30 % of resting effective ventilation in calves at sea level (Bisgard and Vogel, 1971). Another technique used by Bisgard et al (1969) points again to the possibility of a greater role for the aortic bodies. Indeed, they reported that the normal ventilatory response to hypoxia in the calf is reduced by ± 50 % during acute polycythemia which in turn increases arterial oxygen content.

The progressive increase in ventilation that occurs over the ensuing hours and days at high altitude characterizes the ventilatory acclimatization.

Ventilatory acclimatization to hypoxia occurs more rapidly in the awake goat than in other species. It is nearly complete after 4 hours of hypoxic exposure, either isocapnic or poikilocapnic (Smith et al, 1986). There has been great controversy over the underlying mechanism(s) of ventilatory acclimatization to hypoxia. However, it is well established that the carotid body chemoreceptors are required for its normal induction (Busch et al, 1985; Bisgard et al, 1986). In goats, isocapnic hypoxia did not result in hyperventilation on return to normoxia, whereas poikilocapnic hypoxia caused hyperventilation, indicating a different mechanism for the acclimatization and the persistent hyperventilation on return to normoxia in this species (Engwall and Bisgard, 1990).

In ruminants, the gas produced in the rumen may consist of more than 60 % CO_2 (McArthur and Miltimore, 1961). It has been clearly established that the major part of eructed rumen gases is subsequently inhaled (Dougherty et al, 1962a; Dougherty and Cook, 1962b). It has also been shown that this phenomenon significantly influences the pattern of breathing in cattle and that the ventilation in basal condition is characterized by a cyclic variability coupled

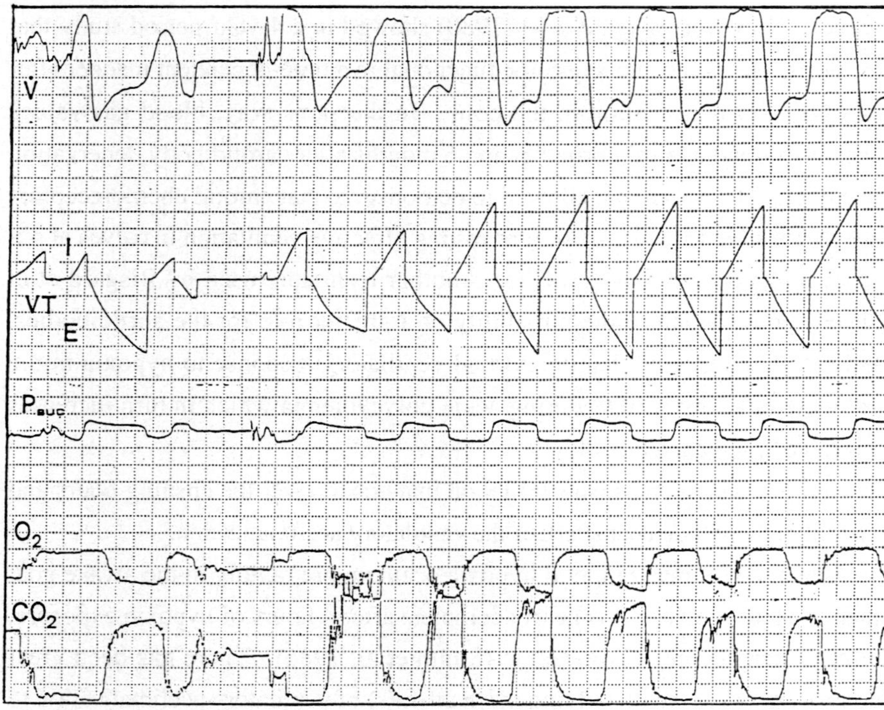

Fig. 6-4. Effect of eructation on the pattern of breathing in cattle. $\dot{V}$: Airflow; V_T : Tidal volume; P_{Buc} : Buccal pressure; O_2 : Oxygen concentration in inspired and expired air; CO_2 : Carbon dioxide concentration in air.

to belching in this species (Fig. 6-4.) (Rollin et al, 1990).

To assess the hypoxic and hypercapnic responses, the rebreathing method is widely used and is much less time-consuming and tiring for animals than classic steady-state methods. For the hypercapnic response, the animal breathes into a reservoir bag filled with a gas mixture containing 7 % CO_2 and 93 % O_2, the volume of which slightly exceeds its vital capacity (Read, 1967). The central chemoreceptors are primarily responsible for the ventilatory response to arterial CO_2 partial pressure elevation because the contribution from the peripheral chemoreceptors is small under hyperoxia. CO_2 sensitivity is assessed by calculating the slope of the linear relationship between respiratory flow and end-tidal CO_2. The same procedure is adopted to test the hypoxic response, except that the bag contains 70 % N_2, 23 % O_2 and 7 % CO_2 (Rebuck and Campbell, 1974).

To specifically study peripheral chemoreceptors responsiveness, single-breath tests are achieved with hypoxic (pure N_2) or hypercapnic gas mixtures (McClean et al, 1988; Caroll et al, 1991). The ventilatory response to these single-breath tests has to be measured before central chemoreceptors enter into activity.

Bisgard et al (1973), studying the ventilatory control in the Hereford calf, found that calves were less sensitive to acute isocapnic hypoxia and to acute hyperoxic hypercapnia than man. They also demonstrated a potentiation between hypoxia and hypercapnia as stimulants to ventilation. The goats appear to be slightly more sensitive to acute hypoxia, when compared to calves (Edelman et al, 1969).

Ventilation, as a measurement of the hypoxic or hypercapnic response, may be influenced by conscious muscle effort or by abnormal mechanical properties of the respiratory system in some circumstances. To palliate this inconvenient, the measurement of inspiratory occlusion pressure at 100 msec ($P_{0.1}$) may represent a useful index of the output of the respiratory centers (Whitelaw et al, 1975). Another method may be the electromyographic analysis of the diaphragmatic activity (Desmecht and Lekeux, 1992).

2.3. Pulmonary and airways receptors

Three kinds of receptors with vagal afferences are located in the lungs and play a role in the ventilatory control.

The *pulmonary stretch receptors* are nerve endings in the tracheal and bronchial smooth muscles. Their activity is enhanced by an enlargement of airway diameter, for example when the lung volume increases, and induces an inhibition of further inspiratory activity. These receptors could be responsible for the adjustment of the pattern of breathing (relation between tidal volume and respiratory frequency for a given minute volume) which minimizes the energetic cost of breathing. They could also prevent a lung overstretching when the ventilatory demand is high, i.e. during heavy exercise.

Irritant receptors have a minor role in the control of breathing. They are located between and below the epithelial cells of the larynx, trachea, bronchi and intrapulmonary airways. They protect the lung against various aggressions by reacting to a variety of stimulations (such as inhalation of irritant gases, dust, release of histamine, ...) and induce tachypnea, bronchospasm, coughing and mucus secretion.

Pulmonary C fibers ramify in the pulmonary interstitium close to the pulmonary capillaries. They may monitor the blood composition or the degree of distention of the interstitium. They are probably responsible for the respiratory adjustments in disease but this remains to be demonstrated in horses.

2.4. Muscle spindle stretch receptors

As other skeletal muscles, the ventilatory muscles have spindle stretch receptors. The density of these receptors variable from one muscle to the other. They are sparse in the diaphragm but numerous in the intercostal muscles. These receptors control the strength of the contraction of the ventilatory muscles.

3. RESPIRATORY CONTROL DURING EXERCISE

Gas exchange requirements, i.e. O_2 uptake and CO_2 output, vary with the metabolic rate. Without doubt, exercise is the most potent stress to the body oxydative machinery, i.e. to the muscle system and to the functions concerning external and alveolar gas exchange, gas transport and tissue respiration. Along with increasing exercise intensity, the O_2 uptake rises linearly up to a maximum termed as $\dot{V}O_2max$. At this level of exercise intensity, all the available aerobic capacities of the muscles are recruited and any further increase in work level requires ATP production by anaerobic pathways.

It is assumed that in horses at maximal exercise, the O_2 uptake may increase more than 40 times, as compared to resting values. Together with other adaptations, this increase is satisfied by an approximately 30-fold increase in the minute volume (Evans and Rose, 1988; Rose et al, 1988; Art et al, 1990). How the ventilatory rate is controlled during exercise is one of the major unresolved questions in respiration physiology. It remains unclear whether the quick and precise adjustments of alveolar ventilation are induced by neural and/or humoral stimuli (Forster and Pan, 1991). In horses, this control seems to be different according to the exercise intensity.

3.1. Respiratory control during low intensity exercise

During moderate exercise, the arterial blood gases and chemical blood composition do not change. This homeostasis occurs because the ventilation rate goes along with the metabolic rate. However, gas tensions are far too stable to explain the increase of ventilation by a simple negative feed-back system existing at rest. Gas tensions are thought to be involved in the control of ventilation during exercise but this mechanism remains controversial. The stimulus for the adjustment of the alveolar ventilation to meet the metabolic demand might be either humoral, i.e. acting through changes in blood-borne agents, or neural, i.e. via changes in neural patways, or neurohumoral, i.e. acting via both pathways (Forster and Pan, 1991).

Other drives which participate also in the control of ventilation are mechano-reflexes originating from motion of the working limbs, changes in cardiac output, thermoregulation, cortical and psychological factors, etc ... (McArdle et al, 1991).

The exercise-induced hyperpnea at mild and moderate exercise intensities has been intensively studied in ponies. These studies show that in this species the hyperpnea is related to an increase in lactacidosis (Erickson et al, 1991) and to spinal afferent information (Pan et al, 1990), but not related to an increase of

arterial or venous CO_2 (Klein et al, 1982; Pan et al, 1983; 1984; Forster et al, 1986; Powers et al, 1987), a decrease of blood pH (Pan et al, 1986), an increased H^+ stimulation of the medullary receptors (Bisgard et al, 1978), a decrease of arterial O_2 partial pressure (Forster et al, 1983), cardio-vascular causes (Pan et al, 1984) nor limb motion (Forster et al, 1984). However, transposition of these observations to horses is questionable because both species differ in their respiratory adjustments. While the horse become hypoxemic and sometimes hypercapnic during heavy exercise, the pony does not become hypoxemic but hypocapnic, with arterial partial pressures in CO_2 as low as 27 mmHg (Parks and Manohar, 1984).
In dogs, it is suggested that fast acting neurogenic mechanisms could be responsible for the major drive to ventilation during low levels of exercise, while humoral factors could become the major stimuli to ventilation during high levels of work (Szlyk et al, 1981). At the onset of exercise, the level of ventilation seems to be preset via potential pre-adaptative adjustments to metabolic needs. During exercise, the pattern of breathing in this species may also be influenced by the thermolytic needs of the body, via thermal polypnea (Flandrois et al, 1971). Therefore, the exercising dog must adapt both its alveolar ventilation and dead space ventilation, in order to meet the metabolic and thermoregulatory requirements, respectively.

3.2. Respiratory control during high intensity short-term exercise

During strenuous exercise, the healthy horse, independently of its sports aptitude and state of fitness, presents a decrease in arterial O_2 partial pressure and pH and sometimes an increase in arterial partial pressure in CO_2. In this specific condition, these chemical regulators are supposed to strongly stimulate the ventilation, but nevertheless they remain insufficient to maintain arterial blood gases homeostasis. This is not the case in other species such as man, dog and pony, which do not show hypoxemia nor hypercapnia during strenuous exercise. However, it must be pointed out that in the elite top-fit human endurance athlete, cardio-vascular and muscular adaptations to training may reach levels so high that the pulmonary system may be stressed maximally or even lag behind the functional capacity of the remaining aerobic system. Such a condition may result in hypoxemia and hypercapnia during high intensity exercise (Dempsey et al, 1984).

In contrast to other species, the horse does not adopt a compensatory hyperpnea, i.e. an hyperventilation which could compensate the gas exchange impairment resulting mainly from diffusion limitation and partly from ventilation/perfusion inequalities (Bayly et al, 1989; Wagner et al, 1989). The reason for this hypercapnic hypoventilation in the horse remains unclear and numerous hypothesises have been put forwards to explain this feature.

3.2.1. Hypothesis to explain the lack of compensatory hyperpnea in heavily exercising horses

3.2.1.1. Influence of the locomotion-respiration coupling on exertional ventilation

The locomotion-respiration coupling has been suggested to be a major constraint to the increase of ventilation. Although there is no doubt that respiratory frequency is totally related to step frequency in galloping horses, several experimental observations rule out the coupling as the unique reason of hypoventilation : (1) standardbred horses present also these blood gas alterations when racing at a trot, i.e. a gait in which a coupling is possible but not compulsory (Thornton et al, 1983); (2) the magnitude of hypercapnia is poorly related to the respiratory frequency (Bayly et al, 1989); (3) the respiratory frequency of the pony is also thightly coupled with its step frequency but this species nevertheless adopts a compensatory hyperventilation and becomes hypocapnic during heavy exercise (Parks and Manohar, 1984).

3.2.1.2. Lesser sensitivity of the receptors

A slight increase of ventilation in horses running at 10 m/sec is observed when CO_2 concentration in the inhaled air increases from 0 to 3 %. However, a further increase in inhaled CO_2 up to 6 % does not induce further changes in ventilation when these horses were not at their maximal ventilation capacity (Landgren et al, 1991). The underlying mechanisms of this observation remain still to be elucidated.

3.2.1.3. Influence of force-velocity characteristics of the ventilatory muscles

Theoretically, the compensatory hyperventilation which would be required for the homeostasis of arterial O_2 partial pressure should be ensured by either (1) a tidal volume of ± 23 L, in combination with a respiratory frequency of about 120 breaths/min, implying a mean respiratory airflow of more than 100 L/sec, or (2) a coupling 2:1 between respiratory frequency and step frequency, which implies that the respiratory frequency should reach values of about 240 breaths/min (Bayly et al, 1989). In terms of respiratory muscle energetics and force-velocity characteristics, such a level of ventilation is likely to be impossible to reach.

3.2.1.4. Negative feed-back mechanisms generated by ventilatory muscle fatigue

The increase of the ventilatory level is accompanied by an exponential increase of both the work of breathing and the O_2 uptake (energetic cost) of the ventilatory muscles. This is mainly caused by the increase in lung volume, in respiratory frequency and in the resistive, elastic and inertial forces (Art et al, 1990). Consequently, the energy demand of the ventilatory muscles becomes substantial and the energy supply may be insufficient to satisfy this demand (Fig. 6-5.). This could result in a negative metabolic balance at the level of the ventilatory muscles, which could lead to fatigue (Leblanc et al, 1988; Fitting, 1991). This phenomenon could control the pattern of breathing by a negative feed-back mechanism acting either on the respiratory centers or directly on the ventilatory muscles (Mador and Acevedo, 1991; Lekeux et al,

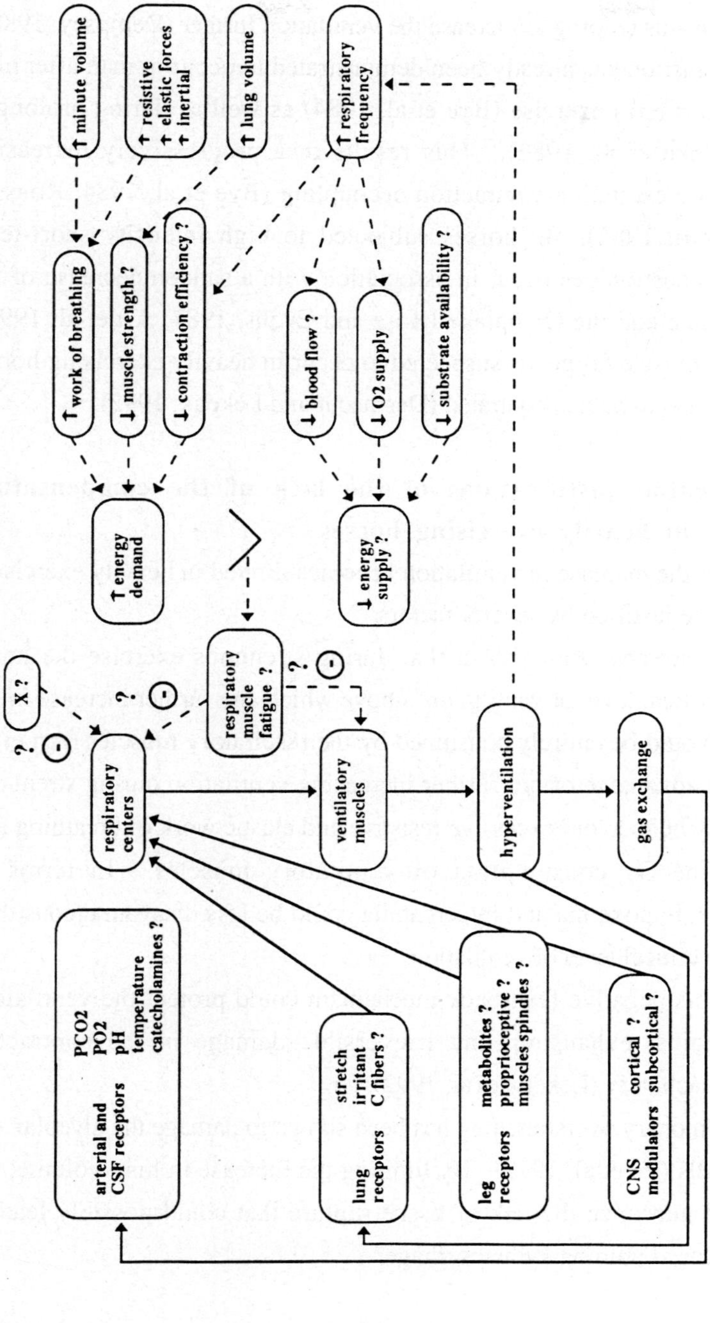

Fig. 6-5. Hypothesis for the control of the ventilatory response in heavily exercising horse.

1992). This negative feed-back would override all the other positive feed-back mechanisms tending to increase the ventilation further (Dempsey, 1988). Muscle exhaustion has already been demonstrated to occur in man after high intensity short term exercise (Bye et al, 1984) as well as during prolonged exercise (Loke et al, 1982). This results in a progressively increasing diaphragmatic excitation-contraction decoupling (Bye et al, 1984; Roussos and Macklem, 1986). In horses subjected to high intensity short-term exercise, exhaustion can occur in association with a sudden decrease of the minute volume and the O_2 uptake (Rose and Evans, 1987; Art et al, 1992). Respiratory muscle fatigue is suspected to occur in heavily exercising horses but this remains to be demonstrated (Desmecht and Lekeux, 1992).

3.2.2. Potential justifications of the lack of the compensatory hyperpnea in heavily exercising horses

The fact that the increase in ventilation becomes limited in heavily exercising horses may be justified by several factors.

First, it has already been shown that during strenuous exercise the horse reaches a "critical level of ventilation" above which any further increase in the O_2 uptake would be entirely consumed by the respiratory muscles (Art et al, 1989). The advantage of not further increasing ventilation during strenuous exercise may be to avoid excessive resistive and elastic work of breathing and to reduce the O_2 consumption of ventilatory muscles. In terms of performance, hypoxemia and hypercapnia could be less disavantageous than reaching the critical level of ventilation.

Secondly, this negative feed-back mechanism could protect the ventilatory muscles against exhaustion and irreversible damage in the contractile oxydative machinery (Lekeux et al, 1992).

Thirdly, pulmonary overstretching has been shown to damage the alveolar and vascular walls (Fu et al, 1992). By limiting the increase in lung volume, the horse could minimize the risk of tissue rupture that could possibly lead to exercise-induced pulmonary hemorrhage.

3.3. Respiratory control during submaximal prolonged exercise

During prolonged heavy -but not maximal- exercise, the impairment of the gas exchange (especially hypercapnia) seems to be progressively compensated after several minutes of exercise (Bayly et al, 1989; Hodgson et al, 1990). This suggests that horses, like man, experience the "second wind" phenomenon, i.e. the relief of hypoventilation which could be induced by diaphragmatic fatigue (Scharf et al, 1984). Several factors are put forwards to explain the improvement of the ventilatory muscle function after a few minutes of exercise : (1) the length of the diaphragm may be modified by recruitment of other ventilatory muscles or by changes in the functional residual capacity, resulting in an increase in its contraction force according to its length-tension characteristics; (2) the contractile function of the diaphragm may be improved; (3) the blood flow in the working diaphragm may be improved and (4) the exercise-induced release of cathecolamines may lead to increased contractility of the diaphragm. These assumptions remain to be confirmed in the horse.

4. CONCLUSIONS

The control of breathing is a complex and controversial mechanism, especially in the heavily exercising horse. In this species, a compensatory hyperpnea is lacking. The mechanism of this phenomenon is not yet elucidated but it could be the result of a compromise between maximalization of alveolar ventilation and minimalization of the work of breathing. This might provide the highest level of oxygen delivery to the locomotor machinery and protect the pulmonary structures against overstretching and irreversible damage.

REFERENCES

ART T, LEKEUX P, GUSTIN P, DESMECHT D., AMORY H., PAIVA M. Inertance of the respiratory system in ponies. *J. Appl. Physiol.* 1989, 67, 534-540.

ART T., ANDERSON L., WOAKES A.J., ROBERTS C., BUTLER P.J., SNOW D.H., LEKEUX P. Mechanics of breathing during strenuous exercise in thoroughbred horses. *Respir. Physiol.* 1990, 82, 279-294.

ART T., VOTION D., Mc ENTEE K., AMORY H., LINDEN A., CLOSE R., LEROY P., LEKEUX P. Influence of training on ventilatory and cardio-respiratory parameters measured during a standardised exercise in thoroughbred horses. In Proceedings : 11th Comparative Respiratory Society Meeting, Urbana (USA), 1992, P1.

BAYLY W.M., HODGSON D.R., SCHULZ D.A., DEMPSEY J.A., GOLLNICK P.D. Exercise-induced hypercapnia in the horse. *J. Appl. Physiol.* 1989, 67, 1958-1966.

BELENKY D.A., STANDAERT T.A., WOODRUM D.E. Maturation of hypoxic ventilatory response of the newborn lamb. *J. Appl. Physiol. : Respirat. Environ. Exercise Physiol.* 1979, 47, 927-930.

BISCOE T.J., PURVES M.J., SAMPSON S.R. Types of nervous activity which may be recorded from the carotid sinus nerve in the sheep foetus. *J. Physiol. London* 1969, 202, 1-23.

BISGARD G.E., ALVAREZ H.G., GROVER R.F. Decreased ventilatory response to hypoxia during acute polycythemia in the calf. *Respir. Physiol.* 1969, 7, 369-382.

BISGARD G.E., VOGEL J.H. Hypoventilation and pulmonary hypertension in calves after carotid body excision. *J. Appl. Physiol.* 1971, 31, 431-437.

BISGARD G.E., RUIZ A.V., GROVER R.F., WILL J.A. Ventilatory control in the Hereford calf. *J. Appl. Physiol.* 1973, 35, 220-226.

BISGARD G.E., FOSTER H.V., ORR J.A., BUSS D.D., RAWLINGS C.A., RASMUSSEN B. Hypoventilation in ponies after carotid body denervation. *J. Appl. Physiol.* 1976, 40, 184-190.

BISGARD G.E., FORSTER H.V., BYRNES B., STANEK K., KLEIN J., MANOHAR M. Cerebrospinal fluid acid-base balance during muscular exercise. *J. Appl. Physiol. : Respirat. Environ. Exercise Physiol.* 1978, 45, 94-101.

BISGARD G.E., FORSTER H.V., KLEIN J.P. Recovery of peripheral chemoreceptor function after denervation in ponies. *J. Appl. Physiol.* 1980, 49, 964-970.

BISGARD G.E., BUSCH M.A., FORSTER H.V. Ventilatory acclimatization to hypoxia is not dependent on cerebral hypocapnic alkalosis. *J. Appl. Physiol.* 1986, 60, 1011-1015.

BUREAU M.A., ZINMAN R., FOULON P., BEGIN R. Diphasic ventilatory response to hypoxia in newborn lambs. *J. Appl. Physiol.* 1984, 56, 84-90.

BUSCH M., BISGARD G.E., FORSTER H.V. Ventilatory acclimatization to hypoxia is not dependent on arterial hypoxemia. *J. Appl. Physiol.* 1985, 58, 1874-1880.

BYE P.T.P., ESAU S.A., WALLEY K.R., MACKLEM P.T., PARDY R.L. Ventilatory muscles during exercise in air and oxygen in normal men. *J. Appl. Physiol. : Respirat. Environ. Exercise Physiol.* 1984, 56, 464-471.

CAROLL J.L., CANET E., BUREAU M.A. Dynamic ventilatory responses to CO_2 in the awake lamb: role of the carotid chemoreceptors. *J. Appl. Physiol.* 1991, 71, 2198-2205.

DEMPSEY J.A., HANSON P.G., HENDERSON K.S. Exercise-induced arterial hypoxaemia in healthy human subjects at sealevel. *J. Physiol. Lond.* 1984, 355, 161-175.

DEMPSEY JA. Problems with the hyperventilatory response to exercise and hypoxia. In : *Oxygen Transfer from Atmosphere to Tissues*, Gonzalez, N.C., Fedde, M.R. (Eds), Plenum Publishing Corporation, 1988, 277-291.

DESMECHT D., LEKEUX P. Respiratory muscle fatigue in large animals. In Proceedings: IXth International Congress of Electromyography and Clinical Neurophysiology, Jerusalem, Israël, June 1992, p347.

DOUGHERTY R.W., STEWART W.E., NOLD M.M., LINDHAL I.L., MULLENAX C.H., LEEK B.F. Pulmonary absorption of eructated gas in ruminants. *Am. J. Vet. Res.* 1962a, 23, 205-212.

DOUGHERTY R.W., COOK H.M. Routes of eructated gas expulsion in cattle - A

quantitative study. *Am. J. Vet. Res.* 1962b, 23, 997-1000.
EDELMAN N.H., CHERNIACK N.S., LAHIRI S., FISHMAN A.P. Response of goats to acute, chronic and life long hypoxia. *Fed. Proc.* 1969, 28, 1223-1227.
ENGWALL M.J., BISGARD G.E. Ventilatory responses to chemoreceptor stimulation after hypoxic acclimatization in awake goats. *J. Appl. Physiol.* 1990, 69, 1236-1243.
ERICKSON B.K., FORSTER H.V., PAN L.G., LOWRY T.F., BROWN D.R., FORSTER M.A., FORSTER A.L. Ventilatory compensation for lactacidosis in ponies: role of carotid chemoreceptors and lung afferents. *J. Appl. Physiol.* 1991, 70, 2619-2626.
EVANS D.L., ROSE R.J. Cardiovascular and respiratory responses to submaximal exercise training in the thoroughbred horse. *Pflügers Arch.* 1988, 411, 316-321.
FITTING J.W. Respiratory muscle fatigue limiting physical exercise ? *Eur. Respir. J.* 1991, 4, 103-108.
FLANDROIS R., LACOUR J.R., OSMAN H. Control of breathing in the exercising dog. *Respir. Physiol.* 1971, 13, 361-371.
FORSTER H.V., BISGARD G.E., KLEIN J.P. Effect of peripheral chemoreceptor denervation on acclimatization of goats during hypoxia. *J. Appl. Physiol. : Respirat. Environ. Exercise Physiol.* 1981, 50, 392-398.
FORSTER H.V., PAN L.G., BISGARD G.E., KAMINSKI R.P., DORSEY S.M., BUSCH M.A. Hyperpnea of exercise at various PIO_2 in normal and carotid body-denervated ponies. *J. Appl. Physiol. : Respirat. Environ. Exercise Physiol.* 1983, 54, 1387-1393.
FORSTER H.V., PAN L.G., BISGARD G.E., FLYNN G., DORSEY S.M., BRITTON M.S. Independence of exercise hypocapnia and limb movement frequency in ponies. *J. Appl. Physiol. : Respirat. Environ. Exercise Physiol.* 1984, 57, 1885-1893.
FORSTER H.V., PAN L.G., BISGARD G.E., FLYNN C., HOFFER R.E. Effect of reducing anatomic dead space on arterial PCO_2 during CO_2 inhalation. *J. Appl. Physiol.* 1986, 61, 728-733.
FORSTER H.V., PAN L.G. Exercise hyperpnea: its characteristics and control. In : *The Lung: Scientific Foundations*, Crystal, R.G., West, J.B. (Eds), Raven Press, New York, 1991, pp 1553-1564.
FU Z., COSTELLO M.L., TSUKIMOTO K., PREDILETTO R., ELLIOTT A.R., MATHIEU-COSTELLO O., WEST J.B. High lung volume increases stress failure in pulmonary capillaries. *J. Appl. Physiol.* 1992, 73, 123-133.
HODGSON D.R., ROSE R.J., KELSO T.B., McCUTCHEON L.J., BAYLY W.M., GOLLNICK P.D. Respiratory and metabolic responses in the horse during moderate and heavy exercise. *Pflügers Arch.* 1990, 417, 73-78.
KLEIN JP, FORSTER HV, BISGARD GE, KAMINSKI R.P., PAN L.G., HAMILTON L.H. Ventilatory response to inspired CO_2 in normal and carotid body-denervated ponies. *J. Appl. Physiol. : Respirat. Environ. Exercise Physiol.* 1982, 52, 1614-1622.
LAHIRI S., EDELMAN N.H., CHERNIACK N.S., FISHMAN A.P. Role of carotid chemoreflex in respiratory acclimatization to hypoxia in goat and sheep. *Respir. Physiol.* 1981a, 46, 367-382.
LAHIRI S., MULLIGAN E., NISHINO T., MOKASHI A., DAVIE R.O. Relative responses of aortic body and carotid body chemoreceptors to carboxyhemoglobinemia. *J. Appl. Physiol.*, 1981b, 50, 580-586.
LANDGREN G.L., GILLESPIE J.R., LEITH D.E. No ventilatory response to CO_2 in thoroughbreds galloping at 14 $m.s^{-1}$. In : *Equine Exercise Physiology 3*, Persson, S.G.B., Lindholm, A., Jeffcott, L.B. (Eds), ICEEP Publications, Davis, California, 1991, pp 59-65.
LEBLANC P., SUMMERS E., INMAN M.D., JONES N.L., CAMPBELL E.J., KILLIAN

K.J. Inspiratory muscles during exercise: a problem of supply and demand. *J. Appl. Physiol.* 1988, 64, 2482-2489.

LEKEUX P., ART T., DESMECHT D. Effect of exercise on equine alveolar ventilation. In Proceedings : 11th Comparative Respiratory Society Meeting, Urbana (USA), 1992, S12.

LOKE J., MAHLER D.A., VIRGULTO J.A. Respiratory muscle fatigue after marathon running. *J. Appl. Physiol.* 1982, 52, 821-824.

MADOR M.J., ACEVEDO F.A. Effect of respiratory muscle fatigue on subsequent exercise performance. *J. Appl. Physiol.* 1991, 70, 2059-2065.

McARDLE W.D., KATCH F.I., KATCH V.L. Exercise Physiology. Energy, nutrition, and human performance, 3rd edn, Lea & Febiger, Philadelphia, 1991.

McARTHUR J.M., MILTIMORE J.E. Rumen gas analysis by gas-solid chromatography. *Can. J. Anim. Sci.* 1961, 41, 187-196.

McCLEAN P.A., PHILLIPSON E.A., MARTINEZ D., ZAMEL N. Single breath of CO_2 as a clinical test of the peripheral chemoreflex. *J. Appl. Physiol.* 1988, 64, 84-89.

PAN L.G., FORSTER H.V., BISGARD G.E., KAMINSKI R.P., DORSEY S.M., BUSCH M.A. Hyperventilation in ponies at the onset of and during steady-state exercise. *J. Appl. Physiol. : Respirat. Environ. Exercise Physiol.* 1983, 54, 1394-1402.

PAN L.G., FORSTER H.V., BISGARD G.E., DORSEY S.M., BUSCH M.A. Cardiodynamic variables and ventilation during treadmill exercise in ponies. *J. Appl. Physiol. : Respirat. Environ. Exercise Physiol.* 1984, 57, 753-759.

PAN L.G., FORSTER H.V., BISGARD G.E., MURPHY C.L., LOWRY T.F. Independence of exercise hyperpnea and acidosis during high-intensity exercise in ponies. *J. Appl. Physiol.* 1986, 60, 1016-1024.

PAN L.G., FORSTER H.V., WURSTER R.D., MURPHY C.L., BRICE A.G., LOWRY T.F. Effect of partial spinal cord ablation on exercise hyperpnea in ponies. *J. Appl. Physiol.* 1990, 69, 1821-1827.

PARKS C.M., MANOHAR M. Blood-gas tensions and acid-base status in ponies during treadmill exercise. *Am. J. Vet. Res.* 1984, 45, 15-19.

PONTE J., PURVES M.J. Types of afferent nervous activity which may be measured in the vagus nerve of the sheep foetus. *J. Physiol. London* 1973, 229, 51-76.

POWERS S.K., BEADLE R.E., THOMPSON D., LAWLER J. Ventilatory and blood gas dynamics at onset and offset of exercise in the pony. *J. Appl. Physiol.* 1987, 62, 141-148.

READ D.J. A clinical method for assessing the ventilatory response to carbon dioxide. *Australas. Ann. Med.* 1967, 16, 20-32.

REBUCK A.S., CAMPBELL E.J. A clinical method for assessing the ventilatory response to hypoxia. *Am. Rev. Respir. Dis.* 1974, 109, 345-350.

ROLLIN F.A., DESMECHT D. J-M., GENICOT B., LINDEN A.S., LEKEUX P.M. Effect of inhalation of the eructed gases on the breathing pattern in cattle. In Proceedings: 9th Comparative Respiratory Society Meeting, Orlando (USA), October 1990, Abstract 21-4.

ROSE R.J., EVANS D.L. Cardiovascular and respiratory function in the athletic horse. In: *Equine Exercise Physiology 2*, Gillespie, J.R., Robinson, N.E. (Eds), ICEEP Publications, Davis, California, 1987, pp 1-24.

ROSE R.J., HODGSON D.R., KELSO T.B., McCUTCHEON L.J., REID T.A., BAYLY W.M. Maximum O_2 uptake, O_2 debt and deficit, and muscle metabolites in thoroughbred horses. *J. Appl. Physiol.* 1988, 64, 781-788.

ROUSSOS C., MACKLEM P.T. Inspiratory muscle fatigue. In : *Handbook of Physiology*, Section 3, The Respiratory System, Volume 3, part 2, Mechanics of

Breathing, Fishman, A.P., Fisher, A.B. (Eds), MD: American Physiological Society, Bethesda, 1986, pp 511-527.

SCHARF S.M., BARK H., HEIMER D., COHEN A., MACKLEM P.T. "Second wind" during inspiratory loading. *Med. Sci. Sports Exerc.* 1984, 16, 87-91.

SMITH C.A., BISGARD G.E., NIELSEN A.M., DARISTOTLE L., KRESSIN N.A., FORSTER H.V., DEMPSEY J.A. Carotid bodies are required for ventilatory acclimatization to moderate and severe chronic hypoxemia. *J. Appl. Physiol.* 1986, 60, 1003-1010.

SZLYK P.C., McDONALD B.W., PENDERGAST D.R., KRASNEY J.A. Control of ventilation during graded exercise in the dog. *Respir. Physiol.* 1981, 46, 345-365.

THORNTON J.R., ESSEN-GUSTAVSSON B., LINDHOLM A. Effects of training and detraining on oxygen uptake, cardiac output, blood gas tensions, pH and lactate concentrations during and after exercise in the horse. In : *Equine Exercise Physiology*, Snow, D.H., Persson, S.G.B., Rose, R.J. (Eds), Granta Editions, Cambridge, 1983, pp 470-486.

WAGNER P.D., GILLESPIE J.R., LANDGREN G.L., FEDDE M.R., JONES B.W., DEBOWES R.M., PIESCHL R.L., ERICKSON H.H. Mechanism of exercise-induced hypoxemia in horses. *J. Appl. Physiol.* 1989, 66, 1227-1233.

WHITELAW W.A., DERENNE J.P., MILIC-EMILI J. Occlusion pressure as a measure of respiratory center output in conscious man. *Respir. Physiol.* 1975, 23, 181-199.

CHAPTER VII

AUTONOMIC REGULATION OF THE PULMONARY FUNCTION

P. Lekeux[1] and P. Gustin[2]

[1] Laboratory for Functional Investigation
[2] Laboratory for Pharmacology and Toxicology
Faculty of Veterinary Medicine
University of Liege

SUMMARY

This paper describes the role of the adrenergic, cholinergic and nonadrenergic noncholinergic pathways in the pulmonary physiology and physiopathology.

KEY WORDS

Respiratory system - Pulmonary function - Autonomic regulation.

1. INTRODUCTION

The pulmonary function is largely influenced by the autonomic nervous system. Most obvious is the autonomic regulation of the tonus of the airway smooth muscle. However, the autonomic control modulates also many other functions of the respiratory system such as the vascular bed, the airway secretions, the mucociliar clearance and the pulmonary blood flow.

Although many researches have been devoted to this subject, the autonomic control remains poorly understood because of its high complexity : various neurotransmitters and receptors, complex interactions between the different neural and humoral mechanisms, species and tissue peculiarities, contradictions between in vitro and in vivo results, dysregulation due to subclinical pathologies, etc ...

However, some evidence for the role of the autonomic control is already available in some animal species. These data can be used for a better understanding of the pulmonary function in these animals and therefore for a better prevention or treatment of their pulmonary dysfunctions.

2. GENERAL ORGANIZATION OF THE AUTONOMIC NERVOUS SYSTEM

The autonomic nervous system works mainly via (1) sensory receptors such as stretch receptors, irritant receptors, C-fiber endings and neuroendocrine cells, (2) upper centers located mainly in the spinal cord, the brain stem and the hypothalamus, and (3) motor innervation (Barnes, 1991a). The latter is generally subdivided into three pathways : the parasympathetic pathway which acts via cholinergic nerves and receptors, the sympathetic pathway which acts via adrenergic receptors, nerves and circulating catecholamines, and the nonadrenergic noncholinergic pathway which seems to act mainly via neuropeptides as neurotransmitters (Fig. 7-1.).

Specific agonists and antagonists have been described for most of the receptors involved in the autonomic control (Table 7-1.). Although their selectivity is rarely absolute, the use of these drugs contributes to a better

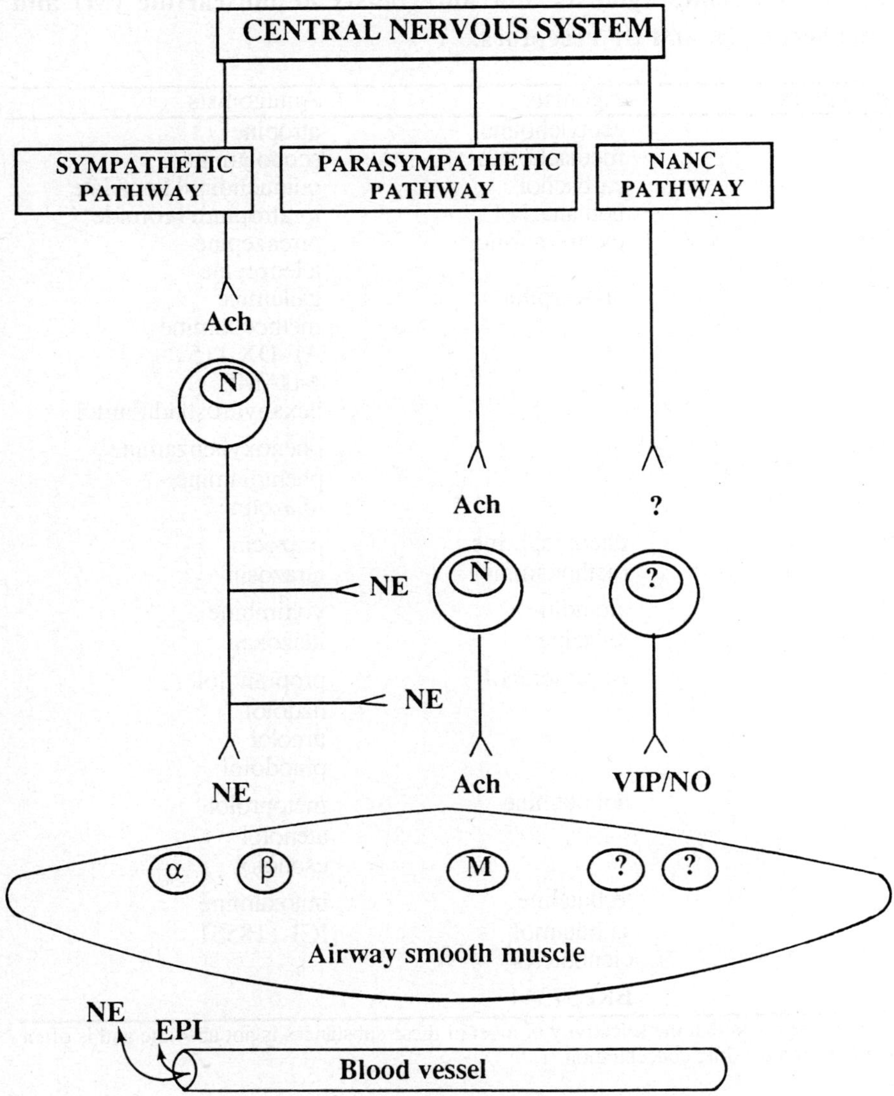

Fig. 7-1. Diagram of the autonomic control of the airway smooth muscle. Ach : Acetylcholine; α : α-receptor; β : β-receptor; EPI : Epinephrine; M : Muscarinic receptor; N : Nicotinic receptor; NANC : Nonadrenergic noncholinergic; NE : Norepinephrine; NO : Nitric oxide; VIP : Vasoactive intestinal peptide (Robinson, 1993).

Table 7-1. Some agonists and antagonists of muscarinic (M) and adrenergic (α and β) receptors.

Receptors	Agonists	Antagonists
M_{1+2+3}	acetylcholine methacholine carbachol bethanachol	atropine scopolamine quinuclidinyl benzilate ipratropium bromide
M_1	oxotremorine	pirenzepine telenzepine
M_2	pilocarpine	gallamine methoctramine AF-DX 115
M_3		4-DAMP hexahydrosiladifenitol
α_{1+2}		phenoxybenzamine phentolamine tolazoline
α_1	phenylephrine methoxamine	prazocin terazosin
α_2	clonidine xylazine	yohimbine idazoxan
β_{1+2}	isoproterenol	propranolol nadolol timolol pinodolol
β_1	dobutamine	metoprolol atenolol esonolol
β_2	terbutaline salbutamol clenbuterol	butoxamine ICI-118551
β_3	BRL37344	

It should be noted that the selectivity of most of these substances is not absolute and is often dependent on the drug concentration.

understanding of the autonomic mechanisms in health and disease and to a better treatment of some pulmonary dysfunctions.

3. AUTONOMIC CONTROL OF AIRWAY SMOOTH MUSCLE

In healthy animals, the tonus of the airway smooth muscle is a compromise between two opposite interests, i.e. relaxation and constriction (Fig. 7-2.). Diffuse relaxation is required in order to increase the airway caliber and therefore decrease the resistance to airflow. Diffuse constriction is required in order to (1) decrease the airway dead space, (2) increase the stiffness of the airways and therefore their resistance to the collapse, and (3) protect the lung against noxious agents.

In diseased animals, autonomic imbalances or abnormalities contribute to pulmonary dysfunctions and result in clinical symptoms observed during airway diseases.

3.1. Cholinergic mechanisms

The cholinergic nerves represent the major neural bronchoconstrictor mechanism. This might be related to the high cholinergic innervation of the mammalian airways (Richardson, 1979). These nerves arise from the vagal nuclei in the brainstem and they reach, via the vagus nerve, the parasasympathetic ganglia located in the walls of the airways. The postganglionic fibers to the smooth muscles are therefore very short. This cholinergic innervation is more dense in large than in small airways and is lacking in the alveolar walls.

Electrical stimulation of the vagus nerve causes bronchoconstriction. This effect can be increased by preventing the degradation of acetylcholine by cholinesterase inhibitors and can be blocked by antagonizing the muscarinic receptors by atropine. The fact that this bronchoconstricton appears and disappears very quickly suggests that it is caused by smooth muscle contraction rather than by wall edema or mucus accumulation (Nadel, 1980).

Cholinergic stimulation induces the release of acetylcholine from the agranular

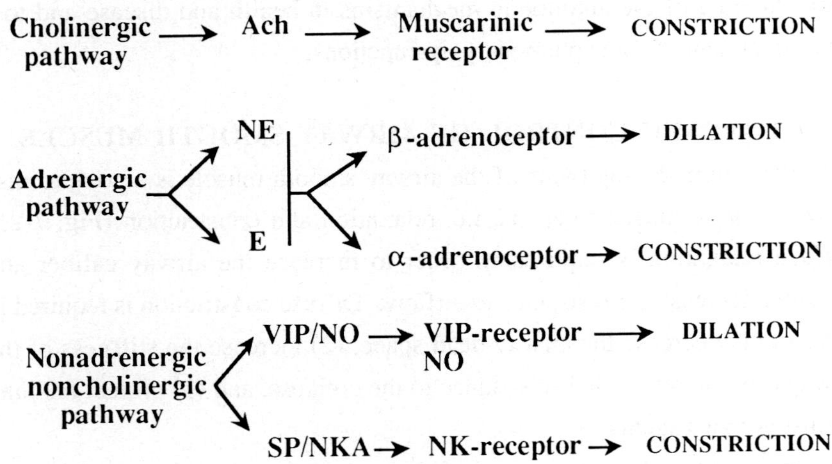

Fig. 7-2. Effects of the stimulation of the several autonomic pathways on the diameter of the airways (Barnes, 1991a). Ach : Acetylcholine; E : Epinephrine; NE : Norepinephrine; NKA : Neurokinin A; NO : Nitric oxide; SP : Substance P; VIP : Vasoactive intestinal peptide.

vesicles of the nerve terminals. This neurotransmitter diffuses to the specific receptors of the target cell and is rapidly broken down by acetylcholinesterase which is stored in the synaptic cleft (Barnes, 1987a).

In most investigated animal species, vagotomy or atropine administration inhibits the resting bronchomotor tone. However, there are species peculiarities concerning its degree. For instance, this physiological bronchomotor tone is more important in cattle which show a significant bronchodilation after vagotomy (Slocombe et al, 1982) and atropine (Gustin et al, 1988), than in horses in which vagotomy (Derksen et al, 1982) and atropine (Broadstone et al, 1988) induce minimal changes.

The cholinergic neurotransmission can be modulated by other mediators. Catecholamines can inhibit the acetylcholine release from postganglionic nerve terminals likely via α_2 presynaptic receptors (Danser et al, 1987). Cholinergic transmission can be inhibited by prostaglandin E_2 (Walters et al, 1984) and potentiated by serotonin (Sheller et al, 1982), thromboxane (Chung et al, 1985) and tachykinins (Hall et al, 1989). Some neuropeptides seem also able to modulate the presynaptic control of the airway smooth muscle (Maclagan, 1987). This is the case for substance P which can induce the release of acetylcholine in the rabbit trachea (Tanaka and Grunstein, 1984).

Acetylcholine released from the preganglionic fibers activates nicotinic receptors, which are stimulated by dimethylphenylpiperazinium and blocked by hexamethonium (Skoogh, 1983).

Acetylcholine released by postganglionic fibers activates muscarinic receptors, which are stimulated by methacholine and blocked by atropine. The smooth muscle contraction resulting from the stimulation of these receptors is due to a receptor-linked phosphoinositide hydrolysis, leading to a calcium release from intracellular stores (Barnes, 1990).

The distribution of muscarinic receptors in the airways is not uniform. The autoradiographic mapping technique shows indeed a higher labeling in large than in small airways (Basbaum et al, 1984).

More recently, different subtypes of muscarinic (M) receptors have been described : three by using radioligand binding assays and functional studies (Eglen and Whiting, 1986) and at least five by using techniques of molecular biology (Kubo et al, 1986).

M_1 receptors are located in the parasympathetic ganglia. They facilitate ganglionic neurotransmission and can be antagonized by pirenzepine (Bloom et al, 1988).

M_2 receptors are located in the postganglionic cholinergic nerves. They inhibit the acetylcholine release and can be antagonized by gallamine (Barnes et al, 1988).

M_3 receptors are located in the airway smooth muscle. They mediate the classical muscarinic effects and can be antagonized by 4-diphenylacetoxy-N-methylpiperidine methiodile (4-DAMP) (Roffel et al, 1990).

The density and relative proportion of these muscarinic receptor subtypes show species peculiarities. For instance, in bovine airways the concentration

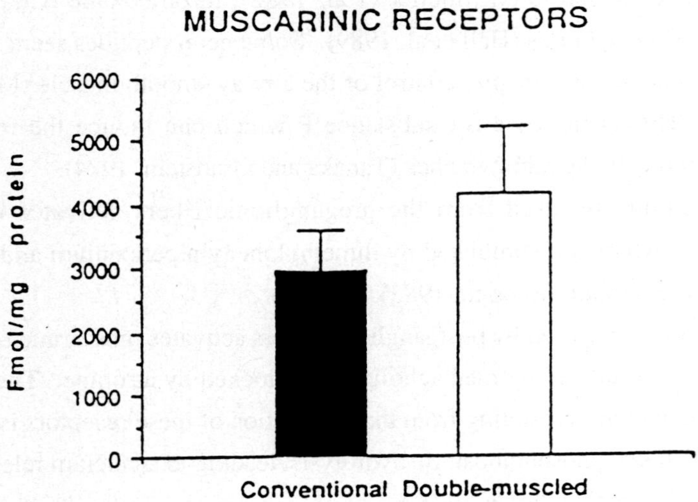

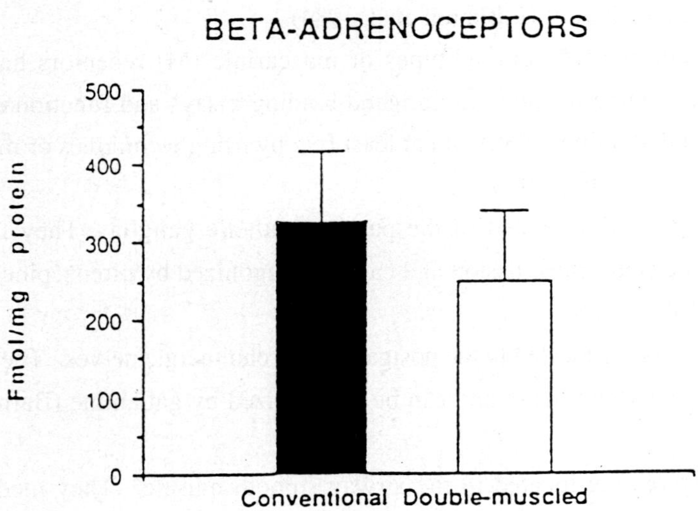

Fig. 7-3. Effect of breed on the autonomic receptor density in bovine tracheal smooth muscle (Roets et al, 1992).

of muscarinic receptors is about 14 times higher than the amount of β_2-adrenergic receptors (Cheng and Townley, 1982). The bovine muscarinic receptors consist of 60 % M_2 receptors and 40 % M_3 receptors (Roets et al, 1992). Furthermore, tracheal smooth muscles from double-muscled cattle have 40 % more muscarinic receptors than these in conventional cattle (Fig. 7-3.) (Roets et al, 1992). In equine airways, M_2 receptors seem not to be present (Yu et al, 1992). This contrasts with the situation in other species such as cats (Blaber et al, 1985) and dogs (Ito and Yoshitomi, 1988).

Inappropriate cholinergic mechanisms have been incriminated during airway obstruction or hyperreactivity caused by airway diseases. This hyperresponsiveness can be explained by several mechanisms, i.e. increase in the discharge of airway afferent receptor, facilitation of parasympathetic neurotransmission and increase in the number or affinity of the muscarinic receptors (Barnes, 1991a).

In cats, feline herpesvirus 1 infection induces a hyperresponsiveness of the tracheal smooth muscle to vagal stimulation, which seems to be presynaptic in origin (Killingsworth et al, 1990).

In horses affected with recurrent airway obstruction, the bronchoconstriction observed during the acute stage of the disease seems to be largely mediated via muscarinic receptors, although there is little evidence of their involvement in the response to histamine given by aerosol (Broadstone et al, 1988).

In cattle, the bronchoconstriction recorded during acute viral respiratory distress syndrome is also largely mediated via muscarinic receptors. This is shown by the airway dilation induced by ipratropium bromide, a non specific antagonist of the muscarinic receptors (Genicot et al, 1992a).

3.2. Adrenergic mechanisms

Adrenergic mechanisms involved in the control of smooth muscle tone of the airways concern both the sympathetic nerves which release norepinephrine and the adrenal medulla which releases mainly epinephrine. These catecholamines activate both α-and β-adrenoreceptors in the airways.

Sympathetic innervation is much less important than the parasympathetic one in the airways, despite the presence of large variations between species (Richardson, 1979). Functional investigations suggest little direct effect of sympathetic nerves on the airway smooth muscle (Barnes, 1987b). However, indirect effects via an inhibitory effect on cholinergic neurotransmission, have been reported in canine bronchi (Danser et al, 1987).

On the other hand, circulating catecholamines seem to play a much more important role in the regulation of the smooth muscle tone of the airways. Epinephrine is a potent bronchodilator and may protect the airways against bronchoconstrictor influences (Barnes, 1987b).

α-Adrenergic receptors are relatively rare in the airways and their role seems to be largely influenced by several factors such as species, clinical status, receptor subtypes, etc ...

In dogs, the insignificant α-adrenergic constriction is increased by pretreatment with some autacoids, probably via a postreceptor mechanism (Kneussl and Richardson, 1978).

In horses, the role of α_1-adrenergic receptors in airway narrowing seems to be lacking in healthy animals and minimal in acutely diseased animals (Scott et al, 1988b). On the other hand, α_2-adrenergic agonists have no effect in healthy ponies and induce a diffuse brochodilation during acute airway obstruction (Broadstone et al, 1992). This could be explained by an inhibition of cholinergic neurotransmission due to stimulation of prejunctional α_2-adrenoreceptors (Grundstrom and Andersson, 1985).

In cattle, the α-adrenergic system seems to play a more important role in the regulation of the bronchomotor tone. This is suggested by the diffuse bronchoconstriction and bronchodilation induced by α_2-agonists and antagonists, respectively (Gustin et al, 1989)

Activation of the β-adrenergic receptors plays an important role in the relaxation of airway smooth muscle. Their direct effects can be potentiated by indirect factors such as decreased release of some mediators (Church and Hiroi, 1987) and reduced cholinergic tone (Rhoden et al, 1988).

The β_1- and β_2-receptors seem to be mainly regulated by adrenergic nerves and circulating epinephrine, respectively (Barnes, 1991a). Their relative density differs with the species and with the age.
In dogs, β_1-subtype represents only 20 % of the total β-receptors in the airways (Barnes et al, 1983). β_3-Receptors could exist in canine bronchial smooth muscles and cause bronchodilation through a cAMP-dependent pathway (Tamaoki et al, 1993).
In cattle, the density of β-receptors seems to be lower than in other species (Cheng and Townley, 1982), even lower in double-muscled than in conventional animals (Fig. 7-3.) (Roets et al, 1992) and also lower in aged than in young animals (Andersson et al, 1978; Roets et al, 1989). β-Agonists are able to induce in healthy calves a bronchodilation (Kotlikoff et al, 1982) which is located mainly at the level of large airways (Gustin et al, 1989). On the other hand, β_2-agonists partly reverse the bronchoconstriction induced by prostaglandine $F_{2\alpha}$ (Nuyten et al, 1986), by subacute but not chronic bronchopneumonia (Hajer, 1988) and by acute respiratory distress syndrome (Genicot et al, 1992b).
In horses, the β-adrenergic system seems to be involved in the control of central airway caliber in diseased but not in healthy animals (Scott et al, 1988a). Histamine-induced airway obstruction is attenuated by β-agonists when given by aerosol (Scott et al, 1991) but not when administered intravenously (Derksen et al, 1987). Although both types of β-receptors exist in the equine airways, the β_2 receptors seem to be primarily involved in the correction of the bronchoconstriction induced by acute airway obstruction (Scott et al, 1991) and by chronic obstructive pulmonary disease (Sasse and Hajer, 1977).

3.3. Nonadrenergic noncholinergic mechanisms

In addition to parasympathetic and sympathetic pathways, other neural mechanisms have been described in the airways (Richardson and Beland, 1976; Andersson and Grundstrom, 1983; Lammers et al, 1992). They include nonadrenergic inhibitory nerves which relax the airway smooth muscle, and noncholinergic excitatory nerves which constrict the airway smooth muscle. Both mechanisms seem to make use, for their neurotransmission, of neuropeptides which could be localized to classical autonomic nerves (Barnes, 1991b; Desmecht et al, 1991).

These nonadrenergic noncholinergic nerves are present in the airways of several animal species. However, a clear demonstration of their role in the control of airway smooth muscle tone in health and disease is still lacking. In the same way, the identification of the neurotransmitters involved in these airway neural pathways is not yet conclusive, although several substances are serious candidates, such as vasoactive intestinal peptide (Matsuzaki et al, 1980) and nitric oxide (Bult et al, 1990; Kannan and Johnson, 1992) for the inhibitory pathway and tachykinins (Grandordy et al, 1988) for the exitatory pathway.

4. AUTONOMIC CONTROL OF VASCULAR BED OF THE AIRWAYS

In contrast with the control of the airway smooth muscle, the sympathetic mechanisms play a more important role than the parasympathetic ones in the control of the airway vascular resistance (Laitinen and Laitinen, 1991).

The adrenergic-induced constrictor effects are mainly mediated via α-adrenoreceptors (Lung et al, 1984).

There is little evidence concerning cholinergic-induced vasodilation at this level. However, in dogs, the vasodilation of tracheal vessels induced by electrical nerve stimulation is halved by atropine, which suggests some contribution of a cholinergic mechanism (Laitinen et al, 1987).

Nonadrenergic noncholinergic nerves have also been described in the airway blood vessels (Burnstock and Griffith, 1983) and several neuropeptides are incriminated as potential neurotransmitters (Polak and Bloom, 1985).

5. AUTONOMIC CONTROL OF AIRWAY SECRETION

All three neural pathways are involved in the control of airway secretion. However, their respective role seems to vary with the species and with the site (Finkbeiner and Widdicombe, 1991).

5.1. Nasal secretion

Cholinergic mechanisms play an important role in the control of nasal secretion. Both parasympathetic nerve stimulation (Wells and Widdicombe, 1986) and parasympathetic agonists (Malm et al, 1983) increase nasal secretion in dogs and in cats (Eccles and Wilson, 1973). In human, the M_3 receptors have the predominant effect (Mullol et al, 1992).

Adrenergic mechanisms could also be involved in the control of nasal secretion. Indeed, sympathetic nerve stimulation, α-adrenergic agonists and β-adrenergic agonists stimulate nasal secretions in cats (Wilson and Yates, 1978), dogs (Malm et al, 1983) and rabbits (Pell et al, 1984), respectively.

Nonadrenergic noncholinergic mechanisms have been suspected, but not yet demonstrated, to contribute to the nasal secretion control. For instance, substance P, but not vasoactive intestinal peptide, is able to increase nasal secretion in dogs (Wells and Widdicombe, 1986).

5.2. Tracheobronchial secretion

Cholinergic agonists stimulate secretion of the tracheobronchial glands in all investigated species, including cats (Gallagher et al, 1975), dogs (Chakrin et al, 1973), pigs (Hartmann et al, 1984) and cattle (Finkbeiner, 1989). This response is inhibited by muscarinic receptor antagonists.

Adrenergic agonists can also stimulate airway secretion in some species such as cats (Phipps et al, 1980) and cattle (Finkbeiner and Basbaum, 1986), but not in dogs (Chakrin et al, 1973).

Nonadrenergic noncholinergic mechanisms influence also the airway secretion, as suggested by the tracheal secretion induced by vasoactive intestinal peptide (Peatfield and Richardson, 1983) and by substance P (Borson et al, 1987).

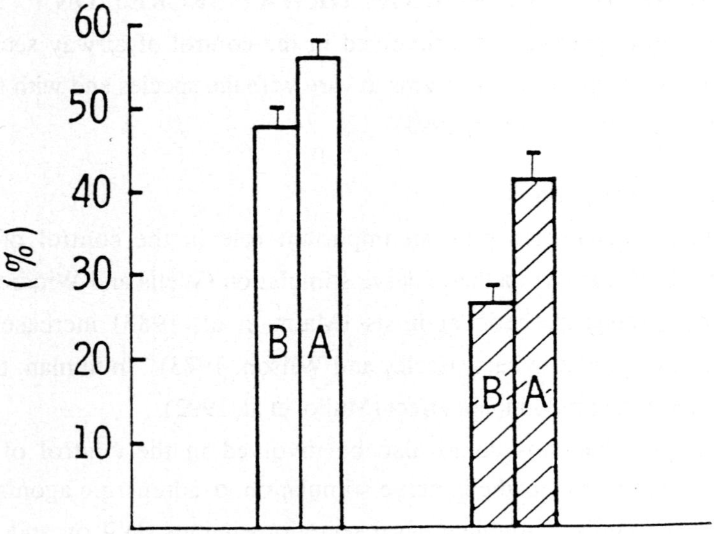

Fig. 7-4. Mucociliar clearance index before (B) and after (A) stimulation of the β_2-receptors in healthy (□) and diseased (▨) horses (Turgut and Sasse, 1989).

5.3. Bronchiolar secretion

Neurohumoral mechanisms modulate also the secretion of the non-ciliated bronchiolar epithelial cells which can be stimulated by muscarinic (Yoneda, 1977), β-adrenergic (Massaro et al, 1979) and α-adrenergic agonists (Massaro et al, 1982).

6. AUTONOMIC CONTROL OF MUCOCILIAR CLEARANCE

Both adrenergic and cholinergic receptors are involved in the regulation of the mucociliar clearance, as suggested by the increase in ciliary beat frequency induced by β_2 and cholinergic agonists (Wong et al, 1988) and by the inhibiting effects induced by β-blockers (Van de Donk and Merkhus, 1982; Pavia et al, 1986) and anticholinergic drugs (Annis et al, 1976; Wong et al, 1988).

β_2 agonists induce an enhancement of mucociliar clearance both in healthy horses (Kiely et al, 1985) and in horses with chronic obstructive pulmonary diseases (Fig. 7-4.) (Turgut and Sasse, 1989), although the required dosage seems to be 2.5 times larger than the dosage recommended for bronchodilation (Pavia et al, 1984).

7. AUTONOMIC CONTROL OF PULMONARY BLOOD FLOW

The pulmonary vasculature is richly innervated with adrenergic and cholinergic nerves (Fisher, 1965). The vascular tone seems to respond to autonomic regulation (Hyman et al, 1991).

When the pulmonary vascular tone is low, the stimulation of α-adrenergic (Kadowitz and Hyman, 1973) and muscarinic (Feeley et al, 1963) receptors causes vasoconstriction and the stimulation of β_2-receptors causes a moderate and frequently masked vasodilation (Hyman et al, 1981). The mediation through α_1-adrenoreceptors is more important than this one through α_2-receptors.

At increased pulmonary vascular tone, the response to α_2- (vasoconstriction) and β_2- (vasodilation) adrenoreceptor stimulation is largely increased (Hyman and Kadowitz, 1986) and the response to muscarinic receptor stimulation is reversed, resulting in vasodilation (Hyman and Kadowitz, 1988).

Nonadrenergic noncholinergic mechanisms are probably also involved in the control of the pulmonary vascular tone. This is suggested by the relaxation of the pulmonary vascular smooth muscle induced by vasoactive intestinal peptide in cats (Nandiwada et al, 1985) and cattle (Barnes, 1986), by substance P in pigs (Adnot et al, 1989) and by nitric oxide in rabbits (Gustafsson et al, 1991).

The vascular permeability is also influenced by autonomic mediators. Recently, it has been shown that acetylcholine can increase this parameter by inducing SP-release from C-fibers and by degranulating mast cells (Delaunois et al, 1993). This could explain the pulmonary edema induced by organophoshates (Delaunois et al, 1992).

8. CONCLUSIONS

Although the mechanisms responsible for the pulmonary autonomic regulation are complex and still poorly understood, it is clear that their appropriate modulation is critical in the treatment of pulmonary dysfunctions. However, these neural mechanisms are not the only factors involved in these dysfunctions, and the humoral and cellular mechanisms must also be taken into account.

REFERENCES

ADNOT S., CIGARINI I., HARF A. Pulmonary vasodilator responses to calcitonin gene-related peptide (CGRP) and substance P (SP). *Am. Rev. Respir. Dis.* 1989, 139, A49.

ANDERSSON R.G.G., KOVESI G., ERICSON E. β-adrenoceptor stimulation and cyclic AMP level in bovine tracheal muscle of old and young animals. *Acta Pharmacol. Toxicol.* 1978, 43, 323-327.

ANDERSSON R.G.G., GRUNDSTROM N. The excitatory non-cholinergic, non-adrenergic nervous system of the guinea-pig airways. *Eur. J. Respir. Dis.* 1983, 64, 141-157.

ANNIS P., LANDA J., LICHTIGER M.C. Effects of atropine on velocity of tracheal mucus in anesthetized patients. *Anesthesiology* 1976, 44, 74-77.

BARNES P.J., NADEL J.A., SKOOGH B.-E., ROBERTS J.M. Characterization of β-adrenoceptor subtypes in canine airway smooth muscle by radioligand binding and physiologic responses. *J. Pharmacol. Exp. Ther.* 1983, 225, 456-461.

BARNES P.J. Nonadrenergic noncholinergic neural control of human airways. *Arch. Int. Pharmacodyn.* 1986, 280, 208-228.

BARNES P.J. Cholinergic control of airway smooth muscle. *Am. Rev. Respir. Dis.* 1987a, 136, S42-S45.

BARNES P.J. Adrenergic regulation of airway function. In : *The Airways: neural Control in Health and Disease*, Kaliner, M.A., Barnes, P.J. (Eds), Marcel Dekker, New York, 1987b, pp 57-85.

BARNES P.J., MINETTE P.A., MACLAGAN J. Muscarinic receptor subtypes in lung. *Trends Pharmacol. Sci.* 1988, 9, 412-416.

BARNES P.J. Muscarinic receptors in airways: recent developments. *J. Appl. Physiol.* 1990, 68, 1777-1785.

BARNES P.J. Neural control of airway smooth muscle. In : *The Lung: Scientific Foundations*, Vol. 1, Crystal, R.G., West, J.B. (Eds), Raven Press, New York, 1991a, pp 903-916.

BARNES P.J. Pharmacology of airway smooth muscle. In : *The Lung: Scientific Foundations*, Vol. 1, Crystal, R.G., West, J.B. (Eds), Raven Press, New York, 1991b, pp 977-985.

BASBAUM C.B., GRILLO M.A., WIDDICOMBE J.H. Muscarinic receptors: evidence for a nonuniform distribution in tracheal smooth muscle and exocrine glands. *J. Neurol. Sci.* 1984, 4, 508-520.

BLABER L.C., FRYER A.D., MACLAGAN J. Neuronal muscarinic receptors attenuate vagally-induced contraction of feline bronchial smooth muscle. *Br. J. Pharmacol.* 1985, 86, 723-728.

BLOOM J.W., BAUMGARTENER-FOLKERTS C., PALMER J.D., YAMAMURA H.I., HALONEN M. A muscarinic receptor subtype modulates vagally stimulated bronchial contraction. *J. Appl. Physiol.* 1988, 85, 2144-2150.

BORSON D.B., CORRALES R., VARSANO S., GOLD M., VIRO N., CAUGHEY G., RAMACHANDRAN J., NADEL J.A. Enkephalinase inhibitors potentiate substance P-induced secretion of $^{35}SO4$-macromolecules from ferret trachea. *Exp. Lung Res.* 1987, 12, 21-36.

BROADSTONE R.V., SCOTT J.S., DERKSEN F.J., ROBINSON N.E. Effects of atropine in ponies with recurrent airway obstruction. *J. Appl. Physiol.* 1988, 65, 2720-2725.

BROADSTONE R.V., GRAY P.R., ROBINSON N.E., DERKSEN F.J. Effects of xylazine on airway function in ponies with recurrent airway obstruction. *Am. J. Vet. Res.* 1992, 53, 1813-1817.

BULT H., BOECKXSTAINS G.E., PELAKMANS P.A., JORDAENS F.H., VAN MAERCKE Y.M., HERMAN A.G. Nitric oxide as an inhibitory nonadrenergic noncholinergic neurotransmitter. *Nature London* 1990, 345, 346-347.

BURNSTOCK G., GRIFFITH, S.G. Neurohumoral control of the vasculature. In: *Biology and Pathology of the Vessel Wall. A modern Appraisal*, Woolf, N. (Ed.), Praeger, Eastbourne, England, 1983, pp 15-40.

CHAKRIN L.W., BAKER A.P., CHRISTIAN P., WARDELL J.R. Jr Effect of cholinergic stimulation on the release of macromolecules by canine trachea in vitro. *Am. Rev. Respir. Dis.* 1973, 108, 69-76.

CHENG Y.C., TOWNLEY R.G. Comparison of muscarinic and β-adrenergic receptors between bovine peripheral lung and tracheal smooth muscles: a striking difference in the receptor concentration. *Life Sci.* 1982, 30, 2079-2086.

CHUNG K.F., EVANS T.W., GRAF P.D., NADEL J.A. Modulation of cholinergic neurotransmission in canine airways by thromboxanemimetic U 46619. *Eur. J. Pharmacol.* 1985, 117, 373-375.

CHURCH M.K., HIROI J. Inhibition of IgE-dependent histamine release from human dispersed lung mast cells by anti-allergic drugs and salbutamol. *Br. J. Pharmacol.* 1987, 90, 421-429.

DANSER A.H.J., VAN DEN ENDE R., LORENZ R.R., FLAVAHAN N.A., VANHOUTTE P.M. Prejunctional β_1-adrenoceptors inhibit cholinergic neurotransmission in canine bronchi. *J. Appl. Physiol.* 1987, 62, 785-790.

DELAUNOIS A., GUSTIN P., ANSAY M. Altered capillary filtration coefficient in parathion- and paraoxon-induced edema in isolated and perfused rabbit lungs. *Toxicol. Appl. Pharmacol.* 1992, 116, 161-169.

DELAUNOIS A., GUSTIN P., ANSAY M. Role of neuropeptides in acetylcholine-induced edema in isolated and perfused rabbit lungs. *J. Pharmacol. Exp. Ther.* 1993, in press.

DERKSEN F.J., ROBINSON N.E., SLOCOMBE R.F., RIEBOLD T.W., BRUNSON D.B. Pulmonary function tests in standing ponies: reproducibility and effect of vagal blockade. *Am. J. Vet. Res.* 1982, 43, 598-602.

DERKSEN F.J., SCOTT J.S., SLOCOMBE R.F., ROBINSON N.E. Effect of clenbuterol on histamine-induced airway obstruction in ponies. *Am. J. Vet. Res.* 1987, 48, 423-426.

DESMECHT D., GUSTIN P., LEKEUX P., ANSAY M. Le système nerveux peptidergique du poumon: physiologie, physiopathologie et perspectives thérapeutiques. *Ann. Méd. Vét.* 1991, 135, 15-31.

ECCLES R., WILSON H. The parasympathetic secretory nerves of the nose of the cat. *J. Physiol. Lond.* 1973, 230, 213-230.

EGLEN R.M., WHITING R.L. Muscarinic receptor subtypes: a critique of the current classification and a proposal for a working nomenclature. *J. Auton. Pharmacol.* 1986, 5, 323-346.

FEELEY J.W., LEE T.D., MILNOR W.R. Active and passive components of pulmonary vascular responses to vasoactive drugs in the dog. *Am. J. Physiol.* 1963, 205, 1193-1199.

FINKBEINER W.E., BASBAUM C.B. β-adrenergic stimulation of cultured bovine tracheal gland serous cells increases intracellular c-AMP. *Am. Rev. Respir. Dis.* 1986, 133, A295.

FINKBEINER W.E. Cell-specific analysis of tracheobronchial secretory cells and secretions (Dissertation). University of California, San Francisco, USA, 1989.

FINKBEINER W.E., WIDDICOMBE J.H. Control of nasal and airway secretions, ion transport, and water movement. In : *Treatise on Pulmonary Toxicology. Comparative Biology of the Normal Lung*, chapter 34, Parent, R.A. (Ed.), CRC Press Inc., Boca Raton, Floride, 1991, pp 633-657.

FISHER A.W.F. The intrinsic innervation of the pulmonary vessels. *Acta Anat.* 1965, 60, 481-496.

GALLAGHER J.T., KENT P.W., PASSATORE M., PHIPPS R.J., RICHARDSON P.S. The composition of tracheal mucus and the nervous control of its secretion in the cat. *Proc. R. Soc. Lond. (Biology)* 1975, 192, 49.

GENICOT B., CLOSE R., MOULIGNEAU F., LEKEUX P. Muscarinic receptors blockade through the inhalation of ipratropium bromide by calves affected by an acute respiratory distress syndrome. *Arch. Int. Physiol. Bioch.* 1992a, 100, P36.

GENICOT B., CLOSE R., MOULIGNEAU F., LEKEUX P. Clinical and pulmonary function changes induced by aerosoltherapy during bovine acute respiratory distress syndrome. In Proceedings : XVIIth World Buiatrics Congress, Saint Paul, USA, 1992b, 3, pp 236-241.

GRANDORDY B.M., FROSSARD N., RHODEN K.J., BARNES P.J. Tachykinin-induced phosphoinositide breakdown in airway smooth muscle and epithelium: relationship to contraction. *Mol. Pharmcol.* 1988, 33, 515-519.

GRUNDSTROM N., ANDERSSON R.G.G. Inhibition of the cholinergic neurotransmission in human airways via prejunctional α-2-adrenoceptors. *Acta Physiol. Scand.* 1985, 125, 513-517.

GUSTAFSSON L.E., LEONE A.M., PERSSON M.G., WIKLUND N.P., MONCADA S. Endogenous nitric oxide is present in the exhaled air of rabbits, guinea pigs and humans. *Biochem. Biophys. Res. Commun.* 1991, 181, 852-857.

GUSTIN P., DHEM A.R., LOMBA F., LEKEUX P., VAN DE WOESTIJNE K.P., LANDSER F.J. Measurement of total respiratory impedance in calves by the forced oscillation technique. *J. Appl. Physiol.* 1988, 64, 1786-1791.

GUSTIN P., DHEM A.R., LEKEUX P., LOMBA F., LANDSER F.J., VAN DE WOESTIJNE K.P. Regulation of bronchomotor tone in conscious calves. *J. vet. Pharmacol. Therap.* 1989, 12, 58-64.

HAJER R. The effects of clenbuterol hydrochloride on the pulmonary function of calves with subacute and chronic bronchopneumonia. *Vet. Rec.* 1988, 123, 370-372.

HALL A.K., BARNES P.J., MELDRUM L.A., MACLAGAN J. Facilitation by tachykinins of neurotransmission in guinea-pig pulmonary parasympathetic nerves. *Br. J. Pharmacol.* 1989, 97, 274-280.

HARTMANN J.F., HUTCHISON C.F., JEWELL M.E. Pig bronchial mucous membrane: a model system for assessing respiratory mucus release in vitro. *Exp. Lung Res.* 1984,

6, 59-70.

HYMAN A.L., NANDIWADA P., KNIGHT D.S., KADOWITZ P.J. Pulmonary vasodilator responses to catecholamines and sympathetic nerve stimulation in the cat. Evidence that vascular β-2 adrenoceptors are innervated. *Circ. Res.* 1981, 48, 407-415.

HYMAN A.L., KADOWITZ P.J. Enhancement of α and β-adrenoceptor responses by elevations in vascular tone in pulmonary circulation. *Am. J. Physiol.* 1986, 250, H1109-H1116.

HYMAN A.L., KADOWITZ P.J. Tone-dependent responses to acetylcholine in the feline pulmonary vascular bed. *J. Appl. Physiol.* 1988, 64, 2002-2009.

HYMAN A.L., DEMPESY C.W., RICHARDSON D.E., LIPPTON H.L. Neural control. In : *The Lung: Scientific Foundations*, Vol. 1, Crystal, R.G., West, J.B. (Eds), Raven Press, New York, 1991, pp 1087-1103.

ITO Y., YOSHITOMI T. Autoregulation of acetylcholine release from vagus nerve terminals through activation of muscarinic receptors in the dog trachea. *Br. J. Pharmacol.* 1988, 93, 636-646.

KADOWITZ P.J., HYMAN A.L. Effect of sympathetic nerve stimulation on pulmonary vascular resistance in the dog. *Circ. Res.* 1973, 32, 221-227.

KANNAN M.S., JOHNSON D.E. Nitric oxide mediates the neural nonadrenergic, noncholinergic relaxation of pig tracheal smooth muscle. *Am. J. Physiol. (Lung Cell. Mol. Physiol. 2)* 1992, 262, L511-L514.

KIELY R.G., JENKINS W.L., MARTENS R.J. Mucociliary transport rate in the horse and its modification with various pharmacologic agents. In Proceedings : 4th Veterinary Respiratory Symposium, Anaheim, California, 1985, pp 7.

KILLINGSWORTH C.R., ROBINSON N.E., ADAMS T., MAES R.K., BERNEY C., ROZANSKI E. Cholinergic reactivity of tracheal smooth muscle after infection with feline herpesvirus I. *J. Appl. Physiol.* 1990, 69, 1953-1960.

KNEUSSL M.P., RICHARDSON J.B. α-adrenergic receptors in human and canine tracheal and bronchial smooth muscle. *J. Appl. Physiol.* 1978, 45, 307-311.

KOTLIKOFF M.I., SLOCOMBE R.F., ROBINSON N.E. Influence of β-adrenergic antagonism on the response of bovine neonatal lungs to intravenous histamine. *Am. J. Vet. Res.* 1982, 43, 984-988.

KUBO T., FUKUDA K., MIKAMI A., MAEDA A., TAKAHASHI H., MISHINA M., HAGA T., HAGA K., ICHIYAMA A., KANGAWA K., KOJIMA M., MATSUO H., HIROSE T., NUMA S. Cloning, sequencing and expression of complementary DNA encoding the muscarinic acetylcholine receptor. *Nature London* 1986, 323, 411-416.

LAITINEN L.A., LAITINEN A., WIDDICOMBE J.G. Parasympathetic nervous control of tracheal vascular resistance in the dog. *J. Physiol. Lond.* 1987, 385, 135-146.

LAITINEN L.A., LAITINEN A. Neural system. In : *The Lung: Scientific Foundations*, Vol. 1, Crystal, R.G., West, J.B. (Eds), Raven Press, New York, 1991, pp 759-765.

LAMMERS J.-W.J., BARNES P.J., CHUNG K.F. Nonadrenergic, noncholinergic airway inhibitory nerves. *Eur. Respir. J.* 1992, 5, 239-246.

LUNG M.A., PHIPPS R.J., WANG J.C.C., WIDDICOMBE J.G. Control of nasal vasculature and airflow resistance in the dog. *J. Physiol. Lond.* 1984, 349, 535-551.

MACLAGAN J. Presynaptic control of airway smooth muscle. *Am. Rev. Respir. Dis.* 1987, 136, S54-S57.

MALM L., McCAFFREY T.V., KERN E.B. α adrenoceptor-mediated secretion from the anterior nasal glands of the dog. *Acta Otolaryngol. (Stockholm)* 1983, 96, 149-155.

MASSARO G.D., PARIS M., THET L.A. In vivo regulation of secretion of bronchiolar Clara cells in rats. *J. Clin. Invest.* 1979, 63, 167-172.

MASSARO G.D., AMADO C., CLERCH L., MASSARO D. Studies on the regulation of secretion in Clara cells with evidence for chemical nonautonomic mediation of the secretory response to increased ventilation in rat lungs. *J. Clin. Invest.* 1982, 70, 608-613.

MATSUZAKI Y., HAMASAKI Y., SAID S.I. Vasoactive intestinal peptide: a possible transmitter of nonadrenergic relaxation of guinea-pig airways. *Science* 1980, 210, 1252-1253.

MULLOL J., BARANIUK J.N., LOGUN C., MERIDA M., HAUSFELD J., SHELHAMER J.H., KALINER M.A. M_1 and M_3 muscarinic antagonists inhibit human nasal glandular secretion in vitro. *J. Appl. Physiol.* 1992, 73, 2069-2073.

NADEL J.A. Autonomic regulation of airway smooth muscle. In : *Physiology and Pharmacology of the Airways*, Nadel, J.A. (Ed.), Marcel Dekker, New York, 1980, pp 217-257.

NANDIWADA P., KADOWITZ P.J., SAID S.I., MOJARAD M., HYMAN A.L. Pulmonary vasodilation responses to vasoactive intestinal peptide in the cat. *J. Appl. Physiol.* 1985, 58, 1723-1728.

NUYTEN J., MUYLLE E., OYAERT W., VAN DEN HENDE C. The influence of clenbuterol on prostaglandin $F_{2\alpha}$-induced dyspnoea in calves. *Vet. Res. Commun.* 1986, 10, 453-461.

PAVIA D., AGNEW J.E., LOPEZ-VIDRIERO M.T., NEWMAN S.P., CLARKE S.W. The effect of metered dose aerosols on the viscoelastic properties and clearance of bronchial secretions. In : *Metered Dose Inhalers*, Epstein, S.W. (Ed.), Astra, Mississauga, 1984, pp 38-48.

PAVIA D., BATEMAN J.R.M., LENNARD-JONES A.M., AGNEW J.E., CLARKE S.W. Effect of selective and non-selective β-blockade on pulmonary function and tracheobronchial mucociliary clearance in healthy subjects. *Thorax* 1986, 41, 301-305.

PEATFIELD A.C., RICHARDSON P.S. Evidence for noncholinergic, nonadrenergic nervous control of mucus secretion into the cat trachea. *J. Physiol. Lond.* 1983, 342, 335-345.

PELL J., PHIPPS R.J., WELLS U.M., WIDDICOMBE J.G. Control of mucoglycoprotein output from the rabbit nose. *J. Physiol. Lond.* 1984, 353, 339-353.

PHIPPS R.J., NADEL J.A., DAVIS B. Effect of α-adrenergic stimulation on mucus secretion and ion transport in cat trachea in vitro. *Am. Rev. Respir. Dis.* 1980, 121, 359-365.

POLAK J.M., BLOOM S.R. Occurrence and distribution of regulatory peptides in the respiratory tract. *Recent Results Cancer Res.* 1985, 99, 1-6.

RHODEN K.J., MELDRUM L.A., BARNES P.J. Inhibition of cholinergic neurotransmission in human airways by β_2-adrenoceptors. *J. Appl. Physiol.* 1988, 65, 700-705.

RICHARDSON J., BELAND J. Non-adrenergic inhibitory nervous system in human airways. *J. Appl. Physiol.* 1976, 41, 764-771.

RICHARDSON J.B. State of art. Nerve supply to the lungs. *Am. Rev. Respir. Dis.* 1979, 119, 785-802.

ROETS E., BURVENICH C., CURVERS P., HOORENS J. Determination of β-adrenoceptors and cAMP in muscle from normal and splayleg Belgian Landrace pigs. *Vet. Res. Commun.* 1989, 13, 273-286.

ROETS E., BURVENICH C., ROBERTS M. Muscarinic receptor subtypes, β-adrenoceptors and cAMP in the tracheal smooth muscle of conventional and double-muscled calves. *Vet. Res. Commun.* 1992, 16, 465-476.

ROFFEL A.F., ELZINGA C.R.S., ZAAGSMA J. Muscarinic M_3-receptors mediate contraction of human central and peripheral airway smooth muscle. *Pulmon. Pharmacol.* 1990, 3, 47-52.

SASSE H.H.L., HAJER R. Enkele veterinair-klinische ervaringen met het gebruik van een

β_2-receptoren stimulerend sympaticomymeticum (NAB 365®) bij paarden met longaandoeningen. *Tijdschr. Diergeneesk.* 1977, 102, 1233-1238.

SCOTT J.S., BROADSTONE R.V., DERKSEN F.J., ROBINSON N.E. β-Adrenergic blockade in ponies with recurrent obstructive pulmonary disease. *J. Appl. Physiol.* 1988a, 64, 2324-2328.

SCOTT J.S., GARON H., BROADSTONE R.V., DERKSEN F.J., ROBINSON N.E. α_1-Adrenergic-induced airway obstruction in ponies with recurrent pulmonary disease. *J. Appl. Physiol.* 1988b, 65, 687-692.

SCOTT J.S., BERNEY C.E., DERKSEN F.J., ROBINSON N.E. β-Adrenergic receptor activity in ponies with recurrent obstructive pulmonary disease. *Am. J. Vet. Res.* 1991, 52, 1416-1422.

SHELLER J.R., HOLTZMAN M.J., SKOOGH B.-E., NADEL J.A. Interaction of serotonin with vagal and acetylcholine-induced bronchoconstriction in canine lungs. *J. Appl. Physiol.* 1982, 52, 964-966.

SKOOGH B.-E. Transmission through airway ganglia. *Eur. J. Respir. Dis. (Suppl.)* 1983, 64, 159-170.

SLOCOMBE R.F., ROBINSON N.E., DERKSEN F.J. Effect of vagotomy on respiratory mechanics and gas exchange in the neonatal calf. *Am. J. Vet. Res.* 1982, 43, 1168-1171.

TAMAOKI J., YAMAUCHI F., CHIYOTANI A., YAMAWAKI I., TAKEUCHI S., KONNO K. Atypical β-adrenoceptor- (β_3-adrenoceptor) mediated relaxation of canine isolated bronchial smooth muscle. *J. Appl. Physiol.* 1993, 74, 297-302.

TANAKA D.T., GRUNSTEIN M.M. Mechanisms of substance P-induced contraction of rabbit airway smooth muscle. *J. Appl. Physiol.: Respirat. Environ. Exercise Physiol.* 1984, 57, 1551-1557.

TURGUT K., SASSE H.H.L. Influence of clenbuterol on mucociliary transport in healthy horses and horses with chronic obstructive pulmonary disease. *Vet. Rec.* 1989, 125, 526-530.

VAN de DONK H.J.M., MERKHUS F.W.H.M. Decrease in ciliary beat frequency due to intranasal administration of propranolol. *J. Pharm. Sci.* 1982, 71, 595-596.

WALTERS E.H., O'BYRNE P.M., FABBRI L.M., GRAF P.D., HOLZMAN M.J., NADEL J.A. Control of neurotransmission by prostaglandins in canine trachealis smooth muscle. *J. Appl. Physiol.* 1984, 57, 129-134.

WELLS U., WIDDICOMBE J.G. Lateral nasal gland secretion in the anaesthetized dog. *J. Physiol. Lond.* 1986, 374, 359-362.

WILSON H., YATES M.S. Sympathetic nerves and nasal secretion in the cat. *Acta Otolaryngol. (Stockholm)* 1978, 85, 426-430.

WONG L.B., MILLER I.F., YEATES D.B. Stimulation of ciliary beat frequency by autonomic agonists: in vivo. *J. Appl. Physiol.* 1988, 65, 971-981.

YONEDA K. Pilocarpine stimulation of the bronchiolar Clara cell secretion. *Lab. Invest.* 1977, 37, 447-452.

YU M., ROBINSON N.E., WANG Z., DERKSEN F.J. Muscarinic receptor subtypes in equine tracheal smooth muscle. *Vet. Res. Commun.* 1992, 16, 301-310.

CHAPTER VIII

AUTACOIDS AND PULMONARY FUNCTION

P. Lekeux and A. Linden

Laboratory for Functional Investigation
Faculty of Veterinary Medicine
University of Liege

SUMMARY

This paper describes the role of the autacoids, i.e. histamine, 5-hydroxytryptamine, bradykinin, eicosanoids, platelet activating factor and the complement system, on the pulmonary physiology and physiopathology.

KEY WORDS

Respiratory system - Pulmonary function - Autacoids.

1. INTRODUCTION

Some endogenous substances, which are normally present or may be formed in the body, are arbitrarily classified under the term autacoid, i.e. "αυτος ακος" in Greek, which means "self medicinal agent". These substances act by humoral regulation and participate in physiological and pathophysiological responses to injuries.

Because these substances usually have a brief lifetime and act near their sites of synthesis, they have often been described as local hormones. However, unlike true hormones which reach their sites of action via the bloodstream, these substances often conduct their affairs closeted from the circulation, such as in the confines of an inflammatory lesion.

The availability of these autacoids (Table 8-1.) and their antagonists (Table 8-2.) has provided some evidences concerning their potential physiological and pathophysiological roles in the respiratory system. This may help for a better understanding and treatment of pulmonary dysfunctions.

Other locally acting substances such as neuropeptides, cytokines and endothelium-derived factors are reviewed elsewhere.

2. HISTAMINE

Histamine is synthetized *in vivo* from histidine and stored in cytoplasmic granules of mast cells and basophils. Various stimuli are able to cause mast cell degranulation. Once released, histamine induces smooth muscle contraction, vascular hyperpermeability and mucus secretion in the lungs. These effects are mediated through specific histamine receptors, i.e. H_1 and H_2. A third histamine receptor has been described in brain tissue (Arrang et al, 1985).

Although the responses vary among species, both inhaled and injected histamine cause bronchospasm in most healthy animals. This response is mediated via H_1 receptors and is exacerbated in diseased animals.

In the dog, constrictor and dilator effects mediated via H_1 and H_2 receptors respectively have been described (Irvin and Dempsey, 1978). Histamine

Table 8-1. Functional effects of some autacoids in the lungs

Autacoids	Airway tonus	Vascular tonus	Vascular permeability	Mucus secretion
Histamine	↗	↘	↗	↗
5-hydroxytryptamine	↗	↗	↗	-
Bradykinin	↗	↘	↗	-
Thromboxane A_2	↗	↗	-	-
Prostaglandin I_2	↘	↘	-	-
Prostaglandin E_2	↘	↗	-	-
Prostaglandin F_2	↗	↗	-	-
Leukotrienes C_4, D_4, E_4	↗	↗	↗	↗
Platelet-activating-factor	↗	↘ or ↗	↗	↗
Complement	↗	↗	↗	-

seems to act both directly and indirectly, via stimulation of irritant receptors (Dixon et al, 1979). The histamine-induced bronchoconstriction in this species is partly due to stimulation of reflex vagal pathways (White and Kaliner, 1991).

In both anesthetized (Slocombe and Robinson, 1981) and unsedated cattle (Gustin et al, 1988), the histamine challenge induces a decrease of the calibre of the large and small airways. These changes are accentuated with aging (Leblanc et al, 1991) and after β-adrenergic blockade (Kotlikoff et al, 1982), and are prevented by H_1 receptor blockade (Slocombe and Robinson, 1981). The histamine-induced bronchoconstriction was showed to be increased after a bovine respiratory syncytial virus infection (Leblanc et al, 1991), suggesting the occurrence of disease-induced hyperresponsiveness in bovine airways.

In the horse, there is a significant correlation between age and sensitivity, but

Table 8-2. Some antagonists of autacoids

Mediators	Antagonists
H_1	Diphenhydramine, Pyrilamine, Chlorpheniramine, Chlorcyclizine, Promethazine, Terfenadine
H_2	Cimetidine, Ranitidine, Famotidine, Nizatidine
H_3	Thioperamide
$5\text{-}HT_{1\text{-}2}$	Methysergide, Mianserin, Spiperone
$5\text{-}HT_2$	Ketanserin, Pirenperone, Metrenperone
$5\text{-}HT_3$	MDL72222, ICS 205930, Zacopride
$B_1\text{-}B_2$	D-Arg(4-OH-Pro^3-D-Phe^7) bradykinin
B_1	des-Arg^9(Leu^8) bradykinin
TXA_2	S-1452, SK&F96148, HN-11500, GR32191
PGD_2	AH 6809, BW A868C, BM 13,177, L-670,596
LTB_4	SC-41930, SM-9064, U-75302, LY 255283
LTC_4/LTD_4	SKF 104,353; SKF 106,203, LY 171,883, ICI 204,219, ICI 198,615, MK-571
PAF	CV 3988, L-652-731, BN 52063, BN 52021, WEB 2086, WEB 2170, WEB 2347, ONO-6240, SRI 63-675, SRI 63-119, SRI 63-441, STY 2108, E 6123, Y-24180
C_{5a}, C_3	SC-41930

H : Histamine; 5-HT : 5-hydroxytryptamine; B : Bradykinin; TX : thromboxane; PG : Prostaglandins; LT : Leukotrienes; PAF : Platelet-activating factor; C : Complement.

not reactivity, to the histamine challenge (Derksen et al, 1982). In horses suffering from recurrent airway obstruction, the bronchoconstrictor response to intravenous histamine was exaggerated during the acute phase of the disease but not during clinical remission (Derksen et al, 1985). Little evidence exists

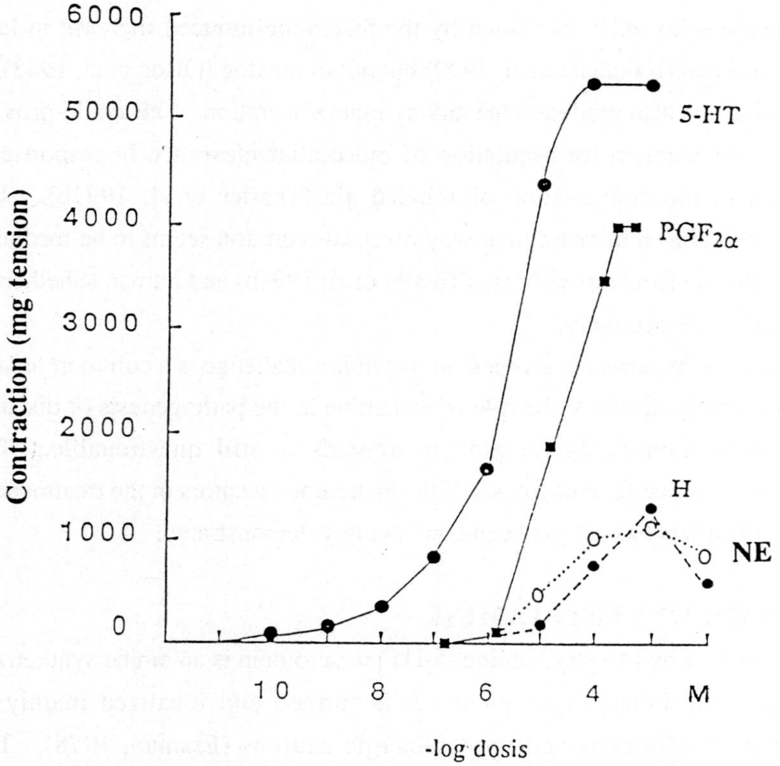

Fig. 8-1. Pressor response to several agonists in bovine pulmonary artery. 5-HT : 5-hydroxytryptamine; H : Histamine; NE : Norepinephrine; $PGF_{2\alpha}$: Prostaglandin $F_{2\alpha}$ (Van de Putte and Burvenich, 1991).

for the involvement of muscarinic (Broadstone et al, 1988) and β-adrenergic receptors (Scott et al, 1988) in the response to histamine challenge in this species.

Histamine may induce constriction of pulmonary vascular smooth muscles, mainly at the level of the pulmonary veins (Fig. 8-1.), and an increased microvascular permeability (White and Kaliner, 1991). This could contribute to pulmonary hemodynamic disorders, pulmonary edema and airway mucosal swelling as observed during some respiratory diseases. However, differences between species exist, as shown by the histamine-induced increase in lung water in sheep (Nakahara et al, 1979) but not in the dog (Olson et al, 1983). Histamine can also modulate the airway mucus secretion. This could provide a direct mechanism for regulation of mucociliar clearance in response to changes in the composition of inhaled air (Tessier et al, 1991b). The histamine-induced increase in airway mucosal secretion seems to be mediated via H_1 and H_2 receptors in horse (Tessier et al, 1991b) and human (Shelhamer et al, 1980), respectively.

Although the hyperresponsiveness to histamine challenge is a common feature of most airway diseases, the role of histamine in the pathogenesis of disease-induced pulmonary dysfunction in animals is still questionable. The usefulness of specific antagonists of the histamine receptors in the treatment of airway disorders has not yet been convincingly demonstrated.

3. 5-HYDROXYTRYPTAMINE

Endogenous 5-hydroxytryptamine (5-HT) or serotonin is an amine synthetized *in vivo* from dietary tryptophan. It is formed and localized mainly in enterochromaffin cells and tryptaminergic neurons (Essman, 1978). The overflow from the enterochromaffin cells is removed by the liver and by the endothelial cells of the pulmonary circulation. Uptake of 5-HT by the smooth muscle cells of the pulmonary arteries has also been described (Lee et al, 1987). 5-HT, escaping the metabolic machinery of the liver and the lungs, is stored as dense granules in circulating thrombocytes and released mainly during platelet aggregation (Movat, 1987).

In the respiratory system, 5-HT is principally localized to nerve terminals and to the dense secretory granules of platelets (Sirek and Sirek, 1970). Mastocytes and neuroepithelial bodies have been proved to be a source for intrapulmonary production of 5-HT in some species (Lauweryns et al, 1973).

5-HT is a potent bronchoconstrictor of airway muscle preparations from guinea pigs (Van Nueten et al, 1982) and horses (Doucet et al, 1990), but it

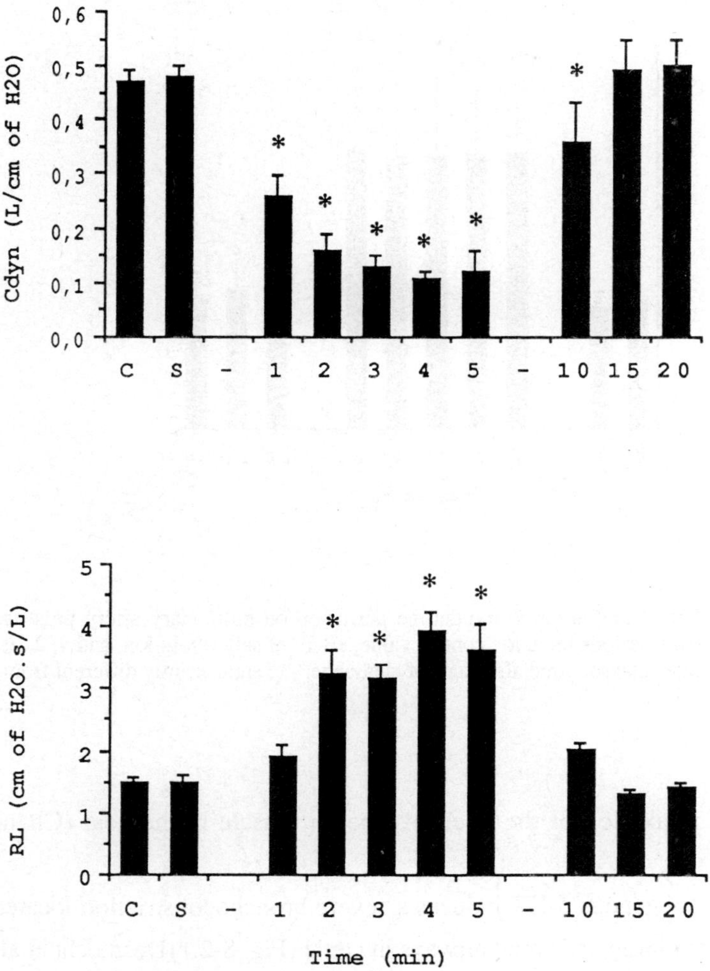

Fig. 8-2. Effect of 5-hydroxytryptamine (5-HT) perfusion on lung dynamic compliance (Cdyn) and total pulmonary resistance (R_L) in healthy calves. Measurements periods include : Control value, effect of saline solution, and 1, 2, 3, 4, 5, 10, 15, 20 minutes elapsed time after start of challenge. * : Significantly different from baseline at $P < 0.05$ level.

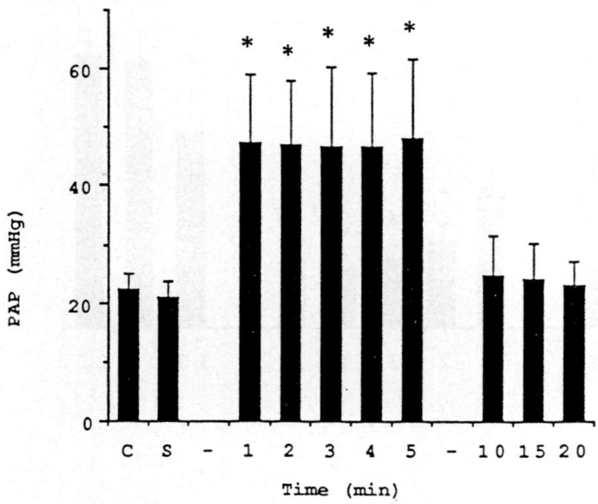

Fig. 8-3. Effect of 5-hydroxytryptamine perfusion on pulmonary artery pressure (PAP). Measurements periods include : control value, effect of saline solution, and 1, 2, 3, 4, 5, 10, 15, 20 minutes elapsed time after start of challenge. * : significantly different from baseline at $P < 0.05$ level.

induces relaxation of the tracheal smooth muscle in the goat (Chand et al, 1979).

In vivo, exogenous 5-HT induces a severe bronchoconstriction located at the level of the large and small airways in cattle (Fig. 8-2.) (Desmecht et al, 1992) and in sheep (Webber et al, 1990) but not in either normal or asthmatic human beings (Cushley et al, 1986).

5-HT is also a potent pulmonary vasoconstrictor (Fig. 8-3.) (Dawson, 1984; Selig et al, 1988; Desmecht et al, 1992). This vasopressor response is potentiated by cyclo-oxygenase blockade (Hofman and Ehrhart, 1987). In addition, 5-HT enhances platelet aggregation and vasoconstriction produced by other vasoactive agents (Gilbert and Newberry, 1987). The mechanism whereby 5-HT operates may be either direct by acting on both vascular and non-vascular smooth muscle (Van Nueten et al, 1982), or indirect by interacting with the cholinergic pathway (Sheller et al, 1982).

These different action pathways of 5-HT may be explained in part by the involvement of different receptor subtypes and effector systems to which the receptors are linked (Roth and Chuang, 1987). At least four general categories of 5-HT receptors have been postulated to exist, i.e. the 5-HT_1, 5-HT_2, 5-HT_3 and 5-HT_4 receptors, some of which having different subtypes (Schmidt and Peroutka, 1989; Frazer et al, 1990). There are species differences in the type of receptors involved in the 5-HT-induced effects. In cat (Ball et al, 1983) and cattle (Van de Putte and Burvenich, 1991), the bronchoconstriction is reported to be mediated via 5-HT_2 receptors, whereas in sheep 5-HT contracts the tracheal smooth muscle by stimulating 5-HT_1-like receptors (Webber et al, 1990).

The blockade of the 5-HT_2 receptors has been shown to have some benefit in human patients with acute respiratory failure (Huval et al, 1984; Vincent et al, 1984). This could partly be explained by a disease-induced decrease in the 5-HT clearance by the lung vascular endothelium (Gillis et al, 1986). The resulting increase in 5-HT concentration in the lung could affect regional smooth muscle tone in blood vessels and airways and enhance leukocyte adherence to the endothelium (Boogaerts et al, 1982).

Animal studies further suggest a role for 5-hydroxytryptamine in several pathologic processes. 5-HT_2 blockade prevents the pulmonary hypertension associated with acid aspiration (Hechtman et al, 1984) and experimental embolization in the dog (Huval et al, 1983). This blockade also attenuates the pulmonary hypertension in ovine (Demling et al, 1985) and porcine (Olson, 1987) endotoxemia.

In cattle, the vasoconstrictor and bronchoconstrictor effects of exogenous 5-HT have been shown to be inhibited by 5-HT_2 blockade (Linden et al, 1993) and the 5-HT concentration was showed to be higher in pneumonic than in healthy lungs (Linden et al, 1991). This could explain the beneficial effect of this blockade as therapeutic measure during the shipping fever syndrome (Genicot et al, 1993a) and during the acute respiratory distress syndrome (Genicot et al, 1993b; 1993c).

4. BRADYKININ AND KALLIDIN

Bradykinin is a nonapeptide formed from plasma precursors as part of the inflammatory response. Kallidin has similar pharmacologic effects (Farmer and Burch, 1991). Bradykinin is generated from high molecular weight kininogen by the enzyme kallikrein which is stored in its inactive form prekallikrein in plasma and in various tissues (Regoli and Barabe, 1980) and may be released by inflammatory cells (Proud et al, 1985).

Once formed, bradykinin acts locally and is rapidly inactivated by the angiotensin-converting enzyme on endothelial cells (Regoli and Barabe, 1980) and by kinase enzymes in plasma and tissues. Neutral endopeptidase is also effective in degrading bradykinin (Dusser et al, 1988).

Bradykinin is a potent vasodilator of pulmonary vascular smooth muscle and it may produce a rise in vascular permeability, partly through the release of eicosanoids (Fuller and Barnes, 1988). Its effects are mediated through specific B_1, B_2 and B_3 receptors (Regoli, 1987; Steranka et al, 1989).

Bradykinin has also a direct effect on airway smooth muscle, although this effect differs in the various species. In guinea pigs, intravenous bradykinin induces bronchoconstriction (Ichinose et al, 1990), while in dogs (Kaufman et al, 1980) and cattle (Slocombe et al, 1982) bradykinin administration has no bronchoconstrictor effect.

Bradykinin causes bronchoconstriction in asthmatic human patients, although it is not effective in normal subjects (Fuller et al, 1987). This bradykinin-induced bronchoconstriction is indirectly mediated through cholinergic mechanisms but not through prostaglandin formation (Fuller et al, 1987).

In sheep, bradykinin seems not be an important mediator of endotoxemia-induced cardiopulmonary dysfunctions (Mann et al, 1991).

5. EICOSANOIDS

Arachidonic acid represents the major fatty acid of lipid membrane that is released during phospholipase A_2-mediated hydrolysis (O'Flaherty, 1987). Once released, arachidonic acid may be converted to a wide variety of biologically active oxygenated products by the cyclooxygenase, the 5-, 12- and 15-lipoxygenase and the monoxygenase pathways (Fig. 8-4.).

5.1. Cyclooxygenase products or prostanoids

Prostanoids act mainly as fine regulators of smooth muscle tone. They seem to play a contributory but not obligatory role in the healthy lung (Robinson and Holgate, 1991). During inflammation, numerous and opposing actions of prostanoids are described. However, the contribution of these substances to the pathogenesis of airway diseases is not clearly established.

5.1.1. Thromboxane A_2 (TxA_2)

Prostaglandin H_2 is converted predominantly to TxA_2 in platelets and perhaps also in macrophages, granulocytes and lung parenchymal cells (Olson et al, 1988). This compound is a powerful constrictor of vascular and airway smooth muscle and leads to aggregation of neutrophils and platelets. Its hydrolysis product TxB_2 is less active in causing smooth muscle contraction or platelet aggregation.

In asthmatic subjects, TxA_2 contributes to the immediate bronchoconstriction induced by inhaled allergen, and this effect is mediated by stimulation of a thromboxane receptor (Beasley et al, 1989). Prophylactic administration of a TxA_2 synthase inhibitor can inhibit the antigen-induced bronchoconstriction and reduce the bronchial hyperresponsiveness (Fujimura et al, 1990).

TxA_2 may be solely responsible for some states of pulmonary hypertension in rabbits (Seeger et al, 1989) and airway hyperreactivity in dogs (O'Byrne et al, 1985).

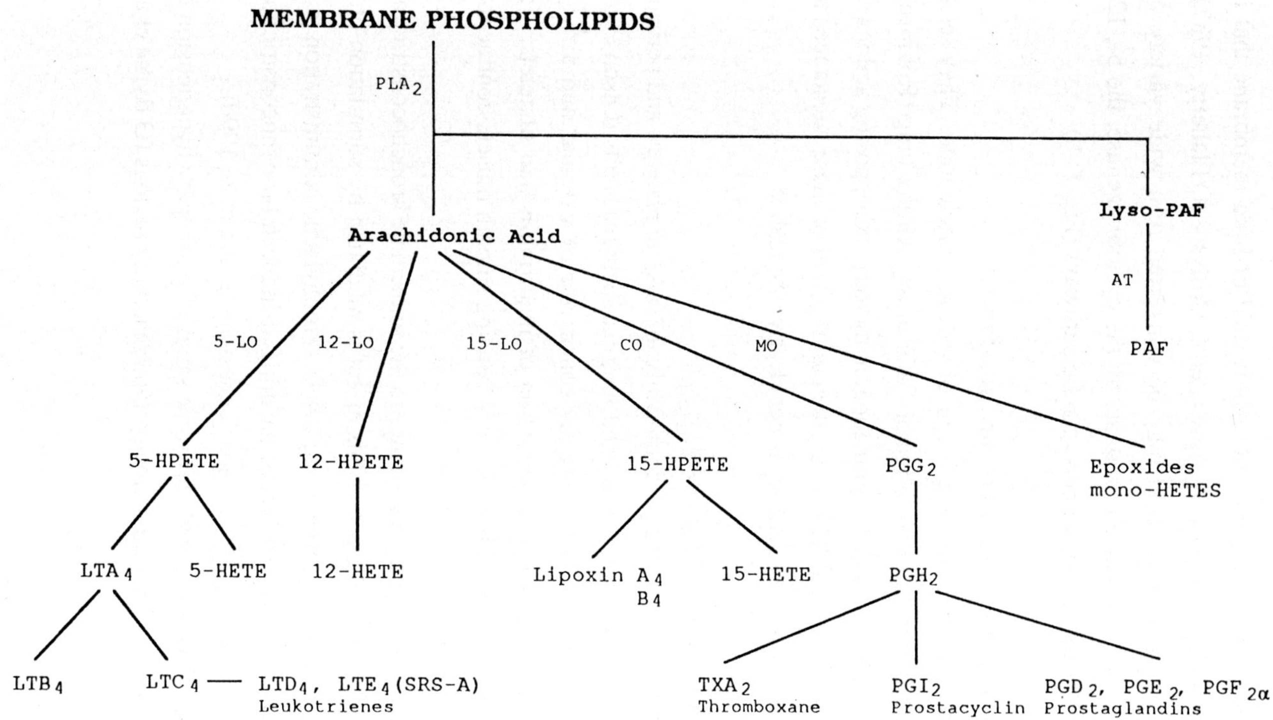

Fig. 8-4. Membrane lipid products. PLA_2 : Phospholipase A_2; AT : Acetyl transferase; LO : Lipoxygenase; CO : Cyclo-oxygenase; MO : Monoxygenase.

5.1.2. Prostacyclin (PGI_2)

PGI_2 is synthetized by vascular endothelial cells. On vascular smooth muscle, PGI_2 has powerful relaxant effects to produce cAMP-dependent vasodilation and it inhibits platelet aggregation (Henderson, 1987). The balance of effects between PGI_2 (vasodilator) and TxA_2 (vasoconstrictor) may play a major role in determining the level of pulmonary vascular tone (Moncada and Vane, 1979). Because PGI_2 is continuously produced and released by the pulmonary circulation, it may be responsible, at least in part for the low physiological levels of arterial pressure and vascular resistance in the pulmonary circulation (Gryglewski, 1980).

In vitro, PGI_2 can produce relaxation of guinea pig tracheal strips (Gardiner and Collier, 1980) whereas it has little or no effect on dynamic compliance or airway resistance in vivo, when inhaled by guinea pigs or dogs (Wasserman et al, 1980). In contrast to its lack of direct airway action in vivo, PGI_2 has been shown to interact with a range of bronchoconstrictor stimuli (Spannhake et al, 1980; Mugridge et al, 1984).

5.1.3. Prostaglandin D_2 (PGD_2)

PGD_2 is unlikely to play a significant role in the control of resting tone in pulmonary smooth muscles.

In asthmatic patients, aerosolized PGD_2 induces a transient cough followed by a bronchoconstriction (Robinson and Holgate, 1991).

5.1.4. Prostaglandin E_2 (PGE_2)

PGE_2 could contribute to the regulation of airway patency under normal conditions, as suggested by its spontaneous release from the bronchi (Robinson and Holgate, 1991).

PGE_2 is able to relax the smooth muscles of the canine airways by a direct effect on the muscle and by an indirect negative effect on acetylcholine release (Walters et al, 1984) but this effect may be reversed at high dosage (Mathé and Hedqvist, 1975).

In horse, airway mucosal PGE_2 production is reduced during chronic obstructive pulmonary disease, suggesting that a relative decrease in this bronchorelaxant substance may be a factor in the pathogenesis of this disease (Gray et al, 1992). However, PGE_2 does not inhibit acetylcholine release in equine airways (Robinson, 1993) and other epithelial-derived relaxant factors could also modulate the contractility of the airway smooth muscles in this species (Tessier et al, 1991a).

5.1.5. Prostaglandin $F_{2\alpha}$ ($PGF_{2\alpha}$)

$PGF_{2\alpha}$ is a potent constrictor of airway smooth muscle (O'Byrne et al, 1984). It may also induce cough by direct stimulation of sensory nerve endings in the airways (Coleridge et al, 1976).

However, its variable and inconstant effects both *in vitro* (Van de Putte and Burvenich, 1989) and after inhalation in diseased patients (Nuytten et al, 1986) suggest that its activity is mediated by much more complex mechanisms.

5.2. 5-Lipoxygenase products or leukotrienes (LT)

Leukotrienes are products of the metabolism of arachidonic acid that are formed mainly in leukocytes and macrophages through the 5-lipoxygenase enzyme pathway. The unstable intermediate LTA_4 can be converted to LTB_4 or to LTC_4. The latter can in turn be metabolized to LTD_4 and then LTE_4.

These last three substances, which are known to represent the slow-reacting substance of anaphylaxis (SRS-A) (Olson et al, 1988), may induce all disorders present during asthmatic-like diseases, i.e. contraction of airway smooth muscle (Dahlen, 1983), airway hyperreactivity (Kaye and Smith, 1990) and enhanced airway mucus secretion (Marom et al, 1982). In the airway, LTC_4 and LTD_4 have been shown to be approximately 1000 times more potent bronchoconstrictors than histamine (Dahlen et al, 1980).

Leukotrienes are also involved in bovine anaphylactic reactions (Burka and Eyre, 1974), porcine endotoxemia (Olson et al, 1990) and human adult respiratory distress syndrome (Bernard et al, 1991), but not in the ovine hypoxic pulmonary vasoconstriction (Pearl and Prielipp, 1991).

5.3. 12-Lipoxygenase products

Although the direct and specific effects of 12-hydroperoxyeicosatetraenoic acid (12-HPETE) or its corresponding hydroxy fatty acid (12-HETE) appear relatively weak, these compounds could act indirectly in lung inflammation, for instance by modulating platelet function (Olson et al, 1990).

5.4. 15-Lipoxygenase products

Leucocytes seem to be able to convert 15-HPETE and 15-HETE to lipoxins A and B (Holtzman, 1991). Increased amounts of these compounds were found to be increased in bronchoalveolar lavage fluid from humans with respiratory diseases (Lee et al, 1990) but not from tracheal epithelium of diseased horses (Gray et al, 1992). Because of the variability in their pulmonary actions, these substances could function as antiinflammatory modulators in the airways (Holtzman, 1991).

5.5. Monoxygenase products

Metabolism of arachidonic acid by cytochrome P-450 monoxygenase leads to ω and ω_1-oxygenated products, as well as epoxy acid (Guengerich and McDonald, 1990). Some of these products have been found in the lung, where they could modulate the local blood flow (Strum et al, 1990).

6. PLATELET-ACTIVATING FACTOR (PAF)

PAF is a biologically active phospholipid with a broad range of cellular targets and responses. It is probably best considered as a mediator acting among a network of mediators involved in inflammatory processes (Chung, 1992). Several actions of PAF in the lungs have been described. Aerosolized PAF induces a potent bronchoconstriction (Rubin et al, 1987), which is reduced by leukotriene blockade but not by blockade of histamine nor thromboxane

(Spencer et al, 1991).

PAF induces also an eicosanoid-independent increase in airway microvascular leakage, which could partly contribute to the PAF-induced narrowing of the airways (Tokuyama et al, 1991).

Mucociliar clearance is impaired by inhaled PAF (Nieminen et al, 1991), although this substance increases the tracheal mucus secretion in vitro (Sasaki et al, 1989).

In sheep, PAF was reported to induce bronchial hyperresponsiveness and pulmonary hypertension in healthy animals (Christman et al, 1988), and to partially mediate endotoxin-induced lung dysfunctions (Christman et al, 1990).

In the hamster, injury of the pulmonary vascular endothelium induced by inhaled bacterial endotoxin was shown to be mediated via PAF (Lantz et al, 1991).

The studies about the effects of specific PAF antagonists in the treatment of human pulmonary disorders do not give clear evidence whether PAF plays a major pathological role in this species (Chung, 1992).

7. COMPLEMENT

The complement system has a major role in the host defense against invading microorganisms. However it can also cause lung tissue injuries and contribute to some pulmonary dysfunctions (Ward et al, 1991). The major active fragments resulting from the activation of the complement cascade are C_{3a}, C_{4a} and C_{5a}, which cause mainly chemotaxis, smooth muscle contraction, airway hyperresponsiveness and increased vascular permeability (Till et al, 1982; Berend, 1988). Evidence for the involvement of complement has been described during naturally acquired bovine respiratory syncytial virus infection (Kimman et al, 1989).

The complement system can also stimulate the release of many other autacoids (Betz and Hansch, 1984; Olson et al, 1988). This hampers the differentiation of its direct and indirect effects during endotoxemia and acute respiratory distress syndrome (Olson and Dodam, 1991).

The proinflammatory properties of the complement system seem to be partly inhibited by agents such as SC-41930 (Fretland et al, 1991).

8. CONCLUSIONS

Although most autacoids have powerful actions on the respiratory system both *in vitro* and *in vivo*, this does not systematically mean that the use of their specific agonists or antagonists may help for the control of pulmonary dysfunctions. The results of each investigation concerning these factors must be analysed very carefully because of the peculiarities due to the species, the challenge, the diseases etc ..., and because of the complex interactions between the humoral, neural and cellular mediators.

Therefore, an appropriate control of the pulmonary dysfunctions in our domestic animals requires a global approach which includes fundamental, applied and clinical investigations, in order to demonstrate whether the most effective treatment of each clinical syndrome is based on the modulation of one specific subtype of receptor or on the inhibition of a complex "soup" of receptors.

REFERENCES

ARRANG J.M., GARBARG M., SCHWARTZ J.C. Autoregulation of histamine release in brain by presynaptic H_3-receptors. *Neuroscience* 1985, 15, 553-562.

BALL H.A., PARRATT J.R., RODGER I.W. The effect of a selective 5-HT_2 antagonist, ketanserin, on the pulmonary responses to *Escherichia coli*. *Br. J. Pharmacol.* 1983, 80, 295-301.

BEASLEY R.C.W., FEATHERSTONE R.L., CHURCH M.K., RAFFERTY P., VARLEY J.G., HARRIS A., ROBINSON C., HOLGATE S. Effect of a thromboxane receptor antagonist on PGD_2- and allergen-induced bronchoconstriction. *J. Appl. Physiol.* 1989, 66, 1685-1693.

BEREND N. Complement. In : *Asthma : Basic Mechanisms and Clinical Management*, Barnes, P.J., Rodger, I.W., Thomson N.C. (Eds), Academic Press, New York, 1988, pp 325-339.

BERNARD G.R., KORLEY V., CHEE P., SWINDELL B., FORD-HUTCHINSON A.W., TAGARI P. Persistent generation of peptido leukotrienes in patients with the adult respiratory distress syndrome. *Am. Rev. Respir. Dis.* 1991, 144, 263-267.

BETZ M., HANSCH G.M. Release of arachidonic acid: a new function of late complement components. *Immunobiol.* 1984, 166, 473-483.
BOOGAERTS M.A., YAMADA O., JACOB H.S., MOLDOW G.F. Enhancement of granulocyte-endothelial cell adherence and granulocyte induced cytoxicity by platelet release products. *Proc. Natl. Acad. Sci. USA* 1982, 79, 7019-7023.
BROADSTONE R.V., SCOTT J.S., DERKSEN F.J., ROBINSON N.E. Effects of atropine in ponies with recurrent airway obstruction. *J. Appl. Physiol.* 1988, 65, 2720-2725.
BURKA J.F., EYRE P. A study of prostaglandins and prostaglandin antagonists in relation to anaphylaxis in calves. *Can. J. Physiol. Pharmacol.* 1974, 52, 942-951.
CHAND N., DE ROTH L., EYRE P. Relaxant response of goat trachea to 5-hydroxytryptamine mediated by D-tryptamine receptors. *Br. J. Pharmacol.* 1979, 66, 331-336.
CHRISTMAN B.W., LEFFERTS P.L., KING G.A., SNAPPER J.R. Role of circulating platelets and granulocytes in PAF-induced pulmonary dysfunction in awake sheep. *J. Appl. Physiol.* 1988, 64, 2033-2041.
CHRISTMAN B.W., LEFFERTS P.L., BLAIR I.A., SNAPPER J.R. Effect of platelet-activating factor receptor antagonism on endotoxin-induced lung dysfunction in awake sheep. *Am. Rev. Respir. Dis.* 1990, 142, 1272-1278.
CHUNG K.F. Platelet-activating factor in inflammation and pulmonary disorders. *Clin. Sci.* 1992, 83, 127-138.
COLERIDGE H.M., COLERIDGE J.C.G., GINZEL K.H., BAKER D.G., BANZETT R.B., MORRISON M.A. Stimulation of irritant receptors and afferent C-fibres in the lungs by prostaglandins. *Nature* 1976, 264, 451-453.
CUSHLEY M.J., WEE L.E., HOLGATE S.T. The effect of inhaled 5-hydroxytryptamine (5-HT, serotonin) on airway calibre in man. *Br. J. Clin. Pharmacol.* 1986, 22, 487-490.
DAHLEN S.-E., HEDQVIST P., HAMMARSTROM S., SAMUELSSON B. Leukotrienes are potent constrictors of human bronchi. *Nature* 1980, 288, 484-486.
DAHLEN S.-E. Pulmonary effects of leukotrienes. *Acta Physiol. Scand. (Suppl.)* 1983, 512, 1-51.
DAWSON C.A. Role of pulmonary vasomotion in physiology of the lung. *Physiol. Rev.* 1984, 64, 544-570.
DEMLING R.H., WONG C., FOX R., HECHTMAN H., HUVAL W. Relationship of increased lung serotonin levels to endotoxin-induced pulmonary hypertension in sheep. *Am. Rev. Respir. Dis.* 1985, 132, 1257-1261.
DERKSEN F.J., SLOCOMBE R.F., ROBINSON N.E. Pulmonary effects of intravenous histamine in the conscious pony: dose-response relationships and reproducibility. *Am. J. Vet. Res.* 1982, 43, 2134-2137.
DERKSEN F.J., SCOTT D., ROBINSON N.E., SLOCOMBE R.F., ARMSTRONG P.J. Intravenous histamine administration in ponies with recurrent airway obstruction (heaves). *Am. J. Vet. Res.* 1985, 46, 774-777.
DESMECHT D.J.-M., LINDEN A.S., ROLLIN F.A., AMORY H., LEKEUX P.M. Effect of intravenous and aerosol administration of 5-hydroxytryptamine on pulmonary function values in healthy calves. *Am. J. Vet. Res.* 1992, 53, 315-320.
DIXON M., JACKSON D.M., RICHARDS I.M. The effect of histamine, acetylcholine, and 5-hydroxytryptamine on lung mechanics and irritant receptors discharge in dogs. *J. Physiol.* 1979, 287, 393-403.
DOUCET M., JONES T.R., FORD-HUTCHINSON A.W. Responses of equine trachealis and lung parenchyma to methacholine, histamine, serotonin, prostanoids, and leukotrienes in vitro. *Can. J. Physiol. Pharmacol.* 1990, 68, 379-383.
DUSSER D.J., NADEL J.A., SEKIZAWA K., GRAF P.D., BORSON D.B. Neutral

endopeptidase and angiotensin converting enzyme inhibitors potentiate kinin-induced contraction of ferret trachea. *J. Pharmacol. Exp. Ther.* 1988, 244, 531-536.

ESSMAN W.B. Serotonin in Health and Disease, Vol. 1, Availability, Localization and Disposition, Spectrum Publications Inc., New York, 1978.

FARMER S.G., BURCH R.M. The pharmacology of bradykinin receptors. In : *Bradykinin Antagonists: Basic and Clinical Research*, Burch, R.M. (Ed.), Marcel Dekker, New York, 1991, pp 1-31.

FRAZER A., MAAYANI S., WOLFE B.B. Subtypes of receptors for serotonin. *Annu. Rev. Pharmacol. Toxicol.* 1990, 30, 307-348.

FRETLAND D.J., WIDOMSKI D.L., ANGLIN C.P., LEVIN S., GAGINELLA T.S. Modulation of the chemotactic properties of complement fragments C_{5a} and C_3 by the anti-inflammatory agent, SC-41930. *Agents and Actions* 1991, 34, 5-7.

FUJIMURA M., NISHIOKA S., KUMABASHIRI I., MATSUDA T., MIFUNE J. Effects of aerosol administration of a thromboxane synthetase inhibitor (OKY-046) on bronchial responsiveness to acetylcholine in asthmatic subjects. *Chest* 1990, 98, 276-279.

FULLER R.W., DIXON C.M.S., CUSS F.M.C., BARNES P.J. Bradykinin-induced bronchoconstriction in humans. *Am. Rev. Respir. Dis.* 1987, 135, 176-180.

FULLER R.W., BARNES P.J. Kinins. In : *Asthma: Basic Mechanisms and Clinical Management*, Barnes, P.J., Rodger, I.W., Thomson, N.C. (Eds), Academic Press, London, 1988, pp 259-272.

GARDINER P.J., COLLIER H.O.J. Specific receptors for prostaglandins in the airways. *Prostaglandins* 1980, 19, 819-841.

GENICOT B., MOULIGNEAU F., ROLLIN F., LINDSEY J.K., CLOSE R., LEKEUX P. Economic, clinical and functional consequences of a treatment using metrenperone during an outbreak of Shipping Fever in cattle. *Vet. Rec.*, 1993a, 132, 245-247.

GENICOT B., MOULIGNEAU F., LINDSEY J.K., LAMBERT P., CLOSE R., LEKEUX P. Efficiency of 5-hydroxytryptamine receptor blockade as therapeutic measure during acute respiratory distress syndrome in double-muscled cattle. *J. Vet. Med. A*, 1993b, 40, 185-193.

GENICOT B., MOULIGNEAU F., LINDSEY J.K., LAMBERT P., CLOSE R., LEKEUX P. Induction of a serotonin-S_2 receptor blockade during early or late stage of acute respiratory distress syndrome in double-muscled calves: a comparative study. *J. Vet. Med. A* 1993c, 40, 241-248.

GILBERT M.J., NEWBERRY N.R. A 5-HT1-like receptor mediates a sympathetic ganglionic hyperpolarisation. *Eur. J. Pharmacol.* 1987, 144, 385-388.

GILLIS C.N., PITT B.R., WIEDEMANN H.P., HAMMOND G.L. Depressed prostaglandin E_1 and 5-hydroxytryptamine removal in patients with adult respiratory distress syndrome. *Am. Rev. Respir. Dis.* 1986, 134, 739-744.

GRAY P.R., DERKSEN F.J., BROADSTONE R.V., ROBINSON N.E., PETERS-GOLDEN M. Decreased airway mucosal prostaglandin E_2 production during airway obstruction in an animal model of asthma. *Am. Rev. Respir. Dis.* 1992, 146, 586-591.

GRYGLEWSKI R.J. The lung as a generator of prostacyclin in metabolic activities of the lung, Ciba Foundation Symposia 78, Excerpta Medica, New York, 1980, pp 147-164.

GUENGERICH F.P., McDONALD T.L. Mechanism of cytochrome P-450 catalysis. *FASEB J.* 1990, 4, 2453-2459.

GUSTIN P., DHEM A.R., LEKEUX P., LOMBA F., LANDSER F.J., VAN DE WOESTIJNE K.P. Investigation of the effects of histamine inhalation on the tracheobronchial tree of calves by the forced oscillation technique. *J. vet. Pharmacol. Therap.* 1988, 11, 374-380.

HECHTMAN H.B., VALERI C.R., SHEPRO D. Role of humoral mediators in adult respiratory distress syndrome. *Chest* 1984, 86, 623-627.

HENDERSON W.R. Eicosanoids and lung inflammation. *Am. Rev. Respir. Dis.* 1987, 135, 1176-1185.

HOFMAN W.F., EHRHART I.C. Effects of cyclooxygenase inhibition on pulmonary vascular responses to serotonin. *J. Appl. Physiol.* 1987, 62, 1192-1200.

HOLTZMAN M.J. Arachidonic acid metabolism. Implications of biological chemistry for lung function and disease. *Am. Rev. Respir. Dis.* 1991, 143, 188-203.

HUVAL W.M., MATHIESON M.A., STEMP L.L., DUNHAM B.M., JONES A.G., SHEPRO D., HECHTMAN H.B. Therapeutic benefits of 5-hydroxytryptamine inhibition following pulmonary embolism. *Ann. Surg.* 1983, 197, 220-225.

HUVAL W.V., LELCUK S., SHEPRO D., HECHTMAN H.D. Role of serotonin in patients with acute respiratory failure. *Ann. Surg.* 1984, 200, 166-172.

ICHINOSE M., BELVISI M.G., BARNES P.J. Bradykinin-induced bronchoconstriction in guinea-pig in vivo: role of neural mechanisms. *J. Pharmacol. Exp. Ther.* 1990, 253, 594-599.

IRVIN C.G., DEMPSEY J.A. Role of H_1 and H_2 receptors in increased small airways resistance in the dog. *Respir. Physiol.* 1978, 35, 161-176.

KAUFMAN M.P., COLERIDGE H.M., COLERIDGE J.C.G., BAKER D.G. Bradykinin stimulates afferent vagal C fibres in intrapulmonary airways of dogs. *J. Appl. Physiol.* 1980, 48, 511-517.

KAYE M.G., SMITH L.J. Effects of inhaled leukotriene D_4 and platelet-activating factor on airway reactivity in normal subjects. *Am. Rev. Respir. Dis.* 1990, 141, 993-997.

KIMMAN T.G., TERPSTRA G.K., DAHA M.R., WESTENBRINK F. Pathogenesis of naturally acquired bovine respiratory syncytial virus infection in calves: evidence for the involvement of complement and mast cell mediators. *Am. J. Vet. Res.* 1989, 50, 694-700.

KOTLIKOFF M.I., SLOCOMBE R.F., ROBINSON N.E. Influence of β-adrenergic antagonism on the response of bovine neonatal lungs to intravenous histamine. *Am. J. Vet. Res.* 1982, 43, 984-988.

LANTZ R.C., KELLER G.E., BURRELL R. The role of platelet-activating factor in the pulmonary response to inhaled bacterial endotoxin. *Am. J. Vet. Res.* 1991, 144, 167-172.

LAUWERYNS J.M., COKELAERE M., THEUNYNCK P. Serotonin producing neuroepithelial bodies in rabbit respiratory mucosa. *Science Wash* 1973, DC180, 410-413.

LEBLANC P.H., BAKER J.C., GRAY P.R., ROBINSON N.E., DERKSEN F.J. Effects of bovine respiratory syncytial virus on airway function in neonatal calves. *Am. J. Vet. Res.* 1991, 52, 1401-1406.

LEE S.L., LONG K., FANBURG B.L. Serotonin uptake by bovine pulmonary artery smooth muscle cells under normoxic and anoxic conditions. *Am. Rev. Respir. Dis.* 1987, 135, A101.

LEE T.H., CREA A.E.G., GANT V., SPUR B.W., MARRON B.E., NICOLAOU K.C., REARDON E., BREZINSKI M., SERHAN C.N. Identification of lipoxin A_4 and its relationship to the sulfidopeptide leukotrienes C_4, D_4, and E_4 in the bronchoalveolar lavage fluids obtained from patients with selected pulmonary diseases. *Am. Rev. Respir. Dis.* 1990, 141, 1453-1458.

LINDEN A., DESMECHT D., AMORY H., WYNANTS J., LEKEUX P. Comparison of 5-hydroxytryptamine concentration in the lungs of healthy and pneumonic calves. In Proceedings : 10th Comparative Respiratory Society Meeting, East Lansing, (U.S.A.), 1991, P-8.

LINDEN A.S., DESMECHT D.J.-M., AMORY H., ROLLIN F.A., MICHAUX C.L., LEKEUX P.M. Pulmonary response to intravenous administration of

5-hydroxytryptamine after type-2 receptor blockade in healthy calves. *Am. J. Vet. Res.* 1993, 54, 168-173..

MANN R., WOODSON L.C., TRABER L.D., HERNDON D.N., TRABER D.L. Role of bradykinin in ovine endotoxemia. *Circ. Shock* 1991, 34, 224-230.

MAROM Z., SHELHAMER J.H., BACH M.K., MORTON D.R., KALINER M. Slow-reacting substances, leukotrienes C_4 and D_4, increase the release of mucus from human airways in vitro. *Am. Rev. Respir. Dis.* 1982, 126, 449-451.

MATHE A.A., HEDQVIST P. Effect of prostaglandins $F_{2\alpha}$ and E_2 on airway conductance in healthy subjects and asthmatic patients. *Am. Rev. Respir. Dis.* 1975, 111, 313-320.

MONCADA S., VANE J.R. Pharmacology and endogenous roles of prostaglandin endoperoxides, thromboxane A_2, and prostacyclin. *Pharmacol. Rev.* 1979, 30, 293-331.

MOVAT H.Z. The role of histamine and others mediators in microvascular changes in acute inflammation. *Can. J. Physiol. Pharmacol.* 1987, 65, 451-457.

MUGRIDGE K.G., HIGGS G.A., MONCADA S. Prostacyclin modulates the response to leukotrienes C_4 and D_4 of guinea pig airway smooth muscle. *Eur. J. Pharmacol.* 1984, 104, 1-5.

NAKAHARA K., OHKUDA K., STRAUB N.C. Effect of infusing histamine into pulmonary or bronchial artery on sheep pulmonary fluid balance. *Am. Rev. Respir. Dis.* 1979, 120, 875-882.

NIEMINEN M.M., MOILANEN E.K., NYHOLM J.-E.J., KOSKINEN M.O., KARVONEN J.I., METSÄ-KETELÄ T.J., VAPAATALO H. Platelet-activating factor impairs mucociliary transport and increases plasma leukotriene B_4 in man. *Eur. Respir. J.* 1991, 4, 551-560.

NUYTTEN J., MUYLLE E., OYAERT W., VAN DEN HENDE C. The influence of clenbuterol on prostaglandin $F_{2\alpha}$-induced dyspnoea in calves. *Vet. Res. Commun.* 1986, 10, 453-461.

O'BYRNE P.M., AIZAWA H., BETHEL R.A., CHUNG K.F., NADEL J.A., HOLTZMAN M.J. Prostaglandin F_{2a} increases responsiveness of pulmonary airways in dogs. *Prostaglandins* 1984, 28, 537-543.

O'BYRNE P.M., LEIKAUF G.D., AIZAWA H., BETHEL R.A., UEKI I.F., HOLTZMAN M.J., NADEL J.A. Leukotriene B_4 causes airway hyperresponsiveness in dogs. *J. Appl. Physiol.* 1985, 59, 1941-1946.

O'FLAHERTY J.T. Platelet-activating factor: mechanism of cellular activation. In : *Platelet-activating Factor and related Lipid Mediators*, Snyder, F. (Ed.), Plenum Press, New York, 1987, pp 283-297.

OLSON N.C., ROBINSON N.E., SCOTT J.B. Effects of histamine on lung water and hemodynamics after β-blockade. *J. Appl. Physiol.: Respirat. Environ. Exercise Physiol.* 1983, 54, 967-971.

OLSON N.C. Role of 5-hydroxytryptamine in endotoxin-induced respiratory failure of pigs. *Am. Rev. Respir. Dis.* 1987, 135, 93-99.

OLSON N.C., SALZER W.L., McCALL C.E. Biochemical, physiological and clinical aspects of endotoxemia. *Molec. Aspects Med.* 1988, 10, 511-629.

OLSON N.C., KRUSE-ELLIOTT K.T., JOHNSON L. Effect of LY171883 on endotoxin-induced lung injury in pigs. *J. Appl. Physiol.* 1990, 69, 1315-1322.

OLSON N.C., DODAM J.R. Inflammatory mediators in the lung. In Proceedings : 10th Comparative Respiratory Society Meeting, East Lansing, USA, 1991, pp 1-17.

PEARL R.G., PRIELIPP R.C. Leukotriene synthesis inhibition and receptor blockade do not inhibit hypoxic pulmonary vasoconstriction in sheep. *Anesth. Analg.* 1991, 72, 169-176.

PROUD D., MAGLASHAN D.W., NEWBALL H.H., SCHULMANS A.,

LICHTENSTEIN L.M. Immunoglobulin E-mediated release of a kininogenase from purified human lung mast cells. *Am. Rev. Respir. Dis.* 1985, 132, 405-406.

REGOLI D., BARABE J. Pharmacology of bradykinin and related kinins. *Pharmacol. Rev.* 1980, 32, 1-46.

REGOLI D. Kinins. *Br. Med. Bull.* 1987, 43, 270-284.

ROBINSON C., HOLGATE S.T. Regulation by prostanoids. In : *The Lung: Scientific Foundations*, Vol. 1, Crystal R.G., West J.B. (Eds), Raven Press, New York, 1991, pp 941-951.

ROBINSON N.E. Le rôle du système nerveux autonome lors de l'obstruction des voies aériennes du cheval. *Ann. Méd. Vét.* 1993, 137, 153-159.

ROTH B.L., CHUANG D. Multiple mechanisms of serotonergic signal transduction. *Life Sci.* 1987, 41, 1051-1064.

RUBIN A.H., SMITH L.J., PATTERSON R. The bronchoconstrictor properties of platelet-activating factor in humans. *Am. Rev. Respir. Dis.* 1987, 136, 1145-1151.

SASAKI T., SHIMURA S., IKADA K., SASAKI H., TAKISHIMA H. Platelet-activating factor increases platelet-dependent glycoconjugate secretion from tracheal submucosal glands. *Am. J. Physiol.* 1989, 257, L373-L378.

SCHMIDT A.W., PEROUTKA S.J. 5-Hydroxytryptamine receptor "families". *FASEB J.* 1989, 3, 2242-2249.

SCOTT J.S., BROADSTONE R.V., DERKSEN F.J., ROBINSON N.E. β-Adrenergic blockade in ponies with recurrent obstructive pulmonary disease. *J. Appl. Physiol.* 1988, 64, 2324-2328.

SEEGER W., WALTER H., SUTTORP N., MUHLY M., BHAKDI S. Thromboxane-mediated hypertension and vascular leakage evoked by low doses of *Escherichia coli* hemolysin in rabbit lungs. *J. Clin. Invest.* 1989, 84, 220-227.

SELIG W.M., BLOOMQUIST M.A., COHEN M.L., FLEISCH J.H. Serotonin-induced pulmonary responses in the perfused guinea-pig lung; evidence for $5HT_2$ receptor-mediated pulmonary vascular and airway smooth muscle constriction. *Pulmonary Pharmacol.* 1988, 1, 93-99.

SHELHAMER J.H., MAROM Z., KALINER M. Immunologic and neuropharmacologic stimulation of mucous glycoprotein release from human airways in vitro. *J. Clin. Invest.* 1980, 66, 1400-1408.

SHELLER J.R., HOLZTMAN M.J., SKOOGH B.-E., NADEL J.A. Interaction of serotonin with vagal- and ACh-induced bronchoconstriction in canine lungs. *J. Appl. Physiol. : Respirat. Environ. Exercise Physiol.* 1982, 52, 964-966.

SIREK A., SIREK O.V. Serotonin: a review. *Can. Med. Ass. J.* 1970, 102, 846-849.

SLOCOMBE R.F., ROBINSON N.E. Histamine H_1, H_2 receptor effects on mechanics of ventilation and gas exchange in neonatal calves. *Am. J. Vet. Res.* 1981, 42, 764-769.

SLOCOMBE R.F., LATTER W., DERKSEN F.J., ROBINSON N.E. Pulmonary response of neonatal calves to intravenous and aerosol bradykinin. *Am. J. Vet. Res.* 1982, 43, 2023-2027.

SPANNHAKE E.W., LEVIN J.L., MELLION B.T., GRUETTER C.A., HYMAN A.L., KADOWITZ P.J. Reversal of 5-HT-induced bronchoconstriction by PGI_2: distribution of central and peripheral actions. *J. Appl. Physiol.* 1980, 49, 521-527.

SPENCER D.A., EVANS J.M., GREEN S.E., PIPER P.J., COSTELLO J.F. Participation of the cysteinyl leukotrienes in the acute bronchoconstrictor response to inhaled platelet activating factor in man. *Thorax* 1991, 46, 441-445.

STERANKA L.R., FARMER S.G., BURCH R.M. Antagonists of B_2 bradykinin receptors. *FASEB J.* 1989, 3, 2019-2025.

STRUM J.M., ITO T., PHILPOT R.M., DESANTI A.M., McDOWELL E.M. The immunocytochemical detection of cytochrome P-450 monooxygenase in the lungs of fetal, neonatal, and adult hamsters. *Am. J. Respir. Cell. Mol. Biol.* 1990, 2, 493-501.

TESSIER G.J., LACKNER P.A., O'GRADY S.M., KANNAN M.S. Modulation of equine tracheal smooth muscle contractility by epithelial-derived and cyclooxygenase metabolites. *Respir. Physiol.* 1991a, 84, 105-114.

TESSIER G.J., TRAYNOR T.R., KANNAN M.S., O'GRADY S.M. Mucosal histamine inhibits Na absorption and stimulates Cl secretion across equine tracheal epithelium. *Am. J. Physiol. (Lung Cell. Mol. Physiol. 5)* 1991b, 261, L456-L461.

TILL G.O., JOHNSON K.J., KUNKEL R., WARD P.A. Intravascular activation of complement and acute lung injury: dependency on neutrophils and toxic oxygen metabolities. *J. Clin. Invest.* 1982, 69, 1126-1135.

TOKUYAMA K., LOTVALL J.O., BARNES P.J., CHUNG K.F. Mechanism of airway narrowing caused by inhaled platelet-activating factor. *Am. Rev. Respir. Dis.* 1991, 143, 1345-1349.

VAN DE PUTTE-VAN MESSOM G., BURVENICH C. Contractility of bovine pulmonary artery: a preliminary study. *Arch. int. Physiol. Bioch.* 1989, 97, P45-P46.

VAN DE PUTTE-VAN MESSOM G., BURVENICH C. The effect of ketanserin on the 5-HT-induced pressor response in the isolated bovine pulmonary artery. *Arch. Int. Physiol. Bioch.* 1991, 99, P23.

VAN NUETEN J.M., LEYSEN J.E., VANHOUTTE P.M., JANSSENS P.A.J. Serotonergic responses in vascular and non-vascular tissues. *Arch. Int. Pharmocodyn. Thér.* 1982, 256, 331-334.

VINCENT J.-L., DEGAUTE J.-P., DOMB M., SIMON P., BERRE J., VANDESTEENE A. Ketanserin, a serotonin antagonist. Administration in patients with acute respiratory failure. *Chest* 1984, 85, 510-513.

WALTERS E.H., O'BYRNE P.M., FABBRI L.M., GRAF P.D., HOLTZMAN M.J., NADEL J.A. Control of neurotransmission by prostaglandins in canine trachealis muscle. *J. Appl. Physiol.* 1984, 57, 129-134.

WARD P.A., MORGANROTH M.L., SENIOR R.M., CAMPBELL E.J. Inflammatory mediators of pulmonary tissue injury. In : *Mediators of Pulmonary Inflammation*, Bray, M.A., Anderson W.H. (Eds), Marcel Dekker, Inc., New York, 1991, pp 533-591.

WASSERMAN M.A., DUCHARME D.W., WENDLING M.G., GRIFFIN R.L., DEGRAFF G.L. Bronchodilator effects of prostacyclin (PGI_2) in dogs and guinea pigs. *Eur. J. Pharmacol.* 1980, 66, 53-63.

WEBBER S.E., SALONEN R.O., WIDDICOMBE J.G. Receptors mediating the effects of 5-hydroxytryptamine on the tracheal vasculature and smooth muscle of sheep. *Br. J. Pharmacol.* 1990, 99, 21-26.

WHITE M.V., KALINER M.A. Regulation by histamine. In : *The Lung: Scientific Foundations*, Vol. 1, Crystal R.G., West J.B. (Eds), Raven Press, New York, 1991, pp 927-939.

CHAPTER IX

PRO-INFLAMMATORY CYTOKINES AND PULMONARY FUNCTION

P. Lekeux and A. Linden

Laboratory for Functional Investigation
Faculty of Veterinary Medicine
University of Liege

SUMMARY
This paper describes the role of pro-inflammatory cytokines in pulmonary physiology and physiopathology.

KEY WORDS
Respiratory system - Pulmonary function - Cytokines.

1. INTRODUCTION

The ability of the body to defend itself against a foreign invading agent depends on its ability to recognize the invader and to mount an organized offensive (Wewers and Gadek, 1991). The cytokines represent one aspect of this response. These substances are mediators which provide messages from cell to cell in order to induce and control the inflammatory reaction of the organism.

The effect of this response is mediated through antigen-stimulated T lymphocytes, which produce proteins that serve to activate various cell populations present in the inflammatory infiltrate (Fig. 9-1.). Some of these cells secrete in turn additional protein mediators that influence the reaction (Pober and Cotran, 1990). These lymphocyte- and mononuclear phagocyte-derived mediators were first called lymphokines and monokines, respectively. When it was discovered that other cells could also secrete similar mediators, these molecules were collectively renamed cytokines (Cohen, 1986).

These substances are secreted not only as part of the immune response to antigens, but also in response to other stimuli such as endotoxins.

The target cell for cytokines may be the cell of origin (i.e. autocrine action), nearby cells (i.e. paracrine action) or distant target cells in other organs (i.e. endocrine action).

Usually, a cytokine induces the secretion of another cytokine from the target cell and so on. This repeated sequence is described as the cytokine cascade. Furthermore, cytokines often modulate the actions of the other cytokines, which may have inhibitory, additive or synergistic interactions. This may result in additional effects not seen with individual cytokine (Pober and Cotran, 1990).

This paper will only focus on some proinflammatory cytokines which are suspected to interfere with the pulmonary function (Fig. 9-2.). However, the available information is still scarce. Other cytokines such as interferons (i.e. IFN-α, β and γ), antiinflammatory cytokines (i.e. interleukins 4 and 10, ...), mitogenic cytokines (i.e. platelet-derived growth factor, fibroblast growth

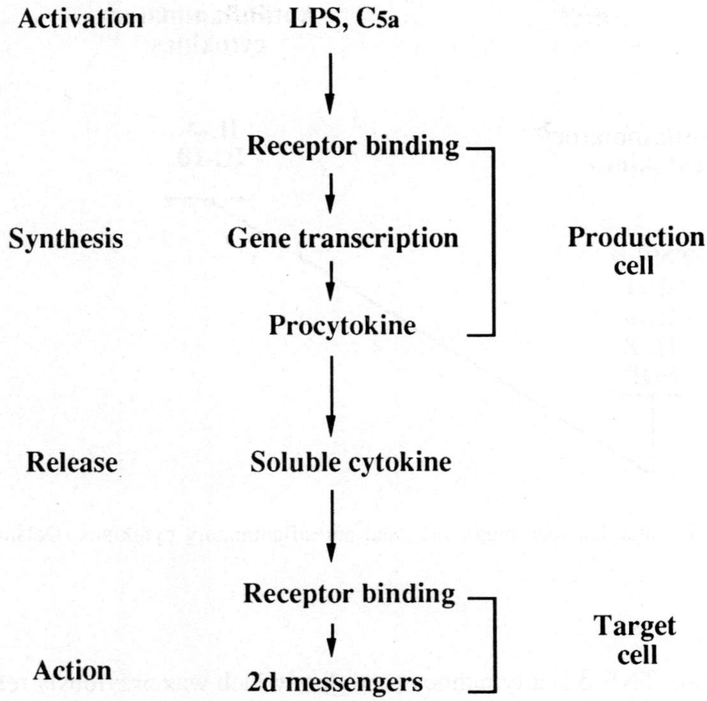

Fig. 9-1. General pathway of proinflammatory cytokine synthesis and action (Delannoy et al, 1993).

factors, insulin-like growth factor, transforming growth factor, epidermal growth factor, etc ...) and myeloid growth factors (i.e. colony-stimulating factors) are not analyzed here and have been reviewed in several textbooks (Demaeyer and Demaeyer-Guignard, 1988; Pastoret et al, 1990; Kelley, 1993).

2. TUMOR NECROSIS FACTOR (TNF)

TNF is a protein which is mainly produced by endotoxin-stimulated macrophages. In fact, TNF exists in two genetic forms. TNF-α is a macrophage product which is predominantly released in response to

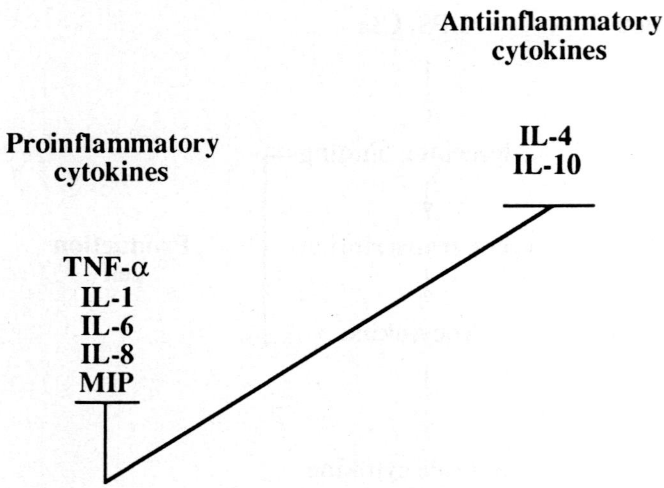

Fig. 9-2. Balance between major pro- and antiinflammatory cytokines (Delannoy et al, 1993).

endotoxin. TNF-β is a lymphocyte product which was previously referred to as lymphotoxin (Wewers and Gadek, 1991). Endothelial and vascular smooth muscle cells are also potential sites of TNF production in the lung (Warner and Libby, 1989).

TNF-α and β apparently share a common receptor which has been characterized on many normal and transformed cells (Aggarwal et al, 1985). The target cells in the lungs are neutrophils (Shalaby et al, 1985), lymphocytes (Yokota et al, 1988), macrophages (Oster et al, 1987), endothelial cells (Collins et al, 1986) and mesenchymal cells (Piguet et al, 1990).

The inhibition or the down-regulation of TNF can be either endogenous, i.e. via interleukin-4 (IL-4) (Essner et al, 1989), IL-6 (Kohase et al, 1986), transforming growth factor (Espevik et al, 1987) and prostaglandin E_2 (Kunkel et al, 1988), or pharmacologic, i.e. via glucocorticoids (Waage, 1987), cyclosporin (Remick et al, 1989) and pentoxifylline (Lilly et al, 1989).

TNF is a multifunctional cytokine which acts on multiple organs by means of direct effects on target cells and indirect effects mediated via TNF-induced secondary cytokines and other inflammatory mediators (Ulich, 1993).

TNF seems not to be expressed under physiological conditions, although a role for TNF has been postulated during normal tissue remodeling (Tracey et al, 1989).

TNF, probably together with IL-1, is considered to be an important mediator of local inflammation and septic shock observed for instance during endotoxemia (Tracey et al, 1987). TNF can also contribute to induce ischemia (Tracey et al, 1986), tumor necrosis (Nawroth and Stern, 1986), cachexia which justified its previous name, i.e. cachectin (Kawakami et al, 1982), and many other effects like fever, sleep, hyperalgesia, depressed cardiac contractility, etc ... (Beutler and Cerami, 1987).

At the level of the lung, the effects of TNF seem to be dose-dependent. Low TNF levels may play a benefical role as suggested by the generation of an appropriate inflammatory response to microorganisms like *Legionella pneumophila* (Blanchard et al, 1988) and by the improvement of the survival rate during hyperoxia, oxygen toxicity (White et al, 1987; Jensen et al, 1992) and infections such as listeriosis (Nakane et al, 1988).

Moderate TNF levels may participate in perpetuating some chronic inflammatory processes such as sarcoidosis (Bachwich et al, 1986).

High TNF levels may contribute to induce pulmonary dysfunctions and bronchial hyperresponsiveness observed during obstructive diseases (Kips et al, 1992) and may lead to acute lung injuries, shock or death observed during acute respiratory distress syndrome (Tracey et al, 1986; 1987). TNF is thus more potent than IL-1 under these circumstances. However, small doses of both cytokines are synergistic in producing lung injuries (Oksusawa et al, 1988).

In dogs, exogenous TNF, but not IL-1, induces acute pulmonary dysfunctions and lung injuries similar to bacterial shock (Fig. 9-3.) (Eichacker et al, 1991). These effects can be reversible or lethal, depending on the perfused dose.

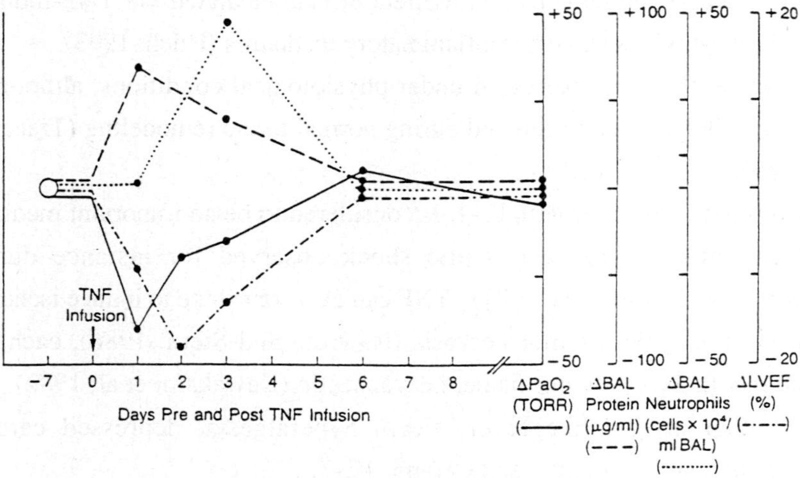

Fig. 9-3. Effect of tumor necrosis factor (TNF) perfusion on mean changes in arterial O_2 partial pressure (PaO_2), in protein and neutrophil concentration from bronchoalveolar lavage (BAL) and in left ventricular ejection fraction (LVEF) in dogs (Eichacker et al, 1991).

In pigs infected with *Pseudomonas aeruginosa*, TNF increases in the plasma during the septicemic phase and its activity correlates with the development of acute lung injury (Leeper-Woodford et al, 1991). These effects are attenuated but not supressed by anti-TNF monoclonal antibodies (Walsh et al, 1992), suggesting the occurrence of other mediators.

In sheep, sublethal doses of TNF induce severe abnormalities in lung mechanics, hemodynamics and gas exchange (Wheeler et al, 1990). These effects are diminished by cyclooxygenase inhibitor (Wheeler et al, 1992) and by platelet-activating factor antagonist (Horvath et al, 1991), which suggests that they are at least partly mediated via lipid mediators.

In horses, cytotoxic activity is detected in the plasma less than one hour after lipopolysaccharide infusion, suggesting that TNF could be an early mediator of the endotoxin-induced effects (McKay et al, 1991).

In cattle, TNF is released from alveolar macrophages stimulated with common

bovine respiratory viruses and bacterial endotoxins (Bienhoff et al, 1992).
In man, acute respiratory distress syndrome induces the presence of TNF in plasma (Romaschin et al, 1992) and in bronchoalveolar lavage fluids (Murch et al, 1992). However, other authors were not able to demonstrate an association between TNF and this syndrome (Parsons et al, 1992). This could be explained by the simultaneous occurrence of TNF inhibitors (Suter et al, 1992).
During lung injury, TNF seems to act mainly through smooth muscle contraction, increasing vascular permeability, neutrophils activation, expression for neutrophils of endothelial cell receptors and activation of other proinflammatory mediators (Wewers and Gadek, 1991).
It is thefore likely that TNF plays a major role in the orchestration of some acute and chronic inflammatory responses in the lung. However, some of the described dysfunctions and injuries are probably due to the indirect effects of TNF, which are mediated via many other cytokines and lipid mediators (Ulich, 1993). Therefore, the relative importance of TNF in the respiratory pathogenesis has to be individually assessed for each respiratory syndrome.

3. INTERLEUKIN 1 (IL-1)

IL-1 is a peptide that is produced by mononuclear phagocytes and by many other cell populations in response to inflammatory stimuli (Allison, 1985). This cytokine exists in two different genetic forms, i.e. IL-1α and IL-1β, which almost completely overlap in function (Rupp et al, 1986). The first one could be the membrane-bound form of IL-1 and the second one, the predominantly released form (Fuhlbrigge et al, 1988).
IL-1 receptors are expressed by many different cells. Binding of IL-1 to its receptor is specific : the particular receptor does not bind other cytokines and other cytokine receptors do not bind IL-1 (Dower et al, 1985). The number of receptors per cell varies considerabily but this does not correlate well with the sensitivity of the cell to IL-1 (Curtis et al, 1989). It appears that there are at least two types of IL-1 receptors and several levels of affinity (Aksamit and

Hunninghake, 1993).

IL-1 inhibitors of various nature and origin have been described : a glycoprotein isolated from the urine of normal subjects (Muchmore et al, 1987), a sequenced protein produced by several cell types (Aksamit and Hunninghake, 1993) and a protein produced by B cells (Giri et al, 1990). On the other hand, monoclonal antibodies (Gershenwald et al, 1990) and corticosteroids (Kern et al, 1988) may also act as IL-1 inhibitors.

The earliest recognized function of IL-1 was its ablity to cause fever which explains its first name, i.e. endogenous pyrogen (Merriman et al, 1977). This process occurs by increasing the synthesis of prostaglandin E_2 in the hypothalamus (Breder et al, 1988). Later, many other effects have been described at the metabolic, endothelial, neurological, hematological, rheumatological and immunological levels (Aksamit and Hunninghake, 1993).

In the healthy lung, IL-1 could play a role in the removal of senescent proteins and in the remodeling of normal tissue (Vlassara et al, 1988).

In the diseased lung, IL-1 seems to act as an important regulator of lung injury and repair and it may induce either favourable or unfavourable effects in both acute and chronic diseases.

In acute lung processes, low levels of IL-1 may enhance the survival rate to some infections (White et al, 1987), which could be explained by an enhanced protection against oxygen toxicity (Tsan et al, 1991).

In chronic lung processes, IL-1 may favorably enhance the production of collagenase and prostaglandin E_2 by the fibroblasts (Dayer et al, 1986).

On the other hand, large amounts of intravenous IL-1 are able to produce an acute respiratory distress syndrome in rabbits (Goldblum et al, 1987) and the use of a recombinant IL-1 antagonist was able to reduce the letality and severity of endotoxinic shock (Ohlsson et al, 1990) and *E. Coli*-induced shock (Wakabayashi et al, 1991). This could be explained by the fact that IL-1 can induce adherence of the neutrophils to endothelial cells (Bevilacqua et al, 1985).

In chronic lung diseases, IL-1 may also partly initiate and maintain the granulomatous inflammation that is typical of some syndromes such as sarcoidosis (Thomas and Hunninghake, 1987).

Its role in the induction of bronchial hyperreactivity has also been suggested (Hernandez et al, 1991)

It is therefore likely that regulated amounts of IL-1 are required for appropriate lung function, host inflammatory reaction and lung tissue repair. However, unregulated large amounts of IL-1 may contribute to pulmonary dysfunctions and injuries in some circumstances. Nevertheless, these effects must not be generalized and the interactions with other mediators have to be taken into account.

4. INTERLEUKIN 2 (IL-2)

IL-2 is a protein product of T-lymphocytes and acts primarily on lymphocytes (Smith, 1988). The regulation of its receptor density seems to occur in a reciprocal fashion that controls T-lymphocyte proliferation (Wewers and Gadek, 1991).

IL-2 has been used during cancer immunotherapy (Rosenberg et al, 1985) because it increases the activity of natural killer cells against selected tumor types (Robinson, 1989). High doses of IL-2 result in pulmonary toxicosis (Farrell, 1992). This effect seems to be mediated through platelet-activating factor (Rabinovici et al, 1992), but could also be explained by the fact that IL-2 may induce the expression of IL-1 (Numerof et al, 1988) and TNF (Mier et al, 1988) by macrophages.

5. INTERLEUKIN 6 (IL-6)

IL-6 is a phosphoglycoprotein produced by many different cells (Ray et al, 1989) by a broad spectrum of stimuli, including viral infection, bacterial endotoxin, agonists of cAMP and other cytokines such as IL-1 and TNF (Ulich, 1993). It is down-regulated by transforming growth factor, glucocorticoids and retinoids (Elias et al, 1991).

IL-6 is likely to play an important role in the pathogenesis of inflammatory lung disorders, as suggested by its potent ability to induce acute phase proteins (Gauldie et al, 1987) and by its presence during severe septic shock (Waage et al, 1989) and interstitial lung disease (Jones et al, 1991). However, many investigations remain to be done to clarify its role in the normal and diseased lung.

6. INTERLEUKIN 8 (IL-8)

IL-8 is a peptide produced by monocytes, alveolar macrophages, endothelial cells, epithelial cells and fibroblasts (Strieter et al, 1993).

It is a potent chemotactic factor for neutrophils which are stimulated to move in a directional fashion, to release oxydants and to degranulate (Wewers and Gadek, 1991).

IL-8 is best elicited by endotoxin and other cytokines such as IL-1 and TNF (Strieter et al, 1989), and could be responsible for the neutrophil accumulation observed during these challenges (Maestrelli et al, 1988) and during clinical sepsis (Hack et al, 1992).

7. MACROPHAGE INFLAMMATORY PROTEINS (MIP)

MIP-1 and MIP-2 are polypeptides secreted by macrophages in response to inflammatory stimuli (Sherry and Cerami, 1991). They appear to contribute, at least in part, to the host responses to infection, neoplastic invasion and tissue injury.

These cytokines seem to act primarily as chemoattractants, activating agents and mitogenic cofactors for neutrophils, fibroblasts and macrophages (Wolpe et al, 1987). They are able to induce fever in a prostaglandin-independent way (Davatelis et al, 1989) and could also enhance the release of superoxyde anion and the degranulation of adherent inflammatory cells during pulmonary diseases (Sherry and Cerami, 1993).

8. CONCLUSIONS

It is too early to conclude that exogenous modulation of some proinflammatory cytokines could help to control some animal pulmonary disorders. However, it has already been established that some of these mediators play a crucial role in lung inflammation and are associated with dysfunctions and injuries. The availability of specific antagonists or antibodies should contribute to a better understanding of the physiological and pathophysiological roles of these substances and to determine the opportunity of their modulation during pathological processes.

REFERENCES

AGGARWAL B.B., EESSALU T.E., HASS P.E. Characterization of receptors for human tumour necrosis factor and their regulation by γ-interferon. *Nature* 1985, 318, 665-667.

AKSAMIT T.R., HUNNINGHAKE G.W. Interleukin-1. In : *Lung Biology in Health and Disease. Cytokines of the Lung*, Kelley, J. (Ed.), Marcel Dekker, Inc., New York, 1993, pp 185-228.

ALLISON A.C. The interleukin-1 family of molecules. *BioEssays* 1985, 3, 260-263.

BACHWICH P.R., LYNCH J.P., LARRICK J., SPENGLER M., KUNKEL S.L. Tumor necrosis factor production by human sarcoid alveolar macrophages. *Am. J. Pathol.* 1986, 125, 421-425.

BEUTLER B., CERAMI A. Cachectin: more than a tumor necrosis factor. *N. Engl. J. Med.* 1987, 316, 379-385.

BEVILACQUA M.P., POBER J.S., WHEELER M.E., COTRAN R.S., GIMBRONE M.A. Jr. Interleukin-1 acts on cultured human vascular endothelium to increase the adhesion of polymorphonuclear leukocytes, monocytes, and related leukocyte cell lines. *J. Clin. Invest.* 1985, 76, 2003-2011.

BIENHOFF S.E., ALLEN G.K., BERG J.N. Release of tumor necrosis factor-α from bovine alveolar macrophages stimulated with bovine respiratory viruses and bacterial endotoxins. *Vet. Immunol. Immunopathol.* 1992, 30, 341-357.

BLANCHARD D.K., DJEU J.Y., KLEIN T.W., FRIEDMAN H., STEWART W.E. Protective effects of TNF in experimental *Legionella pneumophila* infections of mice via activation of PMN function. *J. Leukocyte Biol.* 1988, 43, 429-435.

BREDER C.D., DINARELLO C.A., SAPER C.B. Interleukin-1 immunoreactive innervation of the human hypothalamus. *Science* 1988, 240, 321-324.

COHEN S. Physiologic and pathologic manifestations of lymphokine action. *Hum. Pathol.* 1986, 17, 112-121.

COLLINS T., LAPIERRE L., FIERS W., STROMINGER J.L., POBER J.S. Recombinant human TNF increases mRNA levels and surface expression of HLA-A,B antigens in vascular endothelial cells and dermal fibroblasts in vitro. *Proc. Natl. Acad. Sci. USA* 1986, 83, 446-450.

CURTIS B.M., GALLIS B., OVERELL R.W., McMAHAN C.J., deROOS P., IRELAND R., EISEMAN J., DOWER S.K., SIMS J.E. T-cell interleukin 1 receptor cDNA expressed in Chinese hamster ovary cells regulates functional responses to interleukin-1. *Proc. Natl. Acad. Sci. USA* 1989, 89, 3045-3049.

DAVATELIS G., WOLPE S.D., SHERRY B., DAYER J.-M., CHICHEPORTICHE R., CERAMI A. Macrophage inflammatory protein-1: a prostaglandin-independent endogenous pyrogen. *Science* 1989, 243, 1066-1068.

DAYER J.-M., de ROCHEMONTEIX B., BURRUS B., DEMCZUK S., DINARELLO C.A. Human recombinant interleukin-1 stimulates collagenase and prostaglandin E_2 production by human synovial cells. *J. Clin. Invest.* 1986, 77, 645-648.

DELANNOY I., MIOSSEC P., LEKEUX P. Potentialités de modulation de la réaction inflammatoire. *Ann. Méd. Vét* 1993, 137, 163-194.

DEMAEYER E., DEMAEYER-GUIGNARD J. Interferons and other regulatory cytokines, Wiley (Ed.), New York, 1988.

DOWER S.K., KRONHEIM S.R., MARCH C.J., COLON P.J., HOPP T.P., GILLIS S., URDAL D.L. Detection and characterization of high affinity plasma membrane receptors for human interleukin-1. *J. Exp. Med.* 1985, 162, 501-515.

EICHACKER P.Q., HOFFMAN W.D., FARESE A., BANKS S.M., KUO G.C., McVITTIE T.J., NATANSON C. TNF but not IL-1 in dogs causes lethal lung injury and multiple organ dysfunction similar to human sepsis. *J. Appl. Physiol.* 1991, 71, 1979-1989.

ELIAS J.A., LENTZ V., CUMMINGS P. Transforming growth factor-β regulation of IL-6 production by unstimulated and IL-1 stimulated human fibroblasts. *J. Immunol.* 1991, 146, 3437-3443.

ESPEVIK T., FIGARI I.S., SHALABY M.R., LACKIDES G.A., LEWIS G.D., SHEPARD H.M., PALLADINO M.A. Inhibition of cytokine production by cyclosporin A and TGFβ. *J. Exp. Med.* 1987, 166, 571-576.

ESSNER R., RHOADES K. McBRIDE W.H., MORTON D.L., ECONOMOU J.S. IL-4 downregulates IL-1 and TNF gene expression in human monocytes. *J. Immunol.* 1989, 142, 3857-3861.

FARRELL M.M. The challenge of adult respiratory distress syndrome during interleukin-2 immunotherapy. *Oncol. Nurs. Forum* 1992, 19, 475-480.

FUHLBRIGGE R.C., FINE S.M., UNANUE E.R., CHAPLIN D.D. Expression of membrane interleukin-1 by fibroblasts transfected with murine pro-interleukin 1 α cDNA. *Proc. Natl. Acad. Sci. USA* 1988, 85, 5649-5653.

GAULDIE J., RICHARDS C., HARNISH D., LANDSDORP P., BAUMANN H. Interferon β2/BSF-2 shared identity with monocyte-derived hepatocyte stimulating factor (HSF) and regulates the major acute phase protein responses in liver cells. *Proc. Natl. Acad. Sci. USA* 1987, 84, 7251-7255.

GERSHENWALD J.E., FONG Y., FAHEY T.J., CALVANO S.E., CHIZZONITE R., KILIAN P.L., LOWRY S.F., MOLDAWER L.L. Interleukin-1 receptor blockade attenuates the host inflammatory response. *Proc. Natl. Acad. Sci. USA* 1990, 87, 4966-4970.

GIRI J.G., NEWTON R.C., HORUK R. Identification of soluble interleukin-1 binding protein in cell-free supernants. Evidence for soluble interleukin-1 receptor. *J. Biol. Chem.* 1990, 265, 17416-17419.

GOLDBLUM S.E., JAY M., YONEDA K., COHEN D.A., McCLAIN C.J., GILLESPIE M.N. Monokine-induced acute lung injury in rabbits. *J. Appl. Physiol.* 1987, 63, 2093-2100.

HACK C.E., HART M., VAN SCHIJNDEL R.J., EERENBERG A.J., NUIJENS J.H., THIJS L.G., AARDEN L.A. Interleukin-8 in sepsis: relation to shock and inflammatory mediators. *Infect. Immun.* 1992, 60, 2835-2842.

HERNANDEZ A., OMINI C., DAFFONCHIO L. Interleukin-1 β: a possible mediator of lung inflammation and airway hyperreactivity. *Pharmacol. Res.* 1991, 24, 385-393.

HORVATH C.J., KAPLAN J.E., MALIK A.B. Role of platelet-activating factor in mediating tumor necrosis factor α-induced pulmonary vasoconstriction and plasma-lymph protein transport. *Am. Rev. Respir. Dis.* 1991, 144, 1337-1341.

JENSEN J.C., POGREBNIAK H.W., PASS H.I., BURESH C., MERINO M.J., KAUFFMAN D., VENZON D., LANGSTEIN H.N., NORTON J.A. Role of tumor necrosis factor in oxygen toxicity. *J. Appl. Physiol.* 1992, 72, 1902-1907.

JONES K.P., REYNOLDS S.P., CAPPER S.J., KALINKA S., EDWARDS J.H., DAVIES B.H. Measurement of interleukin-6 in bronchoalveolar lavage fluid by radioimmunoassay: differences between patients with interstitial lung disease and control subjects. *Clin. Exp. Immunol.* 1991, 83, 30-34.

KAWAKAMI M., PEKALA P.H., LANE M.D., CERAMI A. Lipoprotein lipase suppression in 3T3-L1 cells by an endotoxin-induced mediator from exudate cells. *Proc. Natl Acad. Sci. USA* 1982, 79, 912-916.

KELLEY J. Transforming growth factor-β. In: *Lung Biology in Health and Disease. Cytokines of the Lung*, Kelley, J. (Ed.), Marcel Dekker, Inc., New York, 1993, pp 101-137.

KERN J.A., LAMB R.J., REED J.C., DANIELE R.P., NOWELL P.C. Dexamethasone inhibition of interleukin-1 β production by human monocytes: posttranscriptional mechanisms. *J. Clin. Invest.* 1988, 81, 237-244.

KIPS J.C., TAVERNIER J., PAUWELS R.A. Tumor necrosis factor causes bronchial hyperresponsiveness in rats. *Am. Rev. Respir. Dis.* 1992, 145, 332-336.

KOHASE M., HENRIKSEN-DESTEFANO D., MAY L.T., VILCEK J., SEHGAL P.B. Induction of β_2-interferon by TNF: a homeostatic mechanism in the control of cell proliferation. *Cell* 1986, 45, 659-666.

KUNKEL S.L., SPENGLER M., MAY M.A., SPENGLER R., LARRICK J., REMICK D.G. PGE_2 regulates macrophage-derived TNF gene expression. *J. Biol. Chem.* 1988, 263, 5380-5384.

LEEPER-WOODFORD S.K., CAREY P.D., BYRNE K., JENKINS J.K., FISHER B.J., BLOCHER C., SUGERMAN H.J., FOWLER III A.A. Tumor necrosis factor α and β subtypes appear in circulation during onset of sepsis-induced lung injury. *Am. Rev. Respir. Dis.* 1991, 143, 1076-1082.

LILLY C.M., SANDHU J.S., ISHIZAKA A., HARADA H., YONEMARU M., LARRICK J.W., SHI T.X., O'HANLEY P.T., RAFFIN T.A. Pentoxifylline prevents TNF-induced lung injury. *Am. Rev. Respir. Dis.* 1989, 139, 1361-1368.

MAESTRELLI P., TSAI J.-J., CROMWELL O., KAY A.B. The identification and partial characterization of a human mononuclear cell-derived neutrophil chemotactic factor apparently distinct from IL-1, IL-2, GM-CSF, TNF and IFN-γ. *Immunology* 1988, 64, 219-225.

McKAY R.J., MERRITT A.M., ZERTUCHE J.-M., WHITTINGTON M., SKELLEY L.A. Tumor necrosis factor activity in the circulation of horses given endotoxin. *Am. J. Vet. Res.* 1991, 52, 533-538.

MERRIMAN C.R., PULLIAM L.A., KAMPSCHMIDT R.F. Comparison of leukocyte pyrogen and leukocytic endogenous mediator (39642). *Proc. Soc. Exp. Biol. Med.* 1977, 154, 224-227.

MIER J.W., VACHINO G. VAN DER MEER J.W., NUMEROF R.P., ADAMS S., CANNON J.G., BERNHEIM H.A., ATKINS M.B., PARKINSON D.R., DINARELLO C.A. Induction of circulating tumor necrosis factor (TNF α) as the mechanism for the febrile response to interleukin-2 (IL-2) in cancer patients. *J. Clin. Immunol.* 1988, 8, 426-436.

MUCHMORE A.V., SHIFRIN S., DECKER J.M. *In vitro* evidence that carbohydrate derived from uromodulin, an 85,000 dalton immunosuppressive glycoprotein isolated from human pregnancy urine, are immunosuppressive in the absence of intact proteine.

J. Immunol. 1987, 138, 2547-2553.
MURCH S.H., MACDONALD T.T., WOOD C.B., COSTELOE K.L. Tumour necrosis factor in the bronchoalveolar secretions of infants with the respiratory distress syndrome and the effect of dexamethasone treatment. *Thorax* 1992, 47, 44-47.
NAKANE A., MINAGAWA T., KATO K. Endogenous tumor necrosis factor (cachectin) is essential to host resistance against *Listeria monocytogenes* infection. *Infect. Immun.* 1988, 56, 2563-2569.
NAWROTH P.P., STERN D.M. Modulation of endothelial cell hemostatic properties by tumor necrosis factor. *J. Exp. Med.* 1986, 163, 740-745.
NUMEROF R.P., ARONSON F.R., MIER J.W. IL-2 stimulates the production of IL-1 α and IL-1 β by human peripheral blood mononuclear cells. *J. Immunol.* 1988, 141, 4250-4257.
OHLSSON K., BJORK P., BERGENFELDT M., HAGEMAN R., THOMPSON R.C. Interleukin-1 antagonist reduces mortality from endotoxin shock. *Nature* 1990, 348, 550-552.
OKSUSAWA S., GELFAND J.A., IKEJIMA T., CONNOLLY R.J., DINARELLO C.A. Interleukin-1 induces a shock-like state in rabbits: synergism with tumor necrosis factor and the effect of cyclooxygenase inhibition. *J. Clin. Invest.* 1988, 81, 1162-1172.
OSTER W., LINDEMANN A., HORN S., MERTELSMANN R., HERRMANN F. TNFα but not TFNβ induces secretion of colony stimulating factor for macrophages (CSF-1) by human monocytes. *Blood* 1987, 70, 1700-1703.
PARSONS P.E., MOORE F.A., MOORE E.E., IKLE D.N., HENSON P.M., WORTHEN G.S. Studies on the role of tumor necrosis factor in adult respiratory distress syndrome. *Am. Rev. Respir. Dis.* 1992, 146, 694-700.
PASTORET P.-P., GOVAERTS A., BAZIN H. Immunologie Animale, Médecine-Sciences, Flammarion, 1990.
PIGUET P.F., COLLART M.A., GRAU G.E., SAPPINO A.P., VASSALLI P. Requirement of TNF for development of silica-induced pulmonary fibrosis. *Nature* 1990, 344, 245-247.
POBER J.S., COTRAN R.S. Cytokines and endothelial cell biology. *Physiol. Rev.* 1990, 70, 427-451.
RABINOVICI R., SOFRONSKI M.D., RENZ J.F., HILLEGAS L.M., ESSER K.M., VERNICK J., FEUERSTEIN G. Platelet activating factor mediates interleukin-2-induced lung injury in the rat. *J. Clin. Invest.* 1992, 89, 1669-1673.
RAY A., TATTER S.B., SANTHANAM U., HALFGOTT D.C., MAY L.T., SEHGAL P.B. Regulation of expression of interleukin-6. Molecular and clinical studies. *Ann. N.Y. Acad. Sci.* 1989, 557, 353-362.
REMICK D.G., NGUYEN D.T., ESKANDERI M.K., STRIETER R.M., KUNKEL S.L. Cyclosporin inhibits TNF production without decreasing TNF mRNA levels. *Biochem. Biophys. Res. Commun.* 1989, 161, 551-555.
ROBINSON B.W.S. Asbestos and cancer: human natural killer cell activity is suppressed by asbestos fibers but can be restored by recombinant interleukin-2. *Am. Rev. Respir. Dis.* 1989, 139, 897-901.
ROMASCHIN A.D., DEMAJO W.C., WINTON T., D'COSTA M., CHANG G., RUBIN B., GAMLIEL Z., WALKER P.M. Systemic phospholipase A_2 and cachectin levels in adult respiratory syndrome and multiple-organ failure. *Clin. Biochem.* 1992, 25, 55-60.
ROSENBERG S.A., LOTZE M.T., MUUL L.M., LEITMAN S., CHANG A.E., ETTINGHAUSSEN S.E., MATORY Y.L., SKIBBER J.M., SHILONI E., VETTO J.T. Observations on the systemic administration of autologous lymphokine-activated killer cells and recombinant interleukin-2 to patients with metastatic cancer. *N. Engl. J. Med.* 1985, 313, 1485-1492.

RUPP E.A., CAMERON P.M., RANAWAT C.S., SCHMIDT J.A., BAYNE E.K. Specific bioactivities of monocyte-derived interleukin-1 α and interleukin β are similar to each other on cultured murine thymocytes and on cultured human connective tissue cells. *J. Clin. Invest.* 1986, 78, 836-839.

SHALABY M., AGGARWAL B., RINDERKNECHT E., SVEDERSKY L.P., FINKLE B.S., PALLADINO M.A. Activation of human PMN functions by IFNγ and TNF. *J. Immunol.* 1985, 135, 2069-2073.

SHERRY B., CERAMI A. Small cytokine superfamily. *Curr. Opin. Immunol.* 1991, 3, 56-60.

SHERRY B., CERAMI A. Macrophage inflammatory protein-1. In : *Lung Biology in Health and Disease. Cytokines of the Lung*, Kelley, J. (Ed.), Marcel Dekker, Inc., New York, 1993, pp 369-380.

SMITH K.A. Interleukin-2: inception, impact, and implications. *Science* 1988, 2409, 1169-1176.

STRIETER R.M., KUNKEL S.L., SHOWELL H.J., REMICK D.G., PHAN S.H., WARD P.A., MARKS R.M. Endothelial cell gene expression of a neutrophil chemotactic factor by TNF α, LPS, and IL-1 β. *Science* 1989, 243, 1467-1469.

STRIETER R.M., STANDIFORD T.J., ROLFE M.W., KUNKEL S.L. Interleukin-8. In : *Lung Biology in Health and Disease. Cytokines of the Lung*, Kelley, J. (Ed.), Marcel Dekker, Inc., New York, 1993, pp 281-305.

SUTER P.M., SUTER S., GIRARDIN E., ROUX-LOMBARD P., GRAU G.E., DAYER J.-M. High bronchoalveolar levels of tumor necrosis factor and its inhibitors, interleukin-1, interferon, and elastase, in patients with adult respiratory distress syndrome after trauma, shock, or sepsis. *Am. Rev. Respir. Dis.* 1992, 145, 1016-1022.

THOMAS P.D., HUNNINGHAKE G.W. Current concepts of the pathogenesis of sarcoidosis. *Am. Rev. Respir. Dis.* 1987, 135, 747-760.

TRACEY K.J., BEUTLER B., LOWRY S.F., MERRYWEATHER J., WOLPE S., MILSARK I.W., HARIRI R.J., FAHEY III T.J., ZENTELLA A., ALBERT J.D., SHIRES G.B., CERAMI A. Shock and tissue injury induced by recombinant human cachectin. *Science* 1986, 234, 470-474.

TRACEY K.J., FONG Y., HESSE D.G., MANOGUE K.R., LEE A.T., KUO G.C., LOWRY S.F., CERAMI A. Anticachectin/TNF monoclonal antibodies prevent septic shock during lethal bacteriemia. *Nature* 1987, 330, 662-664.

TRACEY K.J., VLASSARA H., CERAMI A. Cachectin/TNF. *Lancet* 1989, 1, 1122-1126.

TSAN M.F., LAWRENCE D., WHITE J.E. Erythrocyte insufflation-induced protection against oxygen toxicity: role of cytokines. *J. Appl. Physiol.* 1991, 71, 1751-1757.

ULICH T.R. Tumor necrosis factor. In : *Lung Biology in Health and Disease. Cytokines of the Lung*, Kelley, J. (Ed.), Marcel Dekker, Inc., New York, 1993, pp 307-332.

VLASSARA H., BROWNLEE M., MANOGUE K.R., DINARELLO C.A., PASAGIAN A. Cachectin/TNF and IL-1 induced by glucose-modified proteins: role in normal tissue remodeling. *Science* 1988, 240, 1546-1548.

WAAGE A. Production and clearance of TNF in rats exposed to endotoxin and dexamethasone. *Clin. Immunol. Immunopathol.* 1987, 45, 348-355.

WAAGE A., BRANTZAEG P., HALSTENSEN A., KIERULF P., ESPEVIK T. The complex pattern of cytokines in serum from patients with meningococcal septic shock. *J. Exp. Med.* 1989, 169, 333-338.

WAKABAYASHI W., GELFAND J.A., BURKE J.F., THOMPSON R.C., DINARELLO C.A. A specific receptor antagonist for interleukin-1 prevents *Escherichia coli*-induced shock in rabbits. *FASEB J.* 1991, 5, 388-343.

WALSH C.J., SUGERMAN H.J., MULLEN P.G., CAREY P.D., LEEPER-WOODFORD

S.K., JESMOK G.J., ELLIS E.F., FOWLER A.A. Monoclonal antibody to tumor necrosis factor α attenuates cardiopulmonary dysfunction in porcine gram-negative sepsis. *Arch. Surg.* 1992, 127, 138-144.

WARNER S.J.C., LIBBY P. Human vascular smooth muscle cells. Target for and source of TNF. *J. Immunol.* 1989, 142, 100-109.

WEWERS M.D., GADEK J.E. Proinflammatory polypeptides. In : *The Lung: Scientific Foundations*, Vol. 1, Crystal, R.G., West, J.B. (Eds), Raven Press, New York, 1991, pp 91-103.

WHEELER A.P., JESMOK G., BRIGHAM K.L. Tumor necrosis factor's effects on lung mechanics, gas exchange and airway reactivity in sheep. *J. Appl. Physiol.* 1990, 68, 2542-2549.

WHEELER A.P., HARDIE W.D., BERNARD G.R. The role of cyclooxygenase products in lung injury induced by tumor necrosis factor in sheep. *Am. Rev. Respir. Dis.* 1992, 145, 632-639.

WHITE C.W., GHEZZI P., DINARELLO C.A., CALDWELL S.A., McMURTRY I.F., REPINE J.E. Recombinant tumor necrosis factor/cachectin and interleukin-1 pretreatment decreases lung oxidized glutathione accumulation, lung injury, and mortality in rats exposed to hyperoxia. *J. Clin. Invest.* 1987, 79, 1868-1873.

WOLPE S.D., DAVATELIS G., SHERRY B., BEUTLER B., HESSE D.G., NGUYEN G.T., MOLDAWER L.L., NATHAN C.F., LOWRY S.F., CERAMI A. Macrophages secrete a novel heparin-binding protein with inflammatory and neutrophil chemokinetic properties. *J. Exp. Med.* 1987, 80, 300-306.

YOKOTA S., GEPPERT T.D., LIPSKY P.E. Enhancement of antigen and mitogen-induced human T lymphocyte proliferation by TNF. *J. Immunol.* 1988, 140, 531-536.

CHAPTER X

NEUROPEPTIDES AND RELATED SUBSTANCES IN THE PULMONARY FUNCTION

P. Lekeux and D. Desmecht

Laboratory for Functional Investigation
Faculty of Veterinary Medicine
University of Liege

SUMMARY

This paper describes the role of the neuropeptides and related substances, such as endothelins and nitric oxide, in the respiratory physiology and physiopathology.

KEY WORDS

Respiratory system - Pulmonary function - Neuropeptides - Endothelins - Nitric oxide.

1. INTRODUCTION

Several peptides released from sensory and autonomic neurons have been identified in the respiratory system. Although their precise physiological roles are not yet known, their effects on airway caliber, bronchial and pulmonary blood flow and airway secretion suggest that these substances could be involved in the physiological regulation of the pulmonary function and in the pathogenesis of dysfunctions.

The purpose of this paper is to analyse the available information about the implication of the neuropeptides in physiological, pathophysiological and therapeutical pulmonary processes. Other substances such as endothelins, which are not released by neurons, and nitric oxide, which is not a peptide, show functional similarities with the neuropeptides in the lung and are also described in this paper.

2. GENERAL CLASSIFICATION

Several systems may be provided for classifying the pulmonary neuropeptides.

According to their origin, neuropeptides can be released in the respiratory system from parasympathetic neurons such as vasoactive intestinal peptide (VIP) and VIP-related peptides, from sympathetic neurons such as neuropeptide Y, and from sensory neurons such as tachykinins and calcitonin gene-related peptide (CGRP).

According to the nervous pathway in which they are supposed to act as neurotransmitter, VIP and nitric oxide (NO) are suspected to mediate the inhibitory nonadrenergic noncholinergic (NANC) pathway, while the tachykinins are suspected to mediate the excitatory-NANC pathway.

According to their action on smooth muscle, endothelin (ET) and CGRP induce a long-lasting contraction and relaxation of the smooth muscle, respectively. Substance P (SP) and NO induce a short-lasting contraction and relaxation of the smooth muscle, respectively.

In addition, pulmonary neuropeptides may also be classified according to their

major sites of action, their mechanisms of action, their power of action, the availability of specific antagonists, etc... (Barnes et al, 1991a).
Table 10-1. summarizes several effects of neuropeptides and related substances on the pulmonary function.

3. VASOACTIVE INTESTINAL PEPTIDE (VIP)

VIP was first isolated from the porcine duodenum (Said and Mutt, 1969) and later from several types of nerves in the respiratory system and in other tissues of different animal species (Barnes et al, 1991a). Immunocytochemic techniques show that VIP-ergic innervation supplies airway and vascular smooth muscles and airway submucosal glands (Dey et al, 1981; Palmer et al, 1985). This innervation is particularly rich at the level of the nasal mucosa and the large airways but decreases toward the bronchioles (Uddman and Sundler, 1979). VIP-immunoreactivity is also present in the autonomic ganglia located along the large airways (Barnes, 1987).
The binding of VIP to its receptors in lung tissues stimulates the production of cyclic AMP through adenylyl cyclase activation (Frandsen et al, 1978). The distribution of VIP receptors seems to be similar in the different species investigated (Lazarus et al, 1986) and is correlated with the distribution of VIP-ergic nerve fibers, except at the level of the alveolar walls where a high density of VIP binding sites is present. Because the VIP is metabolized by the pulmonary capillary endothelium, the alveolar wall receptors could contribute to the uptake of VIP from the circulation.
In vitro, VIP relaxes the airway smooth muscle independently of adrenergic stimulation (Said, 1982). VIP is considered as the most potent endogenous bronchodilator and could contribute to the regulation of large airway tonus (Palmer et al, 1986a). Indeed, these effects are proportional to the airway caliber. They are more important at the level of large than small airways (Carstairs and Barnes, 1986).
In vivo, intravenous administration of VIP induces a severe bronchoconstriction in the cat (Diamond et al, 1983) but not in human beings

Table 10-1. Functional effects of neuropeptides and related substances in the lung (Barnes et al, 1991a).

Peptides	Airway smooth muscle tonus	Vascular smooth muscle tonus	Mucus secretion
VIP	↘↘	↘↘	↗
SP	↗	↘	↗↗
NKA	↗↗	↘	↗
CGRP	↗	↘	↗
NPY	↗	↗↗	↗↗
GRP	↗↗	↗↗	↗↗
CCK	↗↗	-	-
ET	↗↗	↗↗	-
NO	↘↘	↘↘	-

See text for keys.

(Palmer et al, 1986b). Aerosolized VIP protects against histamine-induced bronchoconstriction in cats and dogs (Said, 1982) but not in men (Barnes et al, 1984). This lack of effect in men could be explained by the presence of proteolytic enzymes at the surface of the airway mucosa or by the fact that this mucosa could present a barrier to diffusion (Barnes et al, 1991a).

At the level of pulmonary vessels, VIP induces an important vasodilation which is independent of endothelial cells (Greenberg et al, 1985). The VIP receptors are dense at the level of vascular smooth muscle, which confirms the hypothesis that VIP could act directly, i.e. without an endothelium-released relaxing factor (Barnes et al, 1986b). VIP could therefore contribute to the regulation of pulmonary blood flow.

At the level of bronchial vessels, VIP induces also a vasodilation (Laitinen et al, 1987) and could influence the airway vascular bed. Its vascular effects are more potent on tracheal than on bronchial vessels (Matran et al, 1989).

At the level of nasal vessels, VIP is a powerful vasodilator and may contribute

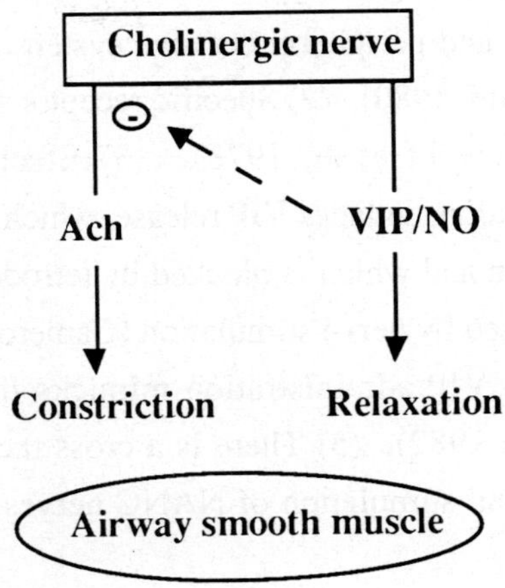

Fig. 10-1. Potential role of vasoactive intestinal peptide (VIP) and nitric oxide (NO) as functional antagonists of cholinergic bronchoconstriction. Ach : Acetylcholine (Barnes et al, 1991a).

to nasal congestion (Lung and Widdicombe, 1987).

Airway secretions are also largely increased by VIP. Mucus glands are more stimulated than serous glands. The resulting VIP-induced hypersecretion is therefore rich in mucous glycoproteins (Lazarus et al, 1986). VIP could also influence the mucociliar clearance as it stimulates the transport of chloride ions and thus increases the water secretion (Nathanson et al, 1983).

At the level of parasympathetic ganglia, VIP could modulate the cholinergic neurotransmission (Fig. 10-1.), which could explain its inhibitory effect on neurally-induced bronchoconstriction (Ellis and Farmer, 1989). On the other hand, VIP coexists with acethylcholine in some cholinergic nerves and could be released after excessive cholinergic stimulation, inducing a functional antagonism (Lundberg, 1981).

At the level of the mast cells, VIP inhibits the release of mediators. This could partly explain its antiinflammatory activity (Undem et al, 1983).

VIP is considered as one of the potential neurotransmitter of the inhibitory-

NANC pathway. This is strongly suggested by several observations. (1) VIP is present in the central and peripheral nervous system, including the nerves within lung (Dey and Said, 1980). (2) Specific receptor for VIP are present in nervous tissues (Robberecht et al, 1978). (3) Electrical stimulation of tracheobronchial preparations induces VIP release, which is proportional to the magnitude of stimulation and which is blocked by tetrodotoxine, proving that this phenomenon is caused by nerve stimulation (Cameron et al, 1983). (4) In several animal species, VIP administration mimicks the effects of NANC nerve stimulation (Said, 1982). (5) There is a cross tachyphylaxia between administration of VIP and stimulation of NANC nerves (Venugopalan et al, 1988).

On the other hand, there is some evidence against the role of VIP as a neurotransmitter of the NANC pathway. The pretreatment of guinea-pig trachea with very high VIP dosages does not inhibit the NANC relaxation (Karlsson et al, 1984). This could be explained by the presence of another neurotransmitter or by the fact that exogenous VIP does not reach all VIP receptors. Furthermore, VIP does not seem to be the inhibitory NANC neurotransmitter in porcine and feline tracheal smooth muscle (Kannan and Johnson, 1992; Fisher et al, 1993).

The availability of potent and specific VIP antagonists should help to clarify the role of this neuropeptide in the NANC pathway.

VIP has also been incriminated in several respiratory disorders. Its insufficient release by nerves (Howarth et al, 1990) or its excessive degradation by mast cell tryptases (Caughey et al, 1988) could be responsible for excessive smooth muscle tonus, airway hyperreactivity or excessive hypoxic vasoconstriction (Venugopalan, 1989). On the other hand, VIP could play a deleterious role in congestive rhinitis (Kurian et al, 1983). In domestic animals, the contribution of the VIP-ergic innervation in pulmonary dysfunctions remains to be investigated further.

4. VIP-RELATED PEPTIDES

Peptide histidine isoleucine (PHI) and peptide histidine methionine (PHM) have a structural similarity with VIP, are encoded by the same gene and are synthetized via the same prohormone (Lundberg et al, 1984a; Richardson and Webber, 1987).

These neuropeptides seem to have a quite similar distribution and similar physiological effects, although PHI is less potent than VIP as a bronchial vasodilator and more potent as a secretion stimulator (Laitinen et al, 1987; Webber, 1988).

Pituitary adenylate cyclase activating peptide (PACAP), which has marked homology with VIP, is also present in the peripheral nervous system and its receptors are dense in lung tissues (Gottschall et al, 1990).

Other VIP-related peptides include peptide histidine valine (Chilvers et al, 1988) and helodermin (Foda et al, 1990).

5. SUBSTANCE P (SP) AND OTHER TACHYKININS

SP and structurally-related peptides, i.e. neurokinin A (NKA) and neurokinin B (NKB), have been identified in the mammalian nervous system and have been called tachykinins because of their quick spasmogenic action (Nawa et al, 1983).

SP is localized to neurons in the airways of many species (Lundberg et al, 1984b). Nerve fibers containing SP are found in the airway epithelium, around blood vessels and in the airway smooth muscle (Barnes et al, 1991a). SP is mainly located in capsaicin-sensitive unmyelinated nerves in the airway. It is mainly synthetized in the vagal ganglia and transported down the vagus to the lung tissues. The location of the other tachykinins seems to be similar (Hua et al, 1985).

The SP receptors are present in high density at the level of the smooth muscle of large and small aiways and, in a lower density, at the level of pulmonary vascular smooth muscles, epithelial cells and submucosal glands (Carstairs and Barnes, 1986). SP, NKA and NKB seem to be the specific agonists of

NK1, NK2 and NK3 receptors, respectively (Lee et al, 1986).

In vitro, tachykinins contract the airway smooth muscle in many species (Karlsson et al, 1984). They are suspected to be the neurotransmitters of the excitatory NANC pathway (Barnes, 1989). NKA is much more potent than SP, suggesting that NK2 receptors are involved in the bronchomotor tonus regulation (Advenier et al, 1987). This is confirmed by the use of specific NK2 agonists (Naline et al, 1989) and antagonists (Maggi et al, 1990). On the other hand, tachykinins potentiate cholinergic neurotransmission at parasympathetic ganglia (Undem et al, 1991) and at postganglionic nerve terminals (Hall et al, 1989) and inhibit the NANC airway relaxation (Stretton et al, 1990).

In vivo, intravenous administration of SP induces a severe bronchospasm in many laboratory animals (Andersson and Persson, 1977) but not in human beings (Fuller et al, 1987). On the other hand, NKA, but not SP, causes bronchoconstriction when given intravenously or by inhalation in asthmatic human beings (Joos et al, 1987; Evans et al, 1988). This constriction seems to be mediated indirectly, because it can be inhibited by pretreatment with cromolyn sodium (Joos et al, 1989).

The effects of tachykinins depend largely on the integrity of the airway epithelium. In fact, an intact epithelium attenuates the bronchoconstrictor effects of these substances, probably because the airway epithelium is the major site of tachykinin metabolism (Frossard et al, 1989). Furthermore, some epithelium-derived relaxant factors may be simultaneously released (Vanhoutte, 1988). Therefore, disease-induced epithelial damages could enhance the tachykinin-induced bronchoconstriction and be partly responsible for the airway hyperresponsiveness. This has been suspected in horses suffering from chronic obstructive pulmonary disease (Sonea and Bowker, 1991b) but remains to be demonstrated.

An important increase in microvascular leakage is observed after intravenous and inhaled SP and after vagus nerve stimulation (Evans et al, 1989; Lötvall et al, 1990). This effect is prevented by pretreatment with NK1 receptor antagonists (Lundberg et al, 1983).

Tachykinins have also important effects on the airway vascular bed. SP and NKA substantially increase the tracheal blood flow in dog and pig (Laitinen et al, 1987). This could be the major physiological effect of the tachykinins.

SP is one of the most potent stimulator of airway mucus secretion (Coles et al, 1984). NK1 receptors are present in high density in airway secretory cells (Rogers et al, 1989). SP also increases the mucociliar clearance by stimulating ion transport in the airway epithelium (Rangachari and McWade, 1985).

Tachykinins have several effects on inflammatory cells. They may degranulate some types of mast cells (Lowman et al, 1988) and eosinophils (Kroegel et al, 1990) and activate monocytes to release inflammatory cytokines (Lotz et al, 1988). This could amplify the inflammatory processes during respiratory disorders and justify a potential inhibition of tachykinin release by specific antagonists.

6. CALCITONIN GENE-RELATED PEPTIDE (CGRP)

CGRP is expressed in sensory neurons under two forms (a and b) (Noguchi et al, 1990). This neuropeptide is colocalized with tachykinins in sensory nerves and is abundant in the respiratory tract (Uddman and Sundler, 1987).

Specific surface CGRP receptors are mainly located in bronchial vessels and airway epithelium (Lundberg et al, 1985). Few CGRP receptors are found in the airway smooth muscle and the airway submucosal glands (Martling et al, 1988).

CGRP is an effective dilator of pulmonary and bronchial vessels, and the resulting increase in blood flow is long-lasting (Salonen et al, 1988; McCormack et al, 1989). CGRP could be the predominant mediator of arterial vasodilation in response to airway sensory nerve stimulation, for instance during airway inflammation (Barnes et al, 1991b). On the other hand, in contrast to SP, CGRP does not affect the airway microvascular leakage (Rogers et al, 1988).

CGRP has little effect on the airway smooth muscle and the constriction

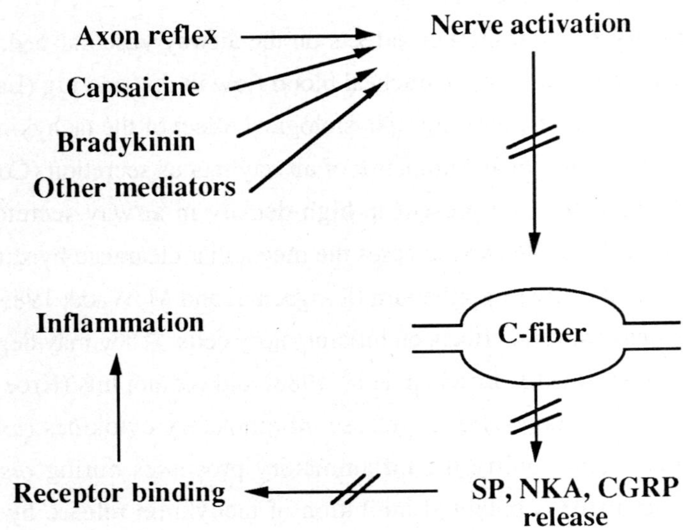

Fig. 10-2. Pathway of neurogenic inflammation. // indicates the potential sites of inhibition.

induced by CGRP could be mediated by other mediators (Palmer et al, 1987). Tachykinins and CGRP have been incriminated in neurogenic inflammation, i.e. antidromic release of neuropeptides from C fibers via an axon reflex (Fig. 10-2.). This could occur during airway diseases (Barnes, 1986a). Therefore, the modulation of neurogenic inflammation has been proposed as a potential treatment of inflammatory airway diseases (Barnes et al, 1990). This modulation could be obtained by several ways : (1) inhibition of sensory neuropeptide effects by specific tachykinin and CGRP receptor antagonists (Snider et al, 1991); (2) inhibition of sensory neuropeptide release by opioids (Belvisi et al, 1988) or GABA (Belvisi et al, 1989); (3) inhibition of sensory nerve activation by local anesthetics (Hirshman et al, 1982), by cromolyn or nedocromil sodium (Verleden et al, 1991) or by inhaled furosemide (Nichol et al, 1990); (4) enhancement of the neutral endopeptidase activity, which is responsible for the clearance of the sensory neuropeptides, by inhaled corticosteroids (Borson et al, 1991), and (5) sensory denervation by local application of capsaicin which depletes sensory neuropeptides (Geppetti et al, 1988).

7. NEUROPEPTIDE Y (NPY)

NPY is mainly a cotransmitter with norepinephrine in adrenergic nerves and is predominantly localized to airway vessels and glands (Sheppard et al, 1984). NPY immunoreactive nerves were also associated with large airway smooth muscle in horses (Sonea and Bowker, 1991a).

NPY is a potent vasoconstrictor in airway vascular beds, acting mainly at the level of resistance arterioles (Salonen et al, 1988). This could contribute to reduce microvascular leakage (Boschetto et al, 1989).

At the level of airway smooth muscle, NPY indirectly induces a bronchoconstriction via the release of prostaglandins (Cadieux et al, 1989). It has also a modulatory effect on cholinergic (Stretton and Barnes, 1988) and excitatory-NANC pathways (Matran et al, 1989).

8. GASTRIN RELEASING PEPTIDE (GRP) AND BOMBESIN-LIKE PEPTIDES

GRP is the mammalian form of bombesin and is localized to neuroendocrine cells in the lower airways (Miller, 1990).

These peptides could play an important role in lung maturation (Spindel et al, 1987). On the other hand, they are able to induce an indirect bronchoconstriction in guinea pigs (Belvisi et al, 1991), a tracheal vasoconstriction in dogs (Salonen et al, 1988) and an airway hypersecretion in cats (Lundgren et al, 1990).

9. CHOLECYSTOKININ (CCK)

CCK is present at low concentration in animal airways (Ghatei et al, 1982). It is binding with specific receptors on airway smooth muscle, causing heavy bronchoconstriction in guinea pigs and human beings (Stretton and Barnes, 1989).

10. SOMATOSTATIN

Somatostatin is present at low concentration in some lung afferent nerves (Holzer, 1988) and seems to potentiate the airway cholinergic neurotransmission (Sekizawa et al, 1989).

11. GALANIN

Galanin appears to be widely distributed in the pulmonary nerves. It is colocalized with VIP in cholinergic nerves (Dey et al, 1990) and with tachykinins and CGRP in sensory nerves (Guiliani et al, 1989). However, no direct functional effect has been described in the lung until now.

12. ENKEPHALINS

Enkephalins are localized to airway neuroendocrine cells (Cutz, 1982) but their functional roles are not yet clarified.

13. NEUROTENSIN

Neurotensin has not been localized to the lung until now, but it might facilitate the airway cholinergic nerve stimulation (Aas and Helle, 1982).

14. ENDOTHELINS (ETS)

ETs are local peptides generated *de novo* by endothelial or epithelial cells in response to various stimuli (Yanagisawa et al, 1988). At least three distinct isoforms of ET and two distinct subtypes of specific receptors have been described until now (Sakurai et al, 1992).

At the vascular level, ETs are the most potent vasoconstrictors described up to now. Their direct long-acting action occur in both arterial and venous smooth muscles (Haynes and Webb, 1992), although the ovine pulmonary veins exhibit greater sensitivity to ET than arteries (Toga et al, 1992). Furthermore,

ET potentiates the vasoconstrictor action of the sympathetic nervous system (Yang et al, 1990). On the other hand, ET3 may cause the release of endothelium-derived relaxing factors, such as prostacyclin and nitric oxide (Warner et al, 1989).

Excessive release of ETs, with or without insufficient release of relaxing factors, is suspected to play a role in pulmonary hypertension (Haynes and Webb, 1992).

At the bronchial level, ET is synthetized by epithelial cells (Black et al, 1989). When given by aerosol, ET induces a potent long-lasting bronchoconstriction (Lagente et al, 1989). This bronchoconstriction could result from a direct effect of ET on specific receptors of bronchial smooth muscle (McKay et al, 1991) or from an indirect effect mediated either by the activation of calcium channels (Grunstein et al, 1991), or by the release of prostaglandins and thromboxanes (Dyson and Kadowitz, 1991). ET also stimulates the production of bronchial chemoattractants for leucocytes (Springall et al, 1991). The increased amount of ET in the bronchial epithelium and in bronchoalveolar lavage fluid during asthmatic bronchoconstriction suggests that this mediator could play a role in some obstructive pulmonary diseases (Nomura et al, 1989).

15. NITRIC OXIDE (NO)

NO is a simple gas which is formed from the amino acid L-arginin by several NO synthases (Palmer et al, 1988). NO seems to play a significant role at the level of the nervous system, the immune system and the inflammatory cells (Snyder, 1992). More important might be its function as physiological mediator of smooth muscle relaxation. Indeed, NO has been recently identified as the endothelium-derived relaxing factor described since many years (Moncada et al, 1988).

At the vascular level, NO is responsible for a short-lasting relaxation by stimulating the formation of cGMP through activation of guanylyl cyclase (Snyder, 1992). NO could balance, together with prostacyclins, the constrictor effects of ETs (Haynes and Webb, 1992).

Inhaled NO is to be able to reverse hypoxic pulmonary vasoconstriction (Frostell et al, 1991), thromboxane-induced vasoconstriction (Rimar and Gillis, 1992) and naturally occurring pulmonary hypertension (Pepke-Zaba et al, 1991). This is promising for the potential use of NO as a therapeutical agent.

At the bronchial level, NO is considered as an unconventional neurotransmitter of the inhibitory NANC pathway (Sanders and Ward, 1992). Indeed, NO is strongly suspected to be the endogenous neurotransmitter of bronchodilator nerves in human beings (Belvisi et al, 1992), guinea pig (Jansen et al, 1992), pig (Kannan and Johnson, 1992) and cat (Fisher et al, 1993). However, it is not yet clear whether NO acts alone or together with other substances such as VIP or other NO-containing molecules.

16. CONCLUSIONS

The discovery of the release of neuropeptides and related substances in the mammalian lung is too recent to provide an integrated analysis of their roles in the pulmonary function and dysfunction. The occurrence of so many mediators and so complex interactions between them complicates the interpretation of experiment. However, if we arrive to better understand the physiological and pathophysiological actions of these compounds, new therapeutical strategies could be developed in order to significantly improve the treatment of several respiratory disorders.

REFERENCES

AAS P., HELLE K.B. Neurotensin receptors in rat bronchi. *Regul. Pept.* 1982, 3, 405-413.

ADVENIER C., NALINE E., DRAPEAU G., REGOLI D. Relative potencies of neurokinins in guinea pig trachea and human bronchus. *Eur. J. Pharmacol.* 1987, 139, 133-137.

ANDERSSON P., PERSSON H. Effect of substance P on pulmonary resistance and dynamic pulmonary compliance in the anesthetized cat and guinea pig. *Acta Pharmacol.*

Toxicol. 1977, 41, 444-448.
BARNES P.J., DIXON C.M.S. The effect of inhaled vasoactive intestinal peptide on bronchial reactivity to histamine in humans. *Am. Rev. Respir. Dis.* 1984, 130, 162-166.
BARNES P.J. Asthma as an axon reflex. *Lancet* 1986a, 1, 242-245.
BARNES P.J. Neural control of human airways in health and disease. *Am. Rev. Respir. Dis.* 1986b, 134, 1289-1314.
BARNES P.J. Neuropeptides in the lung: localization, function, and pathophysiologic implications. *J. Allergy Clin. Immunol.* 1987, 79, 285-295.
BARNES P.J. Airway neuropeptides: roles in fine tuning and in disease. *NIPS* 1989, 4, 116-120.
BARNES P.J., BELVISI M.G., ROGERS D.F. Modulation of neurogenic inflammation: novel approaches to inflammatory diseases. *Trends Pharmacol. Sci.* 1990, 11, 185-189.
BARNES P.J., BARANIUK J.N., BELVISI M.G. Neuropeptides in the respiratory tract. Part I. *Am. Rev. Respir. Dis.* 1991a, 144, 1187-1198.
BARNES P.J., BARANIUK J.N., BELVISI M.G. Neuropeptides in the respiratory tract. Part II. *Am. Rev. Respir. Dis.* 1991b, 144, 1391-1399.
BELVISI M.G., CHUNG K.F., JACKSON D.M., BARNES P.J. Opioid modulation of non-cholinergic neural bronchoconstriction in guinea pig in vivo. *Br. J. Pharmacol.* 1988, 95, 413-418.
BELVISI M.G., ICHINOSE M., BARNES P.J. Modulation of non-adrenergic non-cholinergic neural bronchoconstriction in guinea-pig airways via GABA receptors. *Br. J. Pharmacol.* 1989, 97, 1125-1131.
BELVISI M.G., STRETTON C.D., BARNES P.J. Bombesin-induced bronchoconstriction in the guinea pig: mode of action. *J. Pharmacol. Exp. Ther.* 1991, 255, 36-41.
BELVISI M.G., STRETTON C.D., YACOUB M., BARNES P.J. Nitric oxide is the endogenous neurotransmitter of bronchodilator nerves in humans. *Eur. J. Pharmacol.* 1992, 210, 221-222.
BLACK P.N., GHATEI M.A., TAKAHASHI K., BRETHERTON-WATT D., KRAUSZ T., DOLLERY C.T. Formation of endothelin by cultured airway epithelial cells. *FEBS Lett.* 1989, 255, 129-132.
BORSON D.B., JEW S., GRUENERT D.C. Glucocorticoids induce neutral endopeptidase in transformed human trachea epithelial cells. *Am. J. Physiol.* 1991, 260, L83-L89.
BOSCHETTO P., ROBERTS N.M., ROGERS D.F., BARNES P.J. The effect of antiasthma drugs on microvascular leak in guinea pig airways. *Am. Rev. Respir. Dis.* 1989, 139, 416-421.
CADIEUX A., BENCHEKROUN M.T., St. PIERRE S., FOURNIER A. Bronchoconstrictive action of neuropeptide Y (NPY) on isolated guinea pig airways. *Neuropeptides* 1989, 13, 215-219.
CAMERON A.R., JOHNSTON C.D., KIRKPATRICK C.T., KIRKPATRICK M.C.A. The quest for the inhibitory neurotransmitter in bovine tracheal smooth muscle. *Q. J. Exp. Psychol.* 1983, 68, 413-426.
CARSTAIRS J.R., BARNES P.J. Autoradiographic mapping of substance P receptors in lung. *Eur. J. Pharmacol.* 1986, 127, 295-296.
CAUGHEY G.H., LEIDIG F., VIRO N.F., NADEL J.A. Substance P and vasoactive intestinal peptide degradation by mast cell tryptase and chymase. *J. Pharmacol. Exp. Ther.* 1988, 244, 133-137.
CHILVERS E.R., DIXON C.M.S., YIANGOU Y., BLOOM S.R., IND P.W. Effect of peptide histidine valine on cardiovascular and respiratory function in normal subjects. *Thorax* 1988, 43, 750-755.
COLES S.J., NEILL K.H., REID L.M. Potent stimulation of glycoprotein secretion in

canine trachea by substance P. *J. Appl. Physiol.* 1984, 57, 1323-1327.
CUTZ E. Neuroendocrine cells of the lung - an overview of morphological characteristics and development. *Exp. Lung Res.* 1982, 3, 185-208.
DEY R.D., SAID D.I. Immunochemical localization of VIP-immunoreactive nerves in bronchial walls and pulmonary vessels. *Fed. Proc. Am. Soc. Exp. Biol.* 1980, 39, 1062.
DEY R.D., SHANNON W.A., SAID D.I. Localization of VIP-immunoreactive nerves in airways and pulmonary vessels of dogs, cats and human subjects. *Cell Tissue Res.* 1981, 220, 231-238.
DEY R.D., MITCHELL H.W., COBURN R.F. Organization and development of peptide-containing neurons in the airways. *Am. J. Respir. Cell. Mol. Biol.* 1990, 3, 187-188.
DIAMOND L., SZAREK J.L., GILLESPIE M.N., ALTIERE R.J. *In vivo* bronchodilatory activity of vasoactive intestinal peptide in cat. *Am. Rev. Respir. Dis.* 1983, 128, 827-832.
DYSON M.C., KADOWITZ P.J. Analysis of responses to endothelins 1, 2, and 3 and sarafotoxin 6b in airways of the cat. *J. Appl. Physiol.* 1991, 71, 243-251.
ELLIS J.L., FARMER S.G. Modulation of cholinergic neurotransmission by vasoactive intestinal peptide and peptide histidine isoleucine in guinea pig tracheal smooth muscle. *Pulm. Pharmacol.* 1989, 2, 107-112.
EVANS T.W., DIXON C.M., CLARKE B., CONRADSON T.B., BARNES P.J. Comparison of neurokinin A and substance P on cardiovascular and airway function in man. *Br J. Pharmacol.* 1988, 25, 273-275.
EVANS T.W., ROGERS D.F., AURSUDKIJ B., CHUNG K.F., BARNES P.J. Regional and time-dependent effects of inflammatory mediators on airway microvascular permeability in guinea pigs. *Clin. Sci.* 1989, 76, 479-485.
FISHER J.T., ANDERSON J.W., WALDRON M.A. Nonadrenergic noncholinergic neurotransmitter of feline trachealis: VIP or nitric oxide ? *J. Appl. Physiol.* 1993, 74, 31-39.
FODA H.D., HIGUCHI J., SAID S.I. Helodermin, a VIP-like peptide, is a potent long-acting pulmonary vasodilator (abstract). *Am. Rev. Respir. Dis.* 1990, 141, A486.
FRANDSEN E.K., KRISHINA G.A., SAID S.I. Vasoactive intestinal polypeptide promotes cyclic adenosine 3',5' monophosphate accumulation in guinea pig trachea. *Br. J. Pharmacol.* 1978, 62, 367-369.
FROSSARD N., RHODEN K.J., BARNES P.J. Influence of epithelium on guinea pig airway responses to tachykinins: role of endopeptidase and cyclooxygenase. *J. Pharmacol. Exp. Ther.* 1989, 248, 292-298.
FROSTELL C., FRATACCI M.D., WAIN J.C., JONES R., ZAPOL W.M. Inhaled nitric oxide. A selective pulmonary vasodilator reversing hypoxic pulmonary vasoconstriction. *Circulation* 1991, 83, 2038-2047.
FULLER R.W., MAXWELL D.L., DIXON C.M.S., McGREGOR G.P., BARNES V.F., BLOOM S.R., BARNES P.J. Effects of substance P on cardiovascular and respiratory function in human subjects. *J. Appl. Physiol.* 1987, 62, 1473-1479.
GEPPETTI P., FUSCO B.M., MARABINI S., MAGGI C.A., FANIULLACCI M., SICUTERI F. Secretion, pain, and sneezing with and without allergic rhinitis. *Br. J. Pharmacol.* 1988, 93, 509-514.
GHATEI M.A., SHEPPARD M., O'SHAUNESSY D.J., ADRIAN T.E., McGREGOR G.P., POLAK J.M., BLOOM S.R. Regulatory peptides in the mammalian respiratory tract. *Endocrinology* 1982, 111, 1248-1254.
GOTTSCHALL P.E., TATSUMO I., MIYATA A., ARIMURA A. Characterization and distribution of binding sites for the hypothalamic peptide pituitary adenylate cyclase activating polypeptide. *Endocrinology* 1990, 127, 272-277.

GREENBERG B., ROHDEN K., BARNES P.J. Characteristics of VIP and PHI relaxation of bovine and human pulmonary artery. *Thorax* 1985, 40, 715-716.

GRUNSTEIN M.M., CHUANG S.T., SCHRAMM C.M., PAWLOWSKI N.A. Role of endothelin 1 in regulating rabbit airway contractility. *Am. J. Physiol.* 1991, 260, L75.

GUILIANI S., AMANN R., PAPINI A.M., MAGGI C.A., MELI A. Modulatory action of galanin on responses due to antidromic activation of peripheral terminals of capsaicin sensitive sensory nerves. *Eur. J. Pharmacol.* 1989, 163, 91-96.

HALL A.K., BARNES P.J., MELDRUM L.A., MACLAGAN J. Facilitation of tachykinins of neurotransmission in guinea-pig pulmonary parasympathetic nerves. *Br. J. Pharmacol.* 1989, 97, 274-280.

HAYNES W.G., WEBB D.J. Endothelin: a long-acting local constrictor hormone. *Br. J. Hosp. Med.* 1992, 47, 340-349.

HIRSHMAN C.A., EDELSTEIN G., PEFTZ S., WAYNE R., DOWNES H. Mechanism of action of inhalational anesthesia on airways. *Anesthesiology* 1982, 56, 107-111.

HOLZER P. Local effect or functions of capsaicin-sensitive sensory nerve endings: involvement of tachykinins, calcitonin gene related peptide and other neuropeptides. *Neuroscience* 1988, 24, 739-768.

HOWARTH P.H., BRITTEN K.M., DJUKANOVIC R.J., WILSON J.W., HOLGATE S.T., SPRINGALL D.R., POLAK J.M. Neuropeptide containing nerves in human airways in vivo: a comparative study of atopic asthma, atopic non-asthma and non-atopic non-asthma (abstract). *Thorax* 1990, 45, 786-787.

HUA X.-Y., THODORSSON-NERHEIM E., BRODIN E., LUNDBERG J.M., HOKFELT T. Multiple tachykinins (neurokinin A, neuropeptide K and substance P) in capsaicin-sensitive sensory neurons in the guinea-pig. *Regul. Pept.* 1985, 13, 1-19.

JANSEN A., DRAZEN J., OSBORNE J.A., BROWN R., LOSÇALZO J., STAMLER J.S. The relaxant properties in guinea pig airways of S-nitrosothiols. *J. Pharmacol. Exp. Ther.* 1992, 261, 154-160.

JOOS G., PAUWELS R., VAN DER STRAETEN M.E. Effect of inhaled substance P and neurokinin A in the airways of normal and asthmatic subjects. *Thorax* 1987, 42, 779-783.

JOOS G.F., PAUWELS R.A., VAN DER STRAETEN M.E. Effect of nedocromil sodium on the bronchoconstrictor effect of neurokinin A in subject with asthma. *J. Allergy Clin. Immunol.* 1989, 83, 663-668.

KANNAN M.S., JOHNSON D.E. Nitric oxide mediates the neural nonadrenergic, noncholinergic relaxation of pig tracheal smooth muscle. *Am. J. Physiol.* 1992, 262, L511-L514.

KARLSSON J.-A., FINNEY M.J.B., PERSSON C.G.A., POST C. Substance P antagonist and the role of tachykinins in non cholinergic bronchoconstriction. *Life Sci.* 1984, 35, 2681-2691.

KROEGEL C., GIEMBYCZ M.A., BARNES P.J. Characterization of eosinophil activation by peptides. Differential effects of substance P, melittin, and f-Met-Leu-Phe. *J. Immunol.* 1990, 145, 2581-2587.

KURIAN S.S., BLANK M.A., SHEPPARD M.N. Vasoactive intestinal polypeptide (VIP) in vasomotor rhinitis. *IRCS Med. Sci.* 1983, 11, 425-426.

LAGENTE V., CHABRIER P.E., MENCIA-HUERTA J.M., BRAQUET P. Pharmacological modulation of the bronchopulmonary action of the vasoactive peptide, endothelin, administered by aerosol in the guinea-pig. *Biochem. Biophys. Res. Commun.* 1989, 158, 625-632.

LAITINEN L.A., LAITINEN A., SALONEN R.O., WIDDICOMBE J.G. Vascular actions of airway neuropeptides. *Am. Rev. Respir. Dis.* 1987, 136 (Suppl), 59-64.

LAZARUS S.C., BASBAUM C.B., BARNES P.J., GOLD W.M. Cyclic AMP

immunocytochemistry provides evidence for functional VIP receptors in trachea. *Am. J. Physiol.* 1986, 61, 1322-1328.
LEE C.-M., CAMPBELL N.J., WILLIAMS B.J., IVERSEN L.L. Multiple tachykinin binding sites in peripheral tissues and in brain. *Eur. J. Pharmacol.* 1986, 130, 209-217.
LÖTVALL J.O., LEMEN R.J., HUI K.P., BARNES P.J., CHUNG K.F. Airflow obstruction after substance P aerosol: contribution of airway and pulmonary edema. *J. Appl. Physiol.* 1990, 69, 1473-1478.
LOTZ M., VAUGHN J.H., CARSON D.M. Effect of neuropeptides on production of inflammatory cytokines by human monocytes. *Science* 1988, 241, 1218-1221.
LOWMAN M.A., BENYON R.C., CHURCH M.K. Characterization of neuropeptide-induced histamine release from human dispersed skin mast cells. *Br. J. Pharmacol.* 1988, 95, 131-130.
LUNDBERG J.M. Evidence for coexistence of vasoactive intestinal polypeptide (VIP) and acetylcholine in neurons of cat exocrine glands. Morphological, biochemical and functional studies. *Acta Physiol. Scand.* 1981, 112, 1-57.
LUNDBERG J.M., SARIA A., BRODIN E., ROSELL S., FOLKERS K. A substance P antagonist inhibits vagally induced increase in vascular permeability and bronchial smooth muscle contraction in the guinea-pig. *Proc. Natl. Acad. Sci. USA* 1983, 80, 1120-1124.
LUNDBERG J.M., FAHRENBERG J., HOKFELT T. Coexistence of peptide HI (PHI) and VIP in nerves regulating blood flow and bronchial smooth muscle in various animals, including human. *Peptides* 1984a, 5, 593-606.
LUNDBERG J.M., HOKFELT T., MARTLING C.-R., SARIA A., CUELLO C. Substance P-immunoreactive sensory nerves in the lower respiratory tract of various mammals including man. *Cell Tissue Res.* 1984b, 235, 251-261.
LUNDBERG J.M., FRANCO-CERECEDA A., HUA X., HOKFELT T., FISCHER J.A. Co-existence of substance P and calcitonin gene-related peptide-like immunoreactivities in sensory nerves in relation to cardiovascular and bronchoconstrictor effects of capsaicin. *Eur. J. Pharmacol.* 1985, 108, 315-319.
LUNDGREN J.D., OSTROWSKI N., BARANIUK J.N., SHELHAMER J.H., KALINER M.A. Gastrin releasing peptide stimulates glycoconjugate release from feline tracheal explants. *Am. J. Physiol.* 1990, 258, L68-L74.
LUNG M.A., WIDDICOMBE J.G. Lung reflexes and nasal vascular resistance in the anaesthetized dog. *J. Physiol.* 1987, 386, 465-474.
MAGGI C.A., PATACCHINI R., GIULIANI S., ROVERO P., DION S., REGOLI D., GIACHETTI A., MELI A. Competitive antagonists discriminate between NK2 tachykinin receptor subtypes. *Br. J. Pharmacol.* 1990, 100, 588-592.
MARTLING C.R., SARIA A., FISCHER J.A., HÖKFELT T., LUNDBERG J.M. Calcitonin gene related peptide and the lung: neuronal coexistence and vasodilatory effect. *Reg. Pept.* 1988, 20, 125-139.
MATRAN R., MARTLING C.-R., LUNDBERG J.M. Inhibition of cholinergic and nonadrenergic, noncholinergic bronchoconstriction in the guinea-pig mediated by neuropeptide Y and α_2-adrenoceptors and opiate receptors. *Eur. J. Pharmacol.* 1989, 163, 15-23.
McCORMACK D.G., MAK J.C., COUPE M.O., BARNES P.J. Calcitonin gene-related peptide vasodilation of human pulmonary vessels: receptor mapping and functional studies. *J. Appl. Physiol.* 1989, 67, 1265-1270.
McKAY K.O., BLACK J.L., ARMOUR C.L. The mechanism of action of endothelin in human lung. *Br. J. Pharmacol.* 1991, 102, 422-428.
MILLER Y.E. Bombesin-like peptides: from frog skin to human lung. *Am. Rev. Respir. Cell. Mol. Biol.* 1990, 3, 189-190.

MONCADA S., RADOMSKI M.W., PALMER R.M.J. Endothelium-derived relaxing factor: identification as nitric oxide and role in the control of vascular tone and platelet function. *Biochem. Pharmacol.* 1988, 37, 2495-2501.

NALINE E., DEVILLIER P., DRAPEAU G., TOTY L., BARDACH H., REGOLI D., ADVENIER C. Characterization of neurokinin effects on receptor selectivity in human isolated bronchi. *Am. Rev. Respir. Dis.* 1989, 140, 679-686.

NATHANSON I., WIDDICOMBE J.H., BARNES P.J. Effect of vasoactive intestinal peptide on ion transport across dog tracheal epithelium. *J. Appl. Physiol.* 1983, 545, 1844-1848.

NAWA H., HOROSE T., TAKASHIMA H., INAYAMA S., NAKANISHI S. Nucleotide sequences of cloned cDNAs for two types of bovine brain substance P precursor. *Nature* 1983, 306, 32-36.

NICHOL G.M., ALTON E.W.F.W., NIX A., GEDDES D.M., CHUNG K.F., BARNES P.J. Effect of inhaled furosemide on metabisulfite- and methacholine-induced bronchoconstriction and nasal potential difference in asthmatic subjects. *Am. Rev. Respir. Dis.* 1990, 142, 576-580.

NOGUCHI K., SENBA E., MORITA Y., SATO M., TOHYAMA M. Coexistence of alpha-CGRP and beta-CGRP mRNAs in rat dorsal root ganglion cells. *Neurosci. Lett.* 1990, 108, 1-5.

NOMURA A., UCHIDA Y., KAMEYAMA M., SAOTOME M., OKI K., HASEGAWA S. Endothelin and bronchial asthma. *Lancet* 1989, 2, 747-748.

PALMER J.B., SAMPSON A.P., BARNES P.J. Cholinergic and nonadrenergic inhibitory responses in bovine airways: distribution and functional association. *Am. Rev. Respir. Dis.* 1985, 131, A282.

PALMER J.B., CUSS F.M.C., BARNES P.J. VIP and PHM and their role in non-adrenergic inhibitory responses in isolated human airways. *J. Appl. Physiol.* 1986a, 61, 1322-1328.

PALMER J.B.D., CUSS F.M.C., WARREN J.B., BARNES P.J. The effect of infused vasoactive intestinal peptide on airway function in normal subjects. *Thorax* 1986b, 41, 663-666.

PALMER J.B.D., CUSS F.M.C., MULDERRY P.K., GHATEI M.A., SPRINGALL D.R., CADIEUX A., BLOOM S.R., POLAK J.M., BARNES P.J. Calcitonin gene-related peptide is localized to human airway nerves and potently constricts human airway smooth muscle. *Br. J. Pharmacol.* 1987, 91, 95-101.

PALMER R.M.J., ASHTON D.S., MONCADA S. Vascular endothelial cells synthesize nitric oxide from L-arginine. *Nature London* 1988, 333, 664-666.

PEPKE-ZABA J., HIGENBOTTAM T.W., DINH-XUAN A.T., STONE D., WALLWORK J. Inhaled nitric oxide as a cause of selective pulmonary vasodilatation in pulmonary hypertension. *Lancet* 1991, 338, 1173-1174.

RANGACHARI P.K., McWADE D. Effects of tachykinins on the electrical activity of isolated canine tracheal epithelium: an exploratory study. *Regulatory Peptides* 1985, 12, 9-19.

RICHARDSON P.S., WEBBER S.E. The control of mucous secretion in the airways by peptidergic mechanisms. *Am. Rev. Respir. Dis.* 1987, 136, S72-S76.

RIMAR S., GILLIS C.N. Pulmonary vasodilation by inhaled nitric oxide after endothelial injury. *J. Appl. Physiol.* 1992, 73, 2179-2183.

ROBBERECHT P., DENEEF P., LAMMENS M., DESCHODT-LANCKMAN M., CHRISTOPHE J. Specific binding of vasoactive intestinal peptide to brain membranes from the guinea-pigs. *Eur. J. Biochem.* 1978, 90, 147-154.

ROGERS D.F., BELVISI M.G., AURSUDKIJ B., EVANS T.W., BARNES P.J. Effects and interactions of sensory neuropeptides on airway microvascular leakage in guinea pigs. *Br. J. Pharmacol.* 1988, 95, 1109-1116.

ROGERS D.F., AURSUDKIJ B., BARNES P.J. Effects of tachykinins on mucus secretion on human bronchi in vitro. *Eur. J. Pharmacol.* 1989, 174, 283-286.

SAID S.I., MUTT V. Long acting vasodilator peptide from lung tissue. *Nature* 1969, 224, 699-700.

SAID S.I. Vasoactive peptides in the lung, with special reference to vasoactive intestinal peptide. *Exp. Lung Res.* 1982, 3, 343-348.

SAKURAI T., YANAGISAWA M., MASAKI T. Molecular characterization of endothelin receptors. *TiPS* 1992, 13, 103-108.

SALONEN R.O., WEBBER S.E., WIDDICOMBE J.G. Effects of neuropeptides and capsaicin on the canine tracheal vasculature *in vivo*. *Br. J. Pharmacol.* 1988, 95, 1262-1270.

SANDERS K.M., WARD S.M. Nitric oxide as a mediator of nonadrenergic noncholinergic neurotransmission. *Am. J. Physiol.* 1992, 262, G379-G392.

SEKIZAWA K., GRAF P.D., NADEL J.A. Somatostatin potentiates cholinergic neurotransmission in ferret trachea. *J. Appl. Physiol.* 1989, 67, 2397-2400.

SHEPPARD M.N., POLAK J.M., ALLEN J.M., BLOOM S.R. Neuropeptide tyosine (NPY), a newly discovered peptide, is present in the mammalian respiratory tract. *Thorax* 1984, 39, 326-330.

SNIDER R.M., CONSTANTINE J.W., LOWE III J.A., LONGO K.P., LEBEL W.S., WOODY H.A., DROZDA S.E., DESAI M.C., VINICK F.J., SPENCER R.W., HESS H.J. A potent nonpeptide antagonist of the substance P (NK_1) receptor. *Science* 1991, 251, 435-437.

SNYDER S.H. Nitric oxide: first in a new class of neurotransmitters ? *Science* 1992, 257, 494-496.

SONEA I.M., BOWKER R.M. Distribution of NPY and DBH immunoreactive nerves in the lungs of horses with heaves. In Proceedings : 10th Comparative Respiratory Society Meeting, Urbana, USA, 1991a, P-24.

SONEA I.M., BOWKER R.M. SP-, NKA- and CGRP-like immunoreactivity in the lungs of horses with chronic obstructive pulmonary disease. In Proceedings : 10th Comparative Respiratory Society Meeting, Urbana, USA, 1991b, P-25.

SPINDEL E.R., SUNDAY M.E., HOFLER H., WOLFE H.J., HABENER J.F., CHIN W.W. Transient elevation of mRNAs encoding gastrin releasing peptide (GRP), a putative pulmonary growth factor, in human fetal lung. *J. Clin. Invest.* 1987, 80, 1172-1179.

SPRINGALL D.R., HOWARTH P.H., COUNIHAN H., DJUKANOVIC R., HOLGATE S.T., POLAK J.M. Endothelin immunoreactivity of airway epithelium in asthmatic patients. *Lancet* 1991, 337, 697-701.

STRETTON C.B., BELVISI M.G., BARNES P.J. Sensory nerve depletion potentiates inhibitory NANC nerves in guinea pig airways. *Eur. J. Pharmacol.* 1990, 184, 333-337.

STRETTON D., BARNES P.J. Modulation of cholinergic neurotransmission in guinea pig trachea by neuropeptide Y. *Br. J. Pharmacol.* 1988, 93, 672-678.

STRETTON D., BARNES P.J. Cholecystokinin octa-peptide constricts guinea-pig and human airways. *Br. J. Pharmacol.* 1989, 97, 675-682.

TOGA H., IBE B.O., USHA RAJ J. In vitro responses of ovine intrapulmonary arteries and veins to endothelin-1. *Am. J. Physiol.* 1992, 263, L15-L21.

UDDMAN R., SUNDLER F. Vasoactive intestinal polypeptide nerves in human upper respiratory tract. *Otorhinolaryngol.* 1979, 41, 221-226.

UDDMAN R., SUNDLER F. Neuropeptides in the airways: a review. *Am. Rev. Respir. Dis.* 1987, 136, S3-S8.

UNDEM B.J., DICK E.C., BUCKNER C.K. Inhibition by vasoactive intestinal peptide of antigen-induced histamine release from guinea-pig minced lung. *Eur. J. Pharmacol.* 1983, 88, 247-250.

UNDEM B.J., MYERS A.C., BARTHLOW H., WEINREICH D. Vagal innervation of guinea pig bronchial smooth muscle. *J. Appl. Physiol.* 1991, 69, 1336-1346.

VANHOUTTE P.M. Epithelium-derived relaxing factor: myth or reality ? *Thorax* 1988, 43, 665-668.

VENUGOPALAN C.S., HOLMES E., WILSON V., O'MALLEY N.A. Epithelial role in NANC inhibitory tracheal response. *FASEB J.* 1988, 2, A959.

VENUGOPALAN C.S. Vasoactive intestinal peptide (VIP), a putative neurotransmitter of nonadrenergic noncholinergic (NANC) inhibitory innervation and its relevance to therapy. *J. Vet. Pharmacol.* 1989, 12, 113-123.

VERLEDEN G.M., BELVISI M.G., STRETTON C.D., BARNES P.J. Nedocromil sodium modulates non-adrenergic non-cholinergic bronchoconstrictor nerves in guinea-pig airways *in vitro*. *Am. Rev. Respir. Dis.* 1991, 143, 114-118.

WARNER T.D., MITCHELL J.A., DE NUCCI G., VANE J.R. Endothelin-1 and endothelin-3 release EDRF from isolated perfused arterial vessels of the rat and rabbit. *J. Cardiovasc. Pharmacol.* 1989, 13, S85-S88.

WEBBER S.E. The effects of peptide histidine isoleucine and neuropeptide Y on mucous volume output from ferret trachea. *Br. J. Pharmacol.* 1988, 55, 40-54.

YANAGISAWA M., KURIHARA H., KIMURA S., TOMOBE Y., KOBAYASHI M., MITSUI Y., YAZAKI Y., GOTO K., MASAKI T. A novel potent vasoconstrictor peptide produced by vascular endothelial cells. *Nature London* 1988, 332, 411-415.

YANG Z., RICHARD V., VON SEGESSER L., BAUER E., STULZ P., TURINA M., LUSCHER T.F. Threshold concentrations of endothelin-1 potentiate contractions to norepinephrine and serotonin in human arteries. *Circulation* 1990, 82, 188-195.

CHAPTER XI

FUNCTIONAL EFFECTS OF OBSTRUCTIVE PULMONARY DISEASES

P. Lekeux[1], C. Clercx[2] and T. Art[3]

[1] Laboratory for Functional Investigation
[2] Department of Small Animal Medicine
[3] Equine Sport Medicine Unit
Faculty of Veterinary Medicine
University of Liege

SUMMARY

This paper describes the functional peculiarities of obstructive pulmonary diseases in horses, cattle, pigs, dogs and cats.

KEY WORDS

Respiratory system - Pulmonary function - Obstructive diseases.

1. INTRODUCTION

At a functional point of view, lung diseases are usually divided into obstructive, restrictive, vascular and occupational entities. However, this subdivision is quite theoretical because some diseases, mainly of infectious nature, may induce several types of pulmonary dysfunctions.

Obstructive pulmonary diseases are very common in veterinary medicine. They have been intensively studied and, with a few exceptions, they all have a relatively uniform pattern of functional abnormalities. These diseases are becoming increasingly important as cause of economical losses in production animals and of poor performance, morbidity and mortality in horses and pet animals.

All obstructive pulmonary diseases are characterized by airway obstruction, but the distinction between the various types of obstructive diseases is blurred and this gives rise to difficulties in definition and diagnosis.

This paper attempts to summarize the classification, functional effects and species peculiarities of the various obstructive pulmonary diseases.

2. CLASSIFICATION

2.1. Intraluminal, extraluminal or intramural airway obstruction

Airway radius is the most important determinant of resistance to airflow in the lung. Indeed, the resistance of a cylindrical tube, such as the airway, is inversely proportional to its radius at the fourth power : any decrease in airway radius will dramatically increase its resistance to airflow. The factors that may affect the radius are related to conditions (a) inside the lumen, termed intraluminal causes, (b) within the wall of the airway, termed intramural causes, and (c) in the peripheral region, termed extraluminal causes (Fig. 11-1.).

2.1.1. Intraluminal causes

The lumen may be partly obstructed by excessive secretions, as in chronic obstructive pulmonary disease. A partial obstruction may also occur in heavy

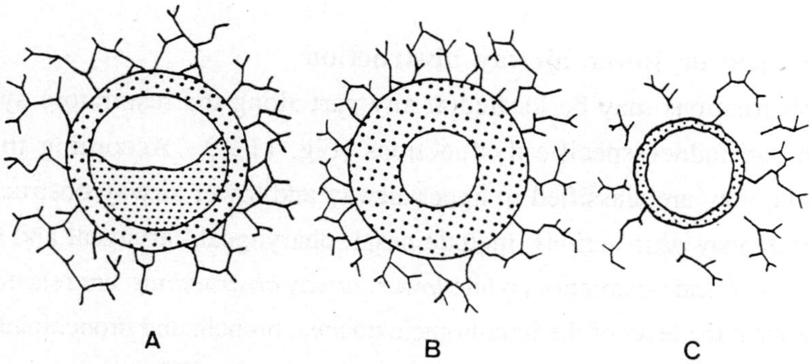

Fig. 11-1. Types of airway obstruction. A : Intraluminal obstruction, e.g. by excessive secretion; B : Intramural obstruction, e.g. by bronchoconstriction; C : Extraluminal obstruction, e.g. by loss of radial traction.

pulmonary edema, after aspiration of fluids or foreign bodies, in exercise-induced pulmonary hemorrhage, or postoperatively with retained secretions.

2.1.2. Intramural causes

Causes located within the wall of the airway include lack of airway enlargement due to a lack of muscle contraction as in laryngeal hemiplegia, excessive contraction of bronchial smooth muscle as in bronchial hyperreactivity, hypertrophy of the mucous glands as in obstructive chronic pulmonary disease, and inflammation and edema of the wall as in laryngitis or bronchitis.

2.1.3. Extraluminal causes

Destruction of lung parenchyma, as seen in emphysema, may cause loss of radial traction and consequent narrowing of the airway. A bronchus may also be compressed by enlarged lymph nodes or neoplasms. Forced expiration as in obstructive chronic pulmonary disease or strenuous exercise may also induce intrathoracic airway narrowing.

2.2. Upper or lower airway obstruction

The obstructions may be located at any part along the respiratory system, which can induce specific dysfunctions (Fig. 11-2.). According to their location, they are classified in upper airway and lower airway obstructions. *Upper airway obstructions* include nasal, pharyngeal, laryngeal and extra-thoracic tracheal obstruction, while *lower airway obstructions* are related with problems at the level of the intrathoracic trachea, bronchi and bronchioles.

There are pathological specificities according to the different species. For example, horses and dogs suffer frequently from laryngeal paralysis and chronic bronchitis, cattle from acute laryngitis and bronchospasm induced by microbiological agents, pigs from atrophic rhinitis, and cats from chronic nasal infections and bronchitis.

There are also some breed peculiarities. Acute laryngitis is more frequent and more severe in double-muscled than in dairy cattle (Lekeux and Art, 1987). Laryngeal paralysis is a hereditary disorder in bouvier dogs while in other canine breeds it is an acquired disorder (Venker-van Haagen, 1980).

Abnormally high resistance at the level of some intrathoracic airways induces inequalities in the regional ventilation, which is commonly termed ventilatory asynchronism. Inhaled air preferentially enters those areas of the lungs that have low resistive airways. This ventilatory asynchronism is moderate in healthy animals and does not have significant effects on gas exchange at low respiratory frequencies. However, this is not the case in patients with significant asynchronism (i.e. subclinical small airway disease) and with a high respiratory frequency (i.e. during exercise or compensatory hyperpnea). Under these conditons, the lobules, which have a long time constant for filling, do not fill adequately before expiration begins. Consequently, ventilation/perfusion mismatching and hypoxemia result. This phenomenon will significantly impair gas exchange.

The interdependence between adjacent lung regions tends to limit the non-

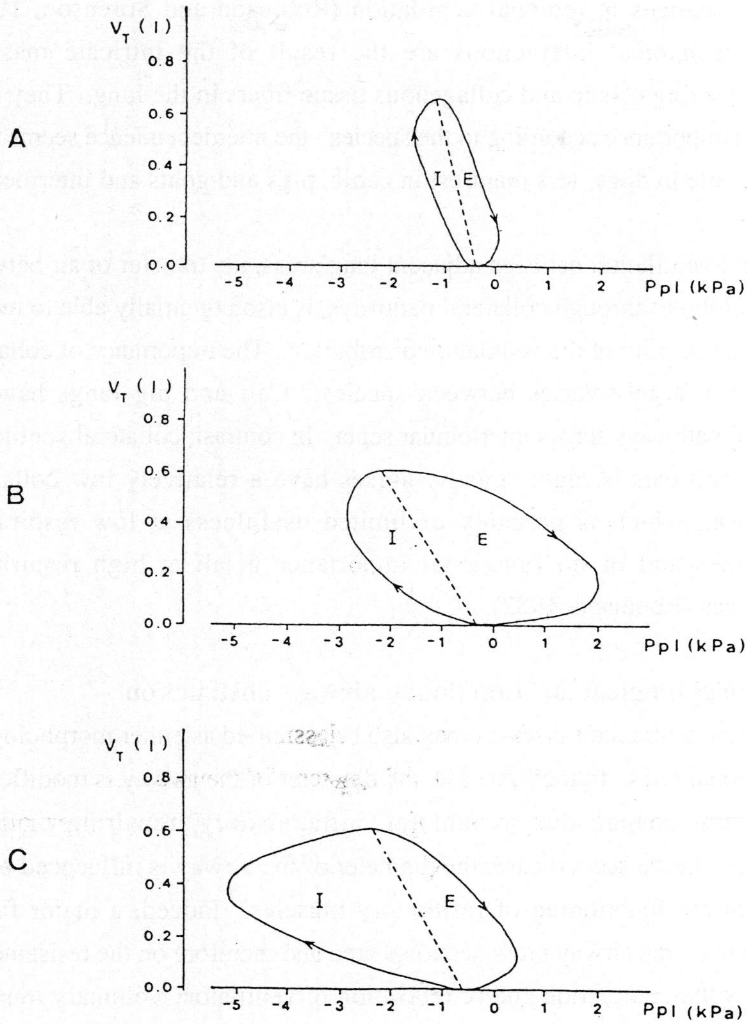

Fig. 11-2. Pressure/volume loops from bovine lungs during normal physiologica conditions (A), during severe intrathoracic airway obstructive disease (B) and during severe extrathoracic airway obstructive disease (C). I : Inspiratory; E : Expiratory; Dashed line Line of compliance (Lekeux and Art, 1987).

uniform changes in regional ventilation (Robinson and Sorenson, 1978). These mechanical interactions are the result of the intricate mash of interconnecting elastic and collagenous tissue fibers in the lung. They have different importance according to the species : the interdependence seems to be considerable in dogs, less manifest in cattle, pigs and goats and intermediate in horses.

Collateral ventilation between adjacent lung areas, i.e. transfer of air between adjacent lobules through collateral pathways, is also potentially able to reduce the non-uniformity of the ventilation distribution. The importance of collateral ventilation largely varies between species. Calf and pig lungs have no collateral pathways across interlobular septa. In contrast, collateral ventilation in dogs and cats is high. Lastly, horses have a relatively low collateral ventilation, which is probably of limited usefulness at low respiratory frequencies and of no functional importance at all at high respiratory frequencies (Robinson, 1982).

2.3. Morphological or functional airway obstruction

Obstructive pulmonary diseases may also be classified as either morphological or functional ones. In the first case, the diameter of the airway is modified by a structural change due to tumoral, inflammatory, repairing or other processes. In the second case, the diameter of the airway is influenced by an inappropriate functioning of respiratory muscles. Indeed, a major factor which acts on the airway cross-sectional area and therefore on the resistance to airflow is the contraction and/or relaxation of ventilatory voluntary muscles and smooth muscles.

At the level of the nares, the pharynx (soft palate) and the larynx, the contraction of voluntary muscles leads to airway enlargement. Therefore, dysfunction of these muscles (paresis, paralysis or fatigue) will invariably induce a rise in pulmonary resistance, generally accompanied by respiratory noises, especially during hyperpnea.

The smooth muscles in the trachea and main bronchi are innervated by the

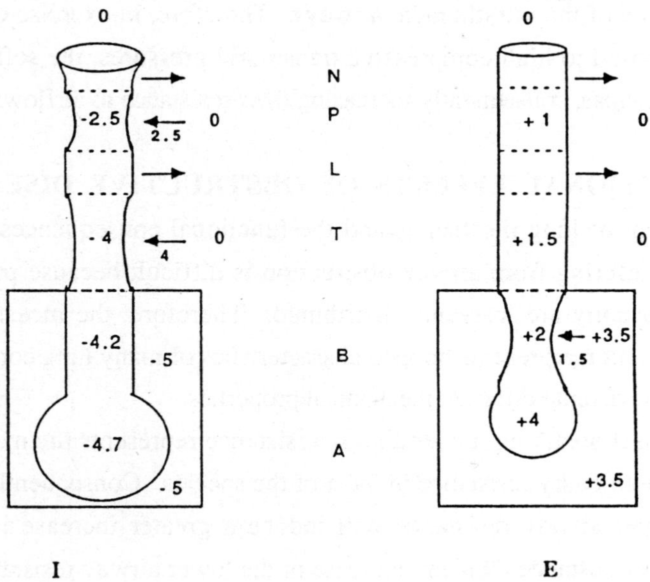

Fig. 11-3. Illustration of the dynamic collapse that may be observed during forced respiration. N : Nasal cavity; P : Pharynx; L : Larynx; T : Extrathoracic trachea; B : Bronchi; A : Alveoli; I : Inspiration; E : Expiration.

autonomic nervous system and modulate the airway diameter by either contracting or relaxing. Dysfunction may result from excessive smooth muscle tonus, as in asthmatic syndromes, or, on the contrary, from unsufficient smooth muscle contraction, leading to a too great airway collapsibility. A decrease in airway rigidity may lead to an increase in pulmonary resistance by the following process. A dynamic partial collapse occurs when the pressure surrounding the airways exceeds the pressure within the lumen (Fig. 11-3.). This occurs in the upper airways during inhalation, when the pressures in the extrathoracic airways are subatmospheric while pressure in the surrounding tissues remains atmospheric. On the opposite, dynamic partial collapse occurs in lower airways during expiration, when the intrathoracic pressure becomes higher than the pressure prevailing inside some of the intrathoracic airways. Therefore, in exercise or diseases, when exposed to high compressive transmural pressures, the soft structures tend to collapse, consequently increasing their resistance to airflow.

3. FUNCTIONAL EFFECTS OF OBSTRUCTIVE DISEASES

Assessment of lung mechanics and the functional consequences thereof in patients suffering from airway obstruction is difficult because pathological changes usually are unevenly distributed. Therefore, the measurement of overall function represents lumped characteristics of many lung compartments that may have quite different mechanical properties.

During nasal breathing, upper airway resistance represents the major part of the total pulmonary resistance in most of the species. Consequently, increase in the upper airway resistance will induce a greater increase in the total pulmonary resistance than any increase in the lower airway resistance. It can therefore be assumed that upper airway obstruction mainly results in an increase in total pulmonary resistance, while lower airway obstruction rather induces a decrease in dynamic pulmonary compliance due to the accompanying ventilatory asynchronism.

Obstruction of the upper airways will result in a dramatic increase of the mechanical work of breathing. This means that animals will spend an abnormally high level of energy to ensure their ventilation. Such a phenomenon may lead to poor performance syndrome in race horses, to reduction of the daily body gain or even weight loss in production animals, and to respiratory muscle fatigue or even failure.

Obstruction of the lower airways may result in uneven ventilatory distribution and ventilation/perfusion mismatching. Hypoxic vasoconstriction and vascular pulmonary hypertension may also occur. Moreover, because of the interdependence between adjacent lung areas, the lobules with increased airflow resistance are stretched and compressed by the surrounding lung parts (Mead et al, 1970). This may induce abnormal stresses on the tissues of these lobules, inducing emphysema or pulmonary hemorrhage (Robinson, 1979). If the ventilatory adjustments to the disease fail to compensate for the obstruction, gas exchange impairment may result. This impairment may be assessed by arterial blood gas analysis and results in a decrease in arterial partial pressure in oxygen, and, in more severe cases, an increase in arterial partial pressure in carbon dioxide.

4. SPECIES PECULIARITIES

Each variation in anatomical structure implies variation in function. These changes can influence the pathogenesis and the sequels of respiratory diseases. These effects are different in the various species. For example, a nasal obstruction can be dramatic in the horse which is a compulsory nasal breather, but this is not the case in the dog. Obstruction of the small airways has less functional impact in dogs in which collateral ventilation and lobar interdependence are high than in cattle in which these morphological specificities are absent.

4.1. Horses

In equine practice, respiratory diseases are as important and common as musculoskeletal diseases. While overt respiratory diseases are obvious and seldom cause a diagnostic challenge, most respiratory diseases are much more subtle and insidious (Morris and Seeherman, 1991). They are liable to impair gas exchange during exercise and therefore to limit the horse's performance primarily by increasing the airway's resistance to airflow and the ventilatory asynchronism.

4.1.1. Nasal disorders

During inspiration, pressure within the nares is subatmospheric and the poorly supported nostrils therefore tend to collapse. This dynamic collapse is prevented or minimized by the nasal muscles. In case of damage to the motor pathways of the facial nerve, the nostrils are paralyzed and the collapse is no

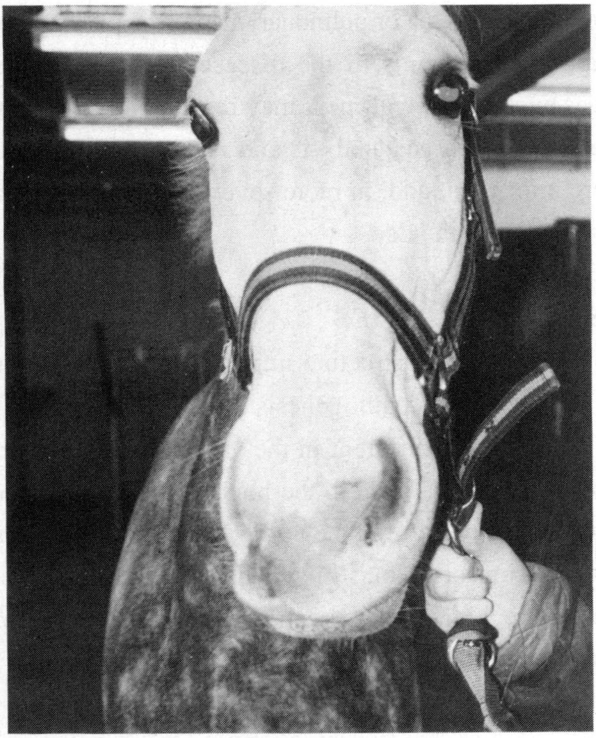

Fig. 11-4. Collapse of the right nostril secondary to facial nerve injury.

longer prevented (Fig. 11-4.). During exercise, the nasal resistance increases (Art et al, 1988). Because the horse is limited to nasal breathing, any partial obstruction at this level will consequently result in exercise intolerance.

4.1.2. Pharyngeal lymphoid hyperplasia

Pharyngeal lymphoid hyperplasia appears to reflect the immature and hyperreactive condition of the submucosal lymphoid tissue present throughout the pharynx (Burrell, 1985). The clinical significance of this condition and its effect on the performance capability of the horse are still controversial. This hyperplasia appears to have little effect on upper airway function (Williams et

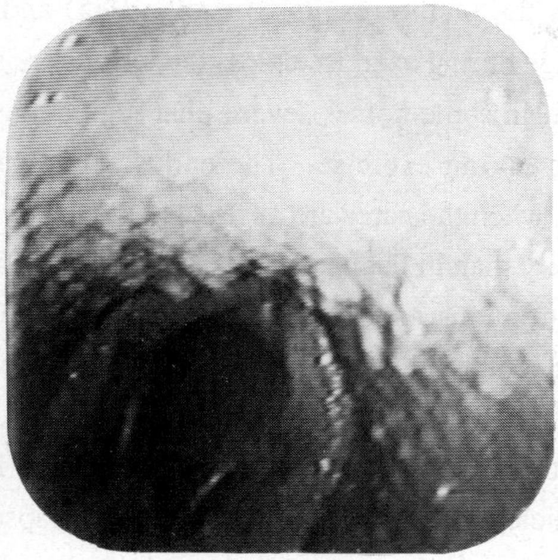

Fig. 11-5. Pharyngeal lymphoid hyperplasia.

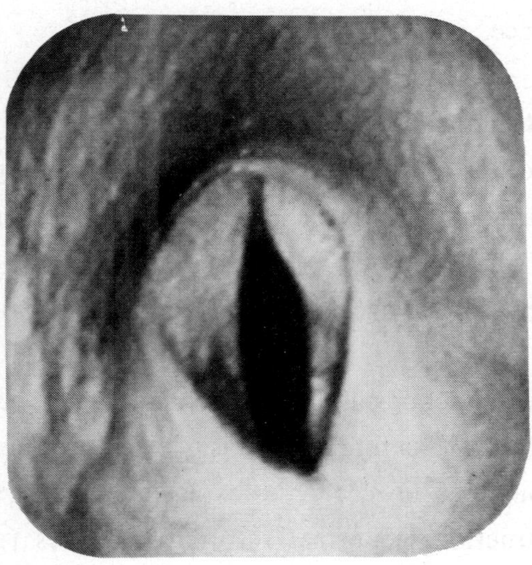

Fig. 11-6. Dorsal displacement of the soft palate and rostral displacement of the palatopharyngeal arch in a horse.

al, 1990a) and on the racing results (Burrell, 1985) and does not seem to impair gas exchange during exercise unless the lesions are severe (Bayly et al, 1984a). However, in some horses severe pharyngitis may induce abnormal inspiratory noises during exercise. The endoscopic examination of these horses shows that, when the nares are obstructed, the pharyngeal walls tend to collapse more easily than in healthy horses (Fig. 11-5.). The same horses re-examined after strenuous exercise show a further hypertrophy, and even hyperemia, of the lymphoid follicles. It can therefore be hypothesized that horses suffering from lymphoid hyperplasia have an abnormally high pharyngeal resistance because the pharyngeal lumen is reduced by the hypertrophied follicles and also because a dynamic collapse of the pharyngeal walls during inspiration further increases the resistance to airflow.
The stimulation of pharyngeal irritant receptors by mediators released by the lymphoid follicles could also result in reflex bronchoconstriction (Robinson, 1979).
It should also be noted that follicular laryngitis can be secondary to problems such as viremia or a poor environment, the latter being the primary cause of exercise intolerance.

4.1.3. Intermittent dorsal displacement of the soft palate

Normally, the soft palate lies ventral to the epiglottis during respiration. In dorsal displacement of the soft palate, the caudal free border of the soft palate is displaced to a position above the epiglottis (Fig. 11-6.). This causes narrowing of the nasopharyngeal airway and turbulence during inspiration and expiration.
Horses with intermittent dorsal displacement of the soft palate generally are asymptomatic at rest and during low intensity exercise. This condition is most frequently encountered in racehorses as an intermittent event that causes temporary obstruction, abnormal respiratory noises (gurgling), mouth breathing and sometimes asphyxia and "chocking down" at high speed.
There are several etiologies for the dorsal displacement of the soft palate. It

may result from or be favoured by (1) anatomical changes, i.e. epiglottic hypoplasia (Haynes, 1981) and malformation of the laryngeal cartilages; (2) functional problems secondary to nervous disorders, guttural pouch infection, pharyngitis and chronic bronchitis, or (3) mechanical actions, i.e. retraction of the tongue which causes both an elevation of the palate and a caudal retraction of the larynx, contraction of the sternohyoid and sternethyroid muscles, and negative intra-pharyngeal pressures during heavy exercise, causing some pharyngeal collapse of the unsupported structures.

Various treatments have been proposed for intermittent dorsal displacement of the soft palate. Preventive techniques include the use of tongue tie and figure-of-eight nose bands preventing opening of the mouth. Surgical treatment consists of resection of the sternohyoid and sternothyroid muscles or resection of cautherization of the caudal free margin of the soft palate. However, the results obviously depend upon effective treatment of the primary cause.

4.1.4. Rostral displacement of the palatopharyngeal arch

In this condition, the caudal margin of the intrapharyngeal ostium is displaced rostrally onto the corniculate processes of the arytenoid cartilages. The rostrally displaced tissue obstructs the laryngeal aperture and forms a sheet which impedes the abduction of the arytenoid cartilages.

The clinical signs resulting from rostral displacement of the palatopharyngeal arch are various. In severely affected horses, it causes dyspnea and dysphagia. In subclinically affected horses, this condition produces airway obstruction and severe exercise intolerance.

4.1.5. Guttural pouch disorders

Diseases of the guttural pouches are rare but may potentially induce secondary problems such as spontaneous epistaxis, damage of some cranial nerves, parotid distension and upper airway dysfunction. Several nerves pass along the guttural pouches, namely the cervical sympathetic trunk and the vagus, glossopharyngeal, hypoglossal, accessory, cranial laryngeal, facial and

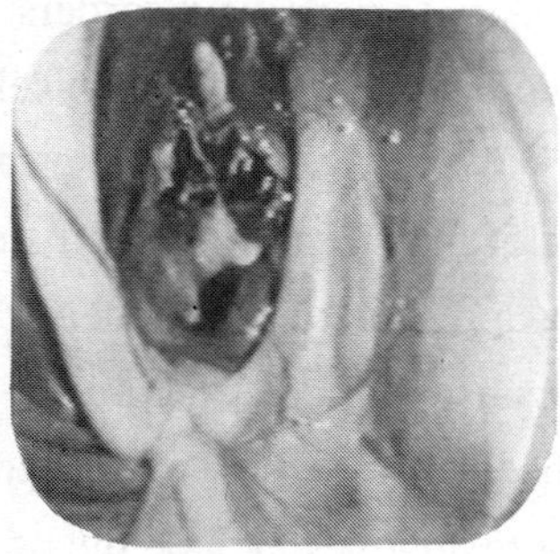

Fig. 11-7. Guttural pouch mycosis.

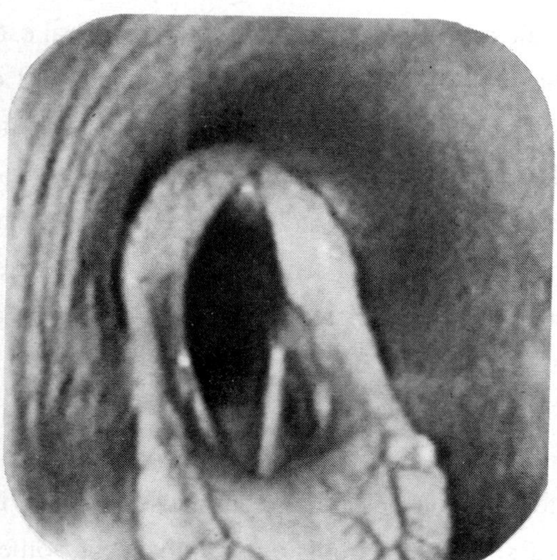

Fig. 11-8. Left laryngeal hemiplegia.

mandibular nerves. Therefore, uni- or bilateral infectious disorders, i.e. empyema and mycosis (Fig. 11-7.), can cause functional disorders such as soft palate displacement and pharyngeal or laryngeal paresis.

4.1.6. Idiopathic laryngeal hemiplegia

The primary lesion associated with left-sided laryngeal hemiplegia is damage to the left recurrent laryngeal nerve. This results in the paralysis or paresis of the dorsal cricoarytenoid muscle. In this condition, the horse cannot fully dilate the larynx on the affected side and there is partial obstruction to airflow, inducing an increase in laryngeal resistance, mainly during inspiration (Derksen et al, 1986; Belknap et al, 1990; Williams et al, 1990a; 1990b). Most horses with laryngeal hemiplegia are presented with a complaint of decreased exercise tolerance and abnormal inspiratory noise during exercise. In galloping horses, laryngeal hemiplegia has been shown to produce a severe hypercapnic hypoxemia (Bayly et al, 1984b; Belknap et al, 1990). Affected ponies have shown a dramatic decrease in athletic ability accompanied by a decoupling of respiratory and step frequencies while galloping (Manohar, 1986).

Laryngeal hemiplegia is not a all-or-none disease : all stages of arytenoid cartilage movement exist, from normal function to paresis and paralysis. Endoscopic examination therefore shows horses with various asynchrony or asymmetry. The following grading system is proposed to objectively describe the movements of the arytenoid cartilages (Hackett et al, 1991). Briefly, grade I represents a normal larynx, showing full and synchronous abduction and adduction. Horses with grade II exhibit asynchronous movements of the arytenoid cartilages at rest, but normal and synchronous movements once they are fully stimulated by nasal occlusion or by exercise. Horses with grade III show asynchronous movements of the arytenoid cartilages even after respiratory stimulation. Horses with grade IV show a marked asymmetry with no movements of the arytenoid cartilage at any stage of the respiratory cycle (Fig. 11-8.). The clinical significance, the functional consequences and the indication for laryngoplasty in cases of grade II and III are sometimes difficult to assess and require functional investigations. In such cases, treadmill endoscopy may allow a rational decision regarding therapy.

4.1.7. Arytenoid chondritis

Arytenoid chondritis is a chronic, progressive condition of the larynx resulting in distortion of either one or both the arytenoid cartilages. This abnormality is characterized by an enlargement of the cartilage causing restriction of normal motion and decreased airway diameter. This results in exercise intolerance and inspiratory noise during exercise (Williams et al, 1990a). In the early stage, it may sometimes be confused with laryngeal hemiplegia. The exact pathogenesis is unknown. Arytenoid chondritis is mainly observed in thoroughbred horses between 2 and 4 years of age.

4.1.8. Epiglottic entrapment

Epiglottic entrapment is the envelopment of the apex and lateral margins of the epiglottis by the ventral epiglottic mucosa and aryepiglottic folds (Fig. 11-9.). This condition has variable effects on exercise tolerance. Sometimes it is found incidentally in horses with no history of respiratory problems, while in other cases severe respiratory distress is present (Linford et al, 1983; Honnas et al, 1990). In these horses, endoscopy of the upper airways during exercise shows a significant reduction of pharyngeal diameter due to billowing of the entrapped fold during expiration.

4.1.9. Tracheal disorders

Tracheal diseases that cause respiratory obstruction in horses are uncommon. Tracheal obstruction, consisting of either dorso-ventral flattening of the cartilage rings or cartilage rings having a scroll-like conformation, have been reported to induce respiratory distress at rest and during exercise (Mair and Lane, 1990). Pathologic tracheal collapse (Fig. 11-10.) sometimes results either from misshapen cartilagenous rings (Carrig et al, 1973) or from

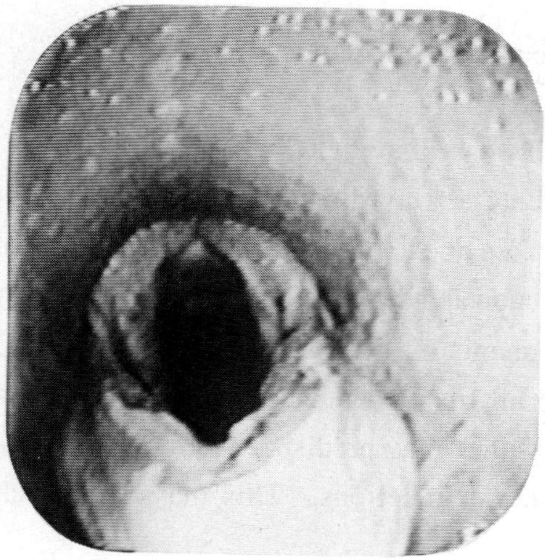

Fig. 11-9. Epiglottic entrapment.

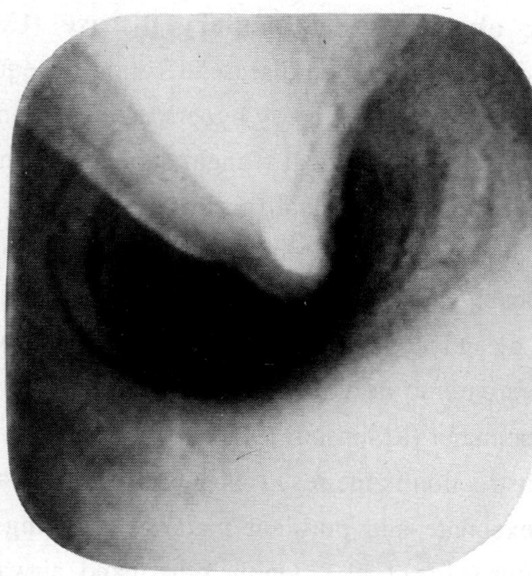

Fig. 11-10. Tracheal collapse.

inflammation of the tracheal membrane (Hardy, 1991).

4.1.10. Acute airway disorders

The etiology of acute airway disorders in horses is generally viral. The functional disorders are due to bronchoconstriction, mucosal edema, epithelial necrosis, hypersecretion and decreased mucociliar clearance caused by damage of the ciliary mechanism (Willoughby et al, 1992). These functional modifications are primarily moderate but, due to an inadequate management of the diseased horses, they may predispose to more deleterious effects caused by secondary bacterial infections. This may lead to chronic respiratory problems.

It has been shown that booster vaccination of thoroughbred horses with an oily adjuvant inactivated vaccine against influenza and rhinopneumonia does not impair their cardio-respiratory and metabolic adjustments to strenuous exercise and to training (Art and Lekeux, 1993).

4.1.11. Chronic obstructive pulmonary disease (C.O.P.D.)

This condition is the most common disease affecting the equine lung. This syndrome is characterized by an airway hyperreactivity to inhaled allergens (Derksen et al, 1985), i.e. biological (fungal spores), chemical (ammonia, hydrogen sulfide, ozone) or physical (airborne particules) irritants. Diet, previous airway infections, poor environmental conditions and genetic predisposition probably are favorising or exacerbating factors.

It is characterized by an inhomogenously distributed lower airway obstruction. The role of the autonomic nervous system in the pathophysiology of the disease seems to be major (Robinson, 1993).

In part, airway obstruction is the result of plugging of airways with mucus, cellular debris, exsudate and purulent material resulting from bacterial secondary infections (Fig. 11-11.). On the other hand, airway obstruction is also caused by airway smooth muscle contraction. Lastly, decrease of the airway lumen may also partly be induced by chronic bronchiolitis with

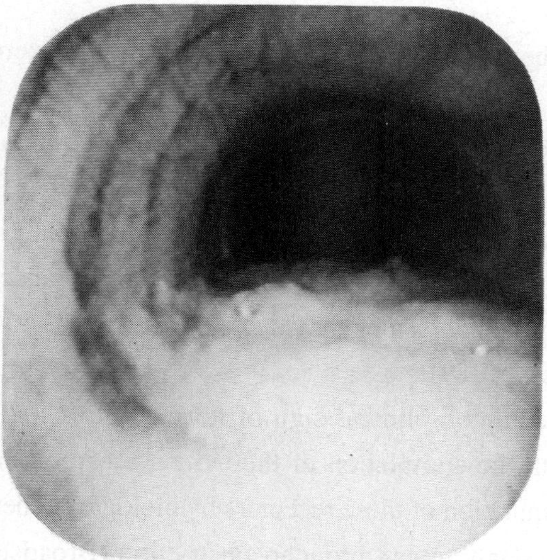

Fig. 11-11. Airway hypersecretion in a horse suffering from C.O.P.D.

hyperplastic epithelium. The alveoli subserved by completely or partially obstructed bronchioles are overinflated (alveolar emphysema). However, bullous interstitial emphysema created by rupture of the alveolar walls is rare in horses with chronic obstructive pulmonary disease.

Horses suffering from this lower airway disorder generally have an increased airway resistance and a decreased dynamic lung compliance (Muylle and Oyaert, 1973) as well as a prolongation of nitrogen washout (Muylle et al, 1972). All these findings are compatible with diffuse airway obstruction. The exacerbated regional differences in small airway resistance and lung compliance result in an uneven distribution of ventilation. The resulting inequalities in ventilation/perfusion ratio may in turn induce hypoxemia (Devous et al, 1980; O'Callaghan, 1991). Moreover, this phenomenon results sometimes in increased pulmonary vascular resistance (Muylle et al, 1982) causing right ventricular hypertrophy and right heart failure in severe and prolonged cases (Dixon et al, 1982). The increase in total pulmonary resistance and the impaired gas exchange decrease the exercise tolerance of affected horses.

In horses suffering from chronic obstructive pulmonary disease, the mucociliary transport rate is significantly lower than in healthy animals (Turgut and Sasse, 1989). It is also suggested that, in bronchiolitis, modification of the rheological properties of the bronchial secretions and loss of cilia due to epithelial lesions may decrease the rate of transport of sputum (Turgut and Sasse, 1989).

Coughing is a common clinical sign of horses with C.O.P.D. The cough reflex starts with the stimulation of the irritant receptors in the respiratory system. The stimulation of these receptors by biological, chemical or physical agents induces coughing and bronchoconstriction (Broadstone et al, 1988). This response is primarily physiological, but in some horses it may be excessive and induce respiratory dysfunction.

4.1.12. Exercise-induced bronchoconstriction

In human subjects, it has been shown that exercise may induce a bronchoconstriction (McFadden and Ingram, 1983; Crimi et al, 1992). This response to exercise depends both on the quality of the inspired air and on the bronchoreactivity of the subject, but the exact sequence of events underlying its pathogenesis is still unclear. Whether or not the same phenomenon occurs in horses remains to be demonstrated.

4.1.13. Exercise-induced dynamic partial collapse of the airways

The importance of the dynamic partial collapse depends on the extent of the compressive transmural pressures and on the shape of the cross-sectional area of the airways (Fig. 11-12.) (Art and Lekeux, 1991a; 1991b).

4.2. Cattle

Functional effects of obstructive diseases have been investigated in cattle (Table 11-1.) (Lekeux et al, 1988). However, most of these syndromes are

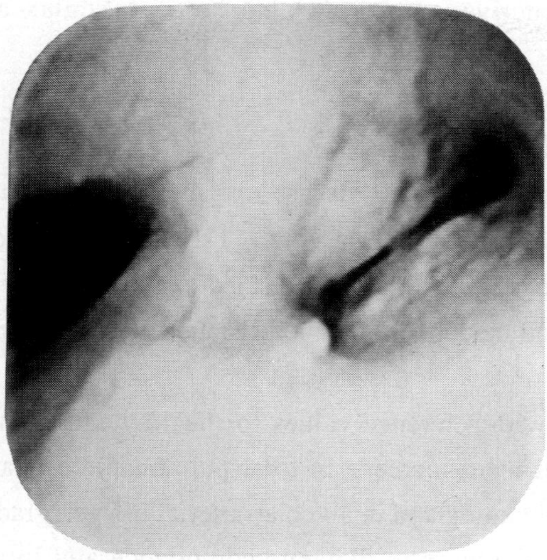

Fig. 11-12. Bronchial collapse in a horse with a severe obstructive disorder.

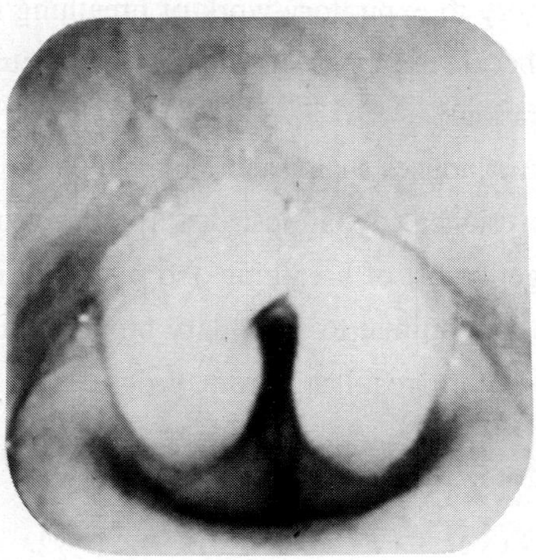

Fig. 11-13. Stridulous laryngitis in a double-muscled calf.

not purely obstructive and show also some vascular and restrictive dysfunctions.

4.2.1. Stridulous laryngitis

A severe obstructive laryngeal disease may be observed during infectious rhinothracheatis or calf diphteria (Fig. 11-13.). This syndrome is more frequent and more severe in double-muscled cattle, probably because of the narrower lumen and the higher airflow resistance of their larynx (Gustin et al, 1987).

When compared with reference values for healthy cattle, infected animals show highly significant increase in total pulmonary resistance, in minute viscous work of breathing and in alveolar-arterial oxygen gradient, as well as highly significant decrease in dynamic compliance and in arterial oxygen tension (Lekeux and Art, 1987). The decrease of dynamic lung compliance in these animals suggests the presence of a concomitant ventilatory asynchronism due to secondary lower airway disease, which is consistent with the post mortem findings which show that bronchopneumonia frequently complicates the necrotic laryngitis (Jensen and Mackey, 1974).

The ratio of inspiratory to expiratory work of breathing is also significantly increased, probably because of a partial collapse of the extrathoracic part of the trachea during inspiration.

This clinical syndrome induces such important changes in pulmonary function that it modifies the tracheal dynamics, disturbs the growing processes by increasing the energetic cost of breathing and by impairing normal feeding, and predisposes the sick animal to secondary broncho-pulmonary infections and to respiratory failure resulting from progressive respiratory muscle fatigue.

4.2.2. Shipping Fever

Shipping Fever is a respiratory syndrome caused by complex interactions between stress factors, environmental conditions and several pathogens in which *Pasteurella haemolytica* plays an important role. Pulmonary function values recorded during the initial stage of this syndrome in feedlot cattle is consistent with an acute obstructive disease located mainly at the level of large airways (Lekeux and Art, 1987; Genicot et al, 1993). The main dysfunctions observed the first day of this syndrome are an increase in respiratory rate, total pulmonary resistance, minute viscous work of breathing and alveolo-arterial oxygen gradient, and a decrease in tidal volume and arterial oxygen tension. If the infection is moderate and the treatment appropriate, these dysfunctions are completely reversible within 2 weeks. This indicates that accurate preventive and curative treatments may avoid the onset of severe pulmonary damage and may reduce the economical losses induced by Shipping Fever.

4.2.3. Verminous bronchitis

Lungworm infection with *Dictyocaulus viviparus* induces a reversible obstructive disease. When compared to normal animals, infected cattle present a significant increase of respiratory frequency, minute ventilation, total pulmonary resistance and minute viscous work, and a significant decrease of tidal volume, dynamic lung compliance and arterial oxygen tension (Lekeux et al, 1985a). Absolute intrapleural pressures are also more negative than in physiological conditions, suggesting an overdistension of the lung and/or the presence of trapped gas in this organ.

Clinical, functional and pathological findings are all consistent with the picture of a peripheral airway obstructive disease.

During experimental infection, most lung parameters show significant changes since the second and third weeks, and maximal changes at the fifth week post infection (Lekeux et al, 1985b). Minute ventilation, dynamic lung compliance, minute viscous work and arterial oxygen tension show the most homogeneous evolution. On the other hand, maximal changes in intrapleural pressure, total pulmonary resistance and viscous work of breathing show higher variability from week to week.

If functional changes observed during bovine verminous bronchitis are

Table 11-1. Effect of bovine obstructive pulmonary diseases on some pulmonary function values.

Values	A	B	C	D	E
f	169*	184*	257*	141	161*
t_I/t_{TOT}	113*	109	113*	100	109*
$\dot{V}$Imax	116*	107	144	136	144
$\dot{V}$Emax	143*	119	153*	164*	156*
V_T	76*	64*	55*	96	87
$\dot{V}_e$	133*	114	151*	134	143*
maxΔPpl	161*	125*	175*	567*	857*
PplFRC	122	124	77*	25*	125
Cdyn	52*	76*	26*	21*	24*
R_L	130*	181*	150*	481*	752*
$\dot{W}$vis	222*	197*	302*	840*	821*
PaO_2	71*	74*	58*	56*	79*
$PaCO_2$	121	90	107	105	107

Data are expressed as the percentage of reference values for healthy cattle. A : Verminous bronchitis; B : Shipping fever; C : Respiratory syncytial virus pneumonia; D : Organophosphate poisoning; E : Necrotic laryngitis; * significantly different from reference values for $P < 0.05$ (one-tailed t-test); f : Respiratory frequency; t_I/t_{TOT} : Inspiratory time/total time of the breathing cycle ratio; $\dot{V}$Imax and $\dot{V}$Emax : Peak inspiratory and expiratory airflow; V_T : Tidal volume; $\dot{V}_e$: Minute volume; maxΔPpl : Peak to peak change in pleural pressure; PplFRC : Ppl at the level of functional residual capacity; Cdyn : Dynamic lung compliance; R_L : Total pulmonary resistance; $\dot{W}$vis : Minute work of breathing; PaO_2 and $PaCO_2$: Arterial oxygen and carbon dioxide tensions.

compared with changes induced in horses by a peripheral airway obstructive disease, cattle show a higher hypoxemia and a lower increase of viscous work of breathing. Decrease of tidal volume and overdistension of the lung are present in this species but not in horses.

The hypoxemia observed during this obstructive disease is probably mainly due to an increase of ventilation/perfusion inequalities resulting from uneven distribution of ventilation.

4.2.4. Respiratory distress induced by organophosphate poisoning

Dichlorvos toxicosis induces a severe respiratory distress due mainly to a hyperacute constriction located in both the large and small airways (Lekeux et al, 1986). Decrease in dynamic lung compliance and arterial oxygen tension and increase in total pulmonary resistance and viscous work of breathing are very important. On the other hand, respiratory rate, tidal volume and carbone dioxide tension are not significantly modified in the early stage of this syndrome.

Atropine reverses promptly and completely all these pulmonary dysfunctions, which suggests the predominence of cholinergic pathways.

4.2.5. Acute bovine respiratory syncytial virus infection

This syndrome may vary from a moderate respiratory disorder to a severe respiratory distress syndrome, depending on the age, sensitivity and immunological status of the patient.

In the acute and early stage of the disease, this syndrome induces mainly a severe obstructive disease located at both large and small airways, as assessed by the large increase in respiratory frequency, maximal change in intrapleural pressure, total pulmonary resistance and alveolo-arterial oxygen gradient, and the large decrease in tidal volume, dynamic compliance and arterial oxygen tension (Lekeux et al, 1985c). These dysfunctions are partly reversed by inhalation of vagolytic and beta-adrenergic drugs, suggesting the occurrence of diffuse bronchoconstriction (Genicot et al, 1992).

On the other hand, this infection may also induce bronchial hyperresponsiveness, as suggested by the hyperreactivity to histamine observed 2 weeks after experimental respiratory syncytial virus infection (Leblanc et al, 1991).

4.3. Pigs

4.3.1. Rhinitis

Rhinitis is a common respiratory disorder in pigs and may be manifested as atrophic rhinitis (Fig. 11-14.) (Pedersen and Nielsen, 1983), inclusion body rhinitis (Kelly, 1967) or necrotic rhinitis (Giles, 1986). Due to the inflammatory processes and the local injuries observed during these diseases, the passage of air through the nasal cavities may be disturbed in some patients. The resulting increase in total pulmonary resistance and viscous work of breathing could partly explain the negative effects of these syndromes on production parameters (Nielsen, 1983).

4.3.2. Exudative bronchopneumonia

Lower airway obstruction may also occur in pigs as a result of several bacterial, mycoplasmal, viral and occupational diseases (Pijoan, 1986). The resulting peribronchiolar cuffing, airway mucosal edema, airway hypersecretion and impaired mucoliliar clearance (Coignoul et al, 1987) increase the work of breathing and the ventilatory asynchronism because the porcine lung has no collateral ventilation (Robinson, 1982). As a consequence, the physiological gas exchanges and production performances are impaired.

4.4. Canine and feline obstructive diseases

4.4.1. Nasal disorders

Because of the well developed turbinates within the nasal cavities of dogs and cats, obstruction of one or both nasal chambers occurs as soon as the conchal mucosa is congested. Dogs and cats with obstructive nasal disease usually exhibit nasal discharge, sneezing, noisy breathing, or open mouth breathing. Nasal permeability is reduced and can be asymmetric. Obstructive nasal diseases are common in dogs and cats. Intranasal causes include nasal tumors, polyps, hypertrophic or inflammatory rhinitis and foreign bodies. In dogs, most of the intranasal masses are malignant tumors, while in cats

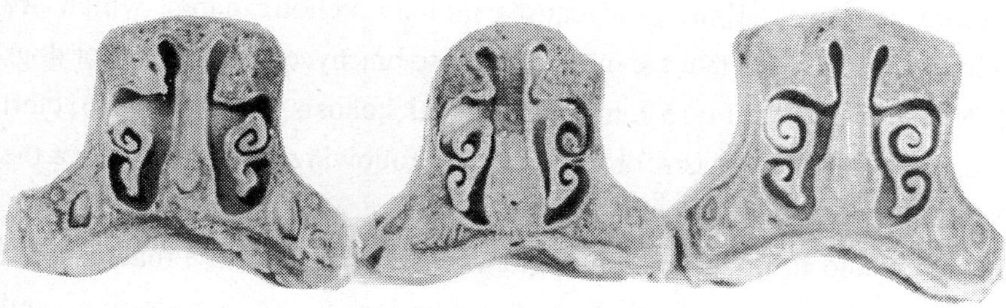

Fig. 11-14. Several degrees of porcine atrophic rhinitis.

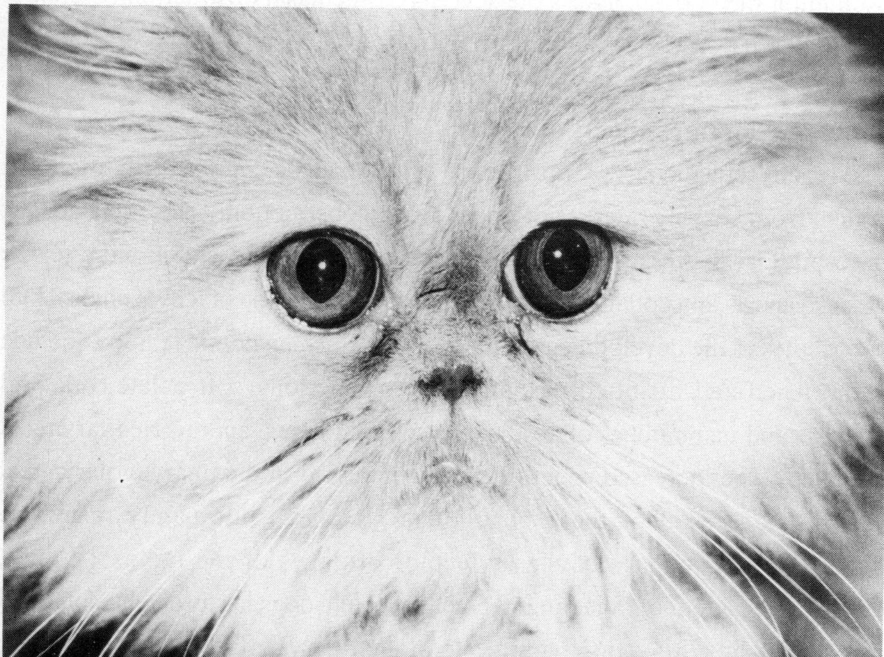

Fig. 11-15. Stenotic nares in a Persian cat.

inflammatory nasopharyngeal polyps originating within the Eustachian tube are more common. Extranasal causes include stenotic nares, which are anatomic abnormalities that are more specific to brachycephalic breeds of dogs and Persian cats (Fig. 11-15.), nasopharyngeal stenosis (Mitten, 1992), cleft palate, soft palate hypoplasia, oro-nasal fistula following dental disease, or the presence of a foreign body behind the soft palate.

Rhinoscopy and thorough mouth exploration usually lead to a macroscopic diagnosis, which can be confirmed or evidenced by histological and micobiological examinations (Venker-van Haagen et al, 1990). Radiography of the nasal cavities and sinuses is also helpful in determining the nasal obstructive problem (Harvey et al, 1979). More recently, CT scan has been used as a diagnostic technique in nasal diseases (Delisle, 1992).

Measurement of the impedance of the total respiratory system by the forced oscillation method can assess the severity of the nasal obstruction (Clercx et al, 1989b).

4.4.2. Nasopharyngeal disorders

The brachycephalic airway obstruction syndrome is a complex condition that results from varying degrees of upper airway obstruction. The signs consist of respiratory distress, stridor, reduced exercise tolerance, and in more severe cases cyanosis and collapse. The inherent anatomy of the brachycephalic skull contributes to the development of these signs. Such anatomic features include a shortened and distorted nasopharynx, an overlong soft palate, bilateral stenosis and inspiratory collapse of the external nares, and everted laryngeal saccules. The increased negative pressure created in the pharyngolaryngeal region, as a result of these obstructing structures, ultimately results in distortion and collapse of the arytenoid cartilages of the larynx (Wykes, 1991). The pattern of breathing in brachycephalic dogs has been characterized using tidal breathing flow-volume loop analysis (Amis and Kurpershoek, 1986).

The English bulldog is a brachycephalic breed subjected to sleep-disordered

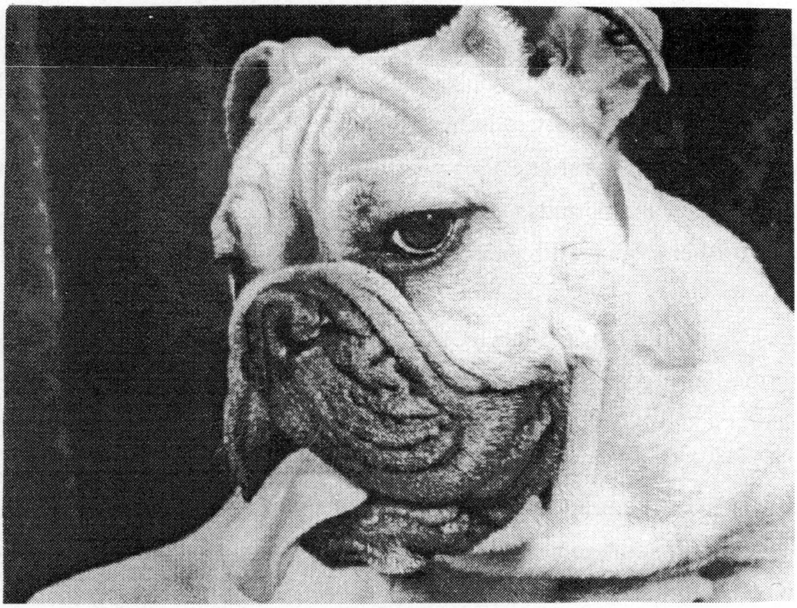

Fig. 11-16. Example of a brachycephalic breed subjected to sleep-disordered breathing.

breathing (Fig. 11-16.) (Hendricks et al, 1991). This could be associated with a specific hyperactivity of the sternohyoid muscle which is an upper airway dilator muscle (Hendricks et al, 1992).

The obstructive dyspnea of the brachycephalic patients can be further complicated by severe restriction of the cranial laryngeal airway caused by the displacement of the glosso-epiglottic mucosal fold (Bedford, 1983), the eversion of the mucosa lining the lateral ventricles, a subsequent inward and downward rotational distortion of parts of the arytenoid cartilages, and a dorsal scrolling of the epiglottis.

4.4.3. Laryngeal disorders

Laryngeal disease is characterized by coughing, altered phonation and varying degrees of obstructive dyspnea. Inspiratory stridor (or in severe cases both inspiratory and expiratory stridor) and exercise intolerance are additional features of obstructive dyspnea of laryngeal origin. This condition can lead to cyanosis and asphyxiation. Observation of the patient at rest is helpful, but exercise may be necessary to induce dyspnea. Satisfactory examination of the larynx requires general anesthesia. However, endoscopy can be performed under sedation and permits an eventual diagnosis of laryngeal paralysis, which can be further evaluated by electromyographic studies (Venker-van Haagen, 1980).

Disease conditions of the larynx include trauma, presence of foreign bodies, infection, laryngeal spasm, paralysis or collapse, and neoplasia. Congenital unilateral and bilateral paralysis has been recorded in the Bouvier des Flandres (Venker-van Haagen, 1980) and the Siberian Husky breeds. Bilateral paralysis is most commonly encountered in elderly dogs of the larger breeds, as the result of neurogenic atrophy of the laryngeal musculature (O'Brien et al, 1973). Quantitative evaluation of airway obstruction in bilateral laryngeal paralysis has been performed using tidal breathing flow-volume loops (Amis et al, 1986).

4.4.4. Tracheal disorders

Obstructive pathologies of the canine trachea include essentially tracheal collapse, congenital hypoplasia, segmental stenosis (Bradley et al, 1987), inflammatory diseases, tumors and extra-luminal compression (mediastinal or intrathoracic masses).

Tracheal collapse is an acquired disease recognized in middle-aged to aged dogs of toy and miniature breeds (Hedlund, 1991). This syndrome is characterized by a chronic "goose honk" cough, associated with paroxysmal features of varying degrees of respiratory distress. The condition is occasionally associated (1) with chronic mitral valvular fibrosis, a condition in which the pressure of the enlarged left atrium upon the left main primary bronchus may aggravate the tracheal cough, even in the absence of heart failure, (2) with hepatomegaly, which can result in decreased ventilatory capacity and compromised respiratory exchange, and (3) with dental tartar.

Diagnosis can be confirmed by tracheoscopy and by both still and motion radiographic studies. During the phase of maximal inspiration, collapse of the cervical tracheal segment and dilation of the thoracic segment are imaged. Conversely, the study made during expiration usually shows a collapse of the thoracic segment, which is more frequently encountered.

Hypoplastic trachea is a congenital disorder recognized primarily in young brachycephalic dogs (Coyne and Fingland, 1992). The condition varies from mild to severe, the severity determining the prognosis for long-term survival of the patient. The condition is associated with chronic respiratory distress and coughing, intermittent acute bronchopneumonia, and recurrent episodes of upper respiratory tract infection. Radiographic determination of the tracheal diameter (Suter et al, 1972; Harvey and Fink, 1982) and radiographic motion studies are helpful in the assessement of the trouble.

Pathologic conditions that are associated with an extraluminal tracheal obstruction include tumor of the larynx, thyroid and parathyroid, enlargement of the mandibular, retropharyngeal or superficial cervical lymph nodes due to infection, neoplasia or granuloma, peritracheal abcesses and cysts, tracheal ring neoplasia, cranial mediastinal masses, thymomas, esophageal tumors or granulomas. Chronic coughing, stertorous breathing, respiratory distress and dyspnea are usually obvious. Pulmonary edema develops in more advanced cases. In most instances, the animal's condition continues to deteriorate despite symptomatic treatment. Radiography and bronchoscopy reveal information relevant for the etiology of the signs of upper airway obstruction.

4.4.5. Lower airway disorders

Patients with bronchial disease commonly are presented with coughing as the major complaint. Other signs of pulmonary disease, such as exercise intolerance, increased respiratory effort, cyanosis and systemic signs can occur as well but are relatively uncommon unless pulmonary parenchyma is also involved. Pneumonia can occur secondary to diseased airways and decreased clearance mechanisms. Auscultation can reveal normal lung sounds, increased bronchial vesicular sounds, wheezes or crackles. Thoracic radiographs inconsistently demonstrate a bronchial pattern when inflammatory disease is present. Inflammation is more effectively assessed by bronchoscopy (Venker-van Haagen, 1979; Amis and McKiernan, 1986) and analysis of bronchial lavage fluid (Hawkins et al, 1990). Septic inflammation is diagnostic for primary or secondary infection. Eosinophilic inflammation occurs with allergic (hypersensitivity) responses or parasitic diseases. Nonseptic chronic inflammation is suggestive of chronic bronchitis. Thoracic radiographs may show evidence of other bronchial diseases, such as bronchial masses, bronchiectasis or bronchial compression.

In feline allergic syndrome (feline asthma), symptoms result from bronchoconstriction, bronchial smooth muscle hypertrophy, inflammatory cell infiltration, increased mucus production and decreased mucus clearance (Moise and Spaulding, 1981; Moise et al, 1989). A type 1 hypersensitivity response is postulated, although the specific mechanisms for the syndrome in cats have not been thoroughly investigated.

Newer methods of diagnostic evaluation include tidal breathing flow-volume loops analysis and lung resistance measurements (McKiernan et al, 1989; Dye and Moise, 1992). Techniques to objectively measure lung function changes in individual cats could provide a better understanding and documentation of the different types of bronchial diseases in this species.

Allergic bronchitis in dogs is not a well-defined clinical entity, because dogs suffering from this condition frequently have co-existing problems, such as chronic bronchitis, bacterial infection or tracheal collapse. However, the dog has been used as an experimental model for allergic bronchitis with hypersensitivity responses created with ragweed and ascarid antigens (Chung et al, 1985).

Measurement of respiratory impedance using the forced oscillation method has been proved useful in detecting histamine-induced bronchospasm in dogs (Clercx et al, in press) and could be a useful tool for the diagnosis and treatment assessment of patients with obstructive lower airway disease.

Chronic bronchitis in dogs is a complex disease that has been well documented by both spontaneous and experimentally induced cases. Small breed adult dogs, often overweight, are most commonly affected.

Loss of cilia, bronchial gland hyperplasia and hypertrophia and increased goblet cells are present together with increased mucus within the airways. Grossly, these alterations result in hyperemic thickened bronchial walls, increased amount of mucus with obstruction of small airways, and sometimes polypoid proliferations of the epithelial surface. Atmospheric pollution, infection, allergic and genetic factors may be involved in initiating these changes (Amis, 1986). The obstructive disease causes air trapping and an abnormal distribution of ventilation and perfusion within the lungs, despite an excellent collateral ventilation in both dogs and cats (Robinson, 1982). The latter troubles can be assessed by lung scintigraphy (Clercx et al, 1989a).

Primary ciliary dyskinesia is a result of one or more defects of ciliary microtubules identifiable by electron microscopy. The disease is genetically transmitted. As a result of this condition, many different clinical features have been recognized in dogs, such as situs inversus, chronic rhinitis and sinusitis, chronic bronchitis, bronchiolitis, bronchiectasis, otitis media, hydrocephalus and male infertility (Edwards et al, 1983; Morrison et al, 1987; Edwards et al, 1989; Hoover et al, 1989).

5. CONCLUSIONS

Obstructive diseases are common in domestic animals. They are frequently responsible for poor performance, impaired gas exchange and sometimes severe respiratory distress syndrome. An accurate evaluation of the functional disorders is essential for an efficient therapeutic strategy.

REFERENCES

AMIS T.C. Chronic bronchitis in dogs. In : *Current Veterinary Therapy IX Small Animal Practice*, Kirk, R.W., Bonagura, J.D. (Eds), W.B. Saunders Company, Philadelphia,

1986, pp 306-313.
AMIS T.C., KURPERSHOEK C. Pattern of breathing in brachycephalic dogs. *Am. J. Vet. Res.* 1986, 47, 2200-2204.
AMIS T.C., McKIERNAN B.C. Systematic identification of endobronchial anatomy during bronchoscopy in the dog. *Am. J. Vet. Res.* 1986, 47, 2649-2657.
AMIS T.C., SMITH M.M., GABER C.E., KURPERSHOEK C. Upper airway obstruction in canine laryngeal paralysis. *Am. J. Vet. Res.* 1986, 47, 1007-1010.
ART T., SERTEYN D., LEKEUX P. Effect of exercise on the partitioning of equine respiratory resistance. *Equine Vet. J.* 1988, 20, 268-273.
ART T., LEKEUX P. Mechanical properties of the isolated equine trachea. *Res. Vet. Sci.* 1991a, 51, 55-60.
ART T., LEKEUX P. The effect of shape, age, and extension on the compliance of equine tracheal segment. *Vet. Res. Commun.* 1991b, 15, 135-146.
ART T., LEKEUX P. Booster vaccination in thoroughbred horses with oily adjuvanted inactived vaccine against influenza and rhinopneumonia. Effect on cardio-respiratory and metabolic adjustments to strenuous exercise and intense training. *J. Vet. Med. A.*, 1993, in press
BAYLY W.M., GRANT B.D., BREEZE R.G. Arterial blood gas tensions and acid base balance during exercise in horses with pharyngeal lymphoid hyperplasia. *Equine Vet. J.* 1984a, 16, 435-438.
BAYLY W.M., GRANT B.D., MODRANSKY P.D. Arterial blood gas tensions during exercise in a horse with laryngeal hemiplegia,.before and after corrective surgery. *Res. Vet. Sci.* 1984b, 36, 256-258.
BEDFORD P.G.C. Displacement of the glosso-epiglottic mucosa in canine asphyxiate disease. *J. Small Anim. Pract.* 1983, 24, 199.
BELKNAP J.K., DERKSEN F.J., NICKELS F.A., STICK J.A., ROBINSON N.E. Failure of subtotal arytenoidectomy to improve upper airway flow mechanics in exercising standardbreds with induced laryngeal hemiplegia. *Am. J. Vet. Res.* 1990, 51, 1481-1487.
BRADLEY R.L., SCHAAF J.P. Tracheal resection and anastomosis for traumatic tracheal collapse in a dog. *Comp. Cont. Educ. Pract. Vet.* 1987, 9, 234-240.
BROADSTONE R.V., SCOTT J.S., DERKSEN F.J., ROBINSON N.E. Effects of atropine in ponies with recurrent airway obstruction. *J. Appl. Physiol.* 1988, 65, 2720-2725.
BURRELL M.H. Endoscopic and virological observations on respiratory disease in a group of young thoroughbred horses in training. *Equine Vet. J.* 1985, 17, 99-103.
CARRIG C., GROENENDYK S., SEAWRIGHT A. Dorsoventral flattening of the trachea in a horse and its attempted surgical correction: a case report. *J. Am. Vet. Radiol. Soc.* 1973, 14, 32-36.
CHUNG K.F., BECKER A.B., LAZARUS S.C., FRICK O.L., NADEL J.A., GOLD W.M. Antigen-induced airway hyperresponsiveness and pulmonary inflammation in allergic dogs. *J. Appl. Physiol.* 1985, 58, 1347-1353.
CLERCX C., VAN DEN BROM W.E., STOKHOF A.A., DE VRIES H.W. Pulmonary scintigraphy in canine lobar and sublobar airway obstruction. *Lung* 1989a, 167, 213-224.
CLERCX C., GUSTIN P., LEKEUX P., HENROTEAUX M., LANDSER F.J. Measurements of total respiratory impedance in dogs during nasal obstruction by the forced oscillation method. In Proceedings : 7th Comparative Respiratory Society Meeting, Liege, 1989b, pp 53.
CLERCX C., GUSTIN P., LANDSER F.J., VAN DE WOESTIJNE K.P. Measurements of total respiratory impedance in dogs by the forced oscillation technique. *Vet. Res.*

Commun., 1993, in press.
COIGNOUL F., MOES J., DEWAELE A. Les mécanismes de défense de l'appareil respiratoire chez le porc. *Rec. Méd. Vét.* 1987, 163, 371-380.
COYNE B.E., FINGLAND R.B. Hypoplasia of the trachea in dogs: 103 cases (1974-1990). *J. Am. Vet. Med. Assoc.* 1992, 201, 768-772.
CRIMI E., BALBO A., MILANESE M., MIADONNA A., ROSSI G.A., BRUSASCO V. Airway inflammation and occurrence of delayed bronchoconstriction in exercise-induced asthma. *Am. Rev. Respir. Dis.* 1992, 146, 507-512.
DELISLE F. Scanner et affections naso-sinusales. In Proceedings : Congrès CNVSPA, Paris, 1992, pp 365-367.
DERKSEN F.J., SCOTT B.S., ROBINSON N.E., SLOCOMBE R.F., ARMSTRONG P.J. Intravenous histamine administration in ponies with recurrent airway obstruction (heaves). *Am. J. Vet. Res.* 1985, 46, 774-777.
DERKSEN F.J., SCOTT E.A., STICK J.A., ROBINSON N.E., SLOCOMBE R.F. Effect of laryngeal hemiplegia and laryngoplasty on upper airway flow mechanics in exercising horses. *Am. J. Vet. Res.* 1986, 47, 16-20.
DEVOUS M.D., THEODORAKIS B.S., HILLIDGE B. Scintigraphic evaluation of pulmonary perfusion and ventilation in equine respiratory disease. *Proc. Ann. Conv. Am. Ass. Equine Pract.* 1980, 25, 373-374.
DIXON P.M., NICHOLLS J.M., McPHERSON E.A., LAWSON G.H., THOMSON J.R., PIRIE H.W., BREEZE R.G. Chronic obstructive pulmonary disease. Anatomical cardiac studies. *Equine Vet. J.* 1982, 14, 80-85.
DYE J.A., MOISE N.S. Feline bronchial disease. In: *Current Veterinary Therapy XI Small Animal Practice*, Kirk, R.W., Bonagura, J.D. (Eds), W.B. Saunders Company, Philadelphia, 1992, pp 803-811.
EDWARDS D.E., PATTON C.S., BEMIS D.A., KENNEDY J.R., SELLER B.A. Immotile cilia syndrome in three dogs from a litter. *J. Am. Vet. Med. Assoc.* 1983, 183, 667-672.
EDWARDS D.E., KENNEDY J.R., PATTON C.S., TOAL R.L., DANIEL G.B., LOTHROP C.D. Familiale-immotile-cilia syndrome in English springer spaniel dogs. *Am. J. Med. Genet.* 1989, 33, 290-298.
GENICOT B., CLOSE R., MOULIGNEAU F., LEKEUX P. Clinical and pulmonary function changes induced by aerosoltherapy during bovine acute respiratory distress syndrome. In Proceedings : XVIIth World Buiatrics Congress, St Paul, USA, 1992, pp 236-241.
GENICOT B., MOULIGNEAU F., ROLLIN F., LINDSEY J.K., CLOSE R., LEKEUX P. Economic, clinical and functional consequences of a treatment with metrenperone during an outbreak of Shipping Fever in cattle. *Vet. Rec.* 1993, 132, 245-247.
GILES C.J. Atropic Rhinitis. In : *Diseases of Swine*, 6th edn, Leman A.D. et al. (Eds), Iowa State University Press, Ames, 1986, pp 455-469.
GUSTIN P., BAKIMA M., LEKEUX P., LOMBA F., VAN DE WOESTIJNE K.P. Partitioning of upper airway resistance in Friesian and double-muscled calves. *Respir. Physiol.* 1987, 69, 299-306.
HACKETT R.P., DUCHARME N.G., FUBINI S.L., ERB H.N. Evaluation of the reliability of endoscopic examination in assessment of arytenoid cartilage movement in horses:1. Subjective and objective laryngeal evaluation. *Vet. Surg.* 1991, 20, 174-179.
HARDY J. Upper respiratory obstruction in foals, weanlings and yearlings. *Vet. Clin. North Am.: Equine Pract.* 1991, 7, 105-122.
HARVEY C.E., BIERY D.N., MORELLO J., O'BRIEN J.A. Chronic nasal disease in the dog: its radiographic diagnosis. *Vet. Radiol.* 1979, 20, 91-98.
HARVEY C.E., FINK E.A. Tracheal diameter: Analysis of radiographic measurements in

brachycephalic and nonbrachycephalic dogs. *J. Am. Anim. Hosp. Assoc.* 1982, 18, 570-576.
HAWKINS E.C., DeNICOLA D.B., KUEHN N.F. Bronchoalveolar lavage in the evaluation of pulmonary disease in the dog and cat. *J. Vet. Intern. Med.* 1990, 4, 267.
HAYNES P.F. Persistent dorsal displacement of the soft palate associated with epiglottic shortening in two horses. *J. Am. Vet. Med. Assoc.* 1981, 179, 677-681.
HEDLUND C.S. Tracheal collapse. *Probl. Vet. Med.* 1991, 3, 229-238.
HENDRICKS J.C., KOVALSKI R.J., KLINE L.R. Phasic respiratory muscle patterns and sleep-disordered breathing during rapid eye movement sleep in Bulldogs. *Am. Rev. Respir. Dis.* 1991, 144, 1112-1120.
HENDRICKS J.C., PETROF B.J., PANCKERI K., PACKJ A.I. Compensatory hyperactivity of an upper airway dilator in Bulldogs. *Am. Rev. Respir. Dis.* 1992, 145, A402.
HONNAS C.M., SCHUMACHER J., DEAN P.W. Epiglottic entrapment: the techniques for diagnosis and surgical treatment. *Vet. Med.* 1990, 613-619.
HOOVER J.P., HOWARD-MARTIN M.O., BARH R.J. Chronic bronchitis, bronchiectasis, bronchiolitis, bronchiolitis obliterans, and bronchopneumonia in a Rottweiler with primary ciliary dyskinesia. *J. Am. Anim. Hosp. Assoc.* 1989, 25, 297-304.
JENSEN R., MACKEY D.R. Diseases of Feedlot Cattle, 2nd edn, Lea & Febiger, Philadelphia, 1974, pp 109-114.
KELLY D.F. Pathology of extranasal lesions in experimental inclusion body rhinitis of pigs. *Res. Vet. Sci.* 1967, 8, 472-478.
LEBLANC P.H., BAKER J.C., GRAY P.R., ROBINSON N.E., DERKSEN F.J. Effects of bovine respiratory syncytial virus on airway function in neonatal calves. *Am. J. Vet. Res.* 1991, 52, 1401-1406.
LEKEUX P., HAJER R., BOON J.H., VERSTEGEN M.W., BREUKINK H.J. Physiological effects of experimental verminous bronchitis in Friesian calves. *Can. J. Comp. Med.* 1985a, 49, 205-207.
LEKEUX P., HAJER R., BREUKINK H.J. Longitudinal study of the effects of lungworm infection on bovine pulmonary function. *Am. J. Vet. Res.* 1985b, 46, 1392-1395.
LEKEUX P., VERHOEFF J., HAJER R., BREUKINK H.J. Respiratory syncytial virus pneumonia in Friesian calves: physiological findings. *Res. Vet. Sci.* 1985c, 39, 324-327.
LEKEUX P., KYAVU A., CLERCX C., ANSAY M. Pulmonary function changes induced by experimental dichlorvos toxicosis in calves. *Res. Vet. Sci.* 1986, 40, 318-321.
LEKEUX P., ART T. Functional changes induced by necrotic laryngitis in double-muscled calves. *Vet. Rec.* 1987, 121, 353-355.
LEKEUX P., ART T., AMORY H. The effect of common bovine respiratory diseases on tidal breathing flow-volume loops. *Vet. Res. Commun.* 1988, 12, 463-473.
LINFORD R.L., O'BRIEN T.R., WHEAT J.D., MEAGHER D.M. Radiographic assessment of epiglottic length and pharyngeal and laryngeal diameters in the thouroughbred. *Am. J. Vet. Res.* 1983, 44, 1660-1666.
MAIR T.S., LANE J.G. Tracheal obstructions in two horses and a donkey. *Vet. Rec.* 1990, 126, 303-304.
MANOHAR M. Right heart pressures and blood-gas tensions in ponies during exercise and laryngeal hemiplegia. *Am. J. Physiol.* 1986, 251, H121-H126.
McFADDEN E.R. Jr, INGRAM R.H. Exercise-induced airway obstruction. *Ann. Rev. Physiol.* 1983, 45, 453-463.
McKIERNAN B.C., DYE J.A., ROZANSKI E.A., JONES S.D., HAYES B. Lung resistance and dynamic compliance in normal cats (abstract). In Proceedings : 8th

Comparative Respiratory Society Meeting, Liege, 1989, P24.
MEAD J., TAKISHIMA T., LEITH D. Stress distribution in lungs: a model of pulmonary elasticity. *J. Appl. Physiol.* 1970, 28, 596-608.
MITTEN R.W. Acquired nasopharyngeal stenosis in cats. In : *Current Veterinary Therapy XI Small Animal Practice*, Kirk, R.W., Bonagura, J.D. (Eds), W.B. Saunders Company, 1992, pp 801-803.
MOISE N.S., SPAULDING G.L. Feline bronchial asthma: pathogenesis, pathophysiology, diagnostics, and therapeutic considerations. *Compend. Cont. Educ. Pract. Vet.* 1981, 3, 1091-1102.
MOISE N.S., WIEDENKELLER D., YEAGER A.E., BLUE J.T., SCARLETT J. Clinical, radiographic, and bronchial cytologic features of cats with bronchial disease: 65 cases (1980-1986). *J. Am. Vet. Med. Assoc.* 1989, 194, 14671473.
MORRIS E.A., SEEHERMAN H.J. Clinical evaluation of poor performance in the racehorse: the results of 275 evaluations. *Equine Vet. J.* 1991, 23, 169-174.
MORRISON W.B., DAGMAR E.G., ROTH J.A., WILSMAN N.J. Assessment of neutrophil function in dogs with primary ciliary dyskinesia. *J. Am. Vet. Med. Assoc.* 1987, 191, 425-430.
MUYLLE E., VAN DEN HENDE C., OYAERT W. Nitrogen clearance in horses as a respiratory function test. *J. Vet. Med. A* 1972, 19, 310-317.
MUYLLE E., OYAERT W. Lung function tests in obstructive pulmonary disease in horses. *Equine Vet. J.* 1973, 5, 37-44.
MUYLLE E., NUYTTEN J., DEPREZ P., VAN DEN HENDE C., OYAERT W. Pulmonary driving pressure as a pulmonary function test in horses. *Equine Vet. Sci.* 1982, 4, 57-59.
NIELSEN N.C. Prevalence and economic significance of atropic rhinitis. Atropic rhinitis of pigs. *Comm. Eur. Communities Rep. EUR 8643 EN*, Luxembourg, 1983, pp 35.
O'BRIEN J.A., HARVEY C.E., KELLY A.M., TUCKERS J.A. Neurogenic atrophy of the laryngeal muscles of the dog. *J. Small Anim. Pract.* 1973, 14, 521-532.
O'CALLAGHAN M.W. Scintigraphic Imaging of Lung Disease in Equine Respiratory Disorders, Beech J. (Ed.), Lea & Febiger, Philadelphia, 1991.
PEDERSEN K.B., NIELSEN N.C. Atropic rhinitis of pigs. *Comm. Eur. Communities Rep. EUR 8643 EN*, Luxembourg, 1983, pp 205.
PIJOAN C. Respiratory system. In : *Diseases of Swine*, 6th edn, Leman, A.D. et al (Eds), Iowa State University Press, Ames, 1986, pp 152-162.
ROBINSON N.E., SORENSON P.R. Collateral flow resistance and time constant in dog and horse lungs. *J. Appl. Physiol.* 1978, 44, 63-68.
ROBINSON N.E. Functional abnormalities caused by upper airway obstruction and heaves: their relationship to the etiology of epistaxis. *Vet. Clin. North Am.: Large Anim. Pract.* 1979, 1, 17-34.
ROBINSON N.E. Some functional consequences of species differences in lung anatomy. *Adv. Vet. Sci. Comp. Med.* 1982, 26, 1-33.
ROBINSON N.E. Rôle du système nerveux autonome dans l'obstruction des voies aériennes du cheval. *Ann. Méd. Vét.* 1993, 137, 153-159.
SUTER P.F., COLGROVE D.J., EWING G.O. Congenital hypoplasia of the canine trachea. *J. Am. Anim. Hosp. Assoc.* 1972, 8, 120-127.
TURGUT K., SASSE H.H.L. Influence of clenbuterol on mucociliary transport in healthy horses and horses with chronic obstructive pulmonary disease. *Vet. Rec.* 1989, 125, 526-530.
VENKER-VAN HAAGEN A.J. Bronchoscopy of the normal and abnormal canine. *J. Am. Anim. Hosp. Assoc.* 1979, 15, 397-410.
VENKER-VAN HAAGEN A.J. Investigations on the pathogenesis of hereditary laryngeal

paralysis in the Bouvier. Thesis, Utrecht University, 1980.
VENKER-VAN HAAGEN A.J., VAN OOSTERHOUT I.C.A.M., MEIJ B.P., CLERCX C. L'examen rhinoscopique en clinique des petits animaux: analyse de 233 rhinoscopies. *Prat. Méd. Chir. Anim. Comp.* 1990, 25, 79-87.
WILLIAMS J.W., MEAGHER D.M., PASCOE J.R., HORNOF W.J. Upper airway function during maximal exercise in horses with obstructive upper airway lesions. Effect of surgical treatment. *Vet. Surg.* 1990a, 19, 142-147.
WILLIAMS J.W., PASCOE J.R., MEAGHER D.M., HORNOF W.J. Effects of left recurrent laryngeal neurectomy, prosthetic laryngoplasty, and subtotal arytenoidectomy on upper airway pressure during maximal exertion. *Vet. Surg.* 1990b, 19, 136-141.
WILLOUGHBY R., ECKER G., McKEE S., RIDOLLS L., VERNAILLEN C., DUBOUI E., LEIN D., MAHONY J.B., CHERNESKY M., MAGY E. The effects of equine rhinovirus, influenza virus and herpesvirus infection on tracheal clearance rate in horses. *Can. J. Vet. Res.* 1992, 56, 115-121.
WYKES P.M. Brachycephalic airway obstructive syndrome. *Probl. Vet. Med.* 1991, 3, 188-197.

CHAPTER XII

FUNCTIONAL EFFECTS OF VASCULAR PULMONARY DISEASES

P. Lekeux[1], C. Clercx[2] and T. Art[3]

[1] Laboratory for Functional Investigation
[2] Department of Small Animal Medicine
[3] Equine Sport Medicine Unit
Faculty of Veterinary Medicine
University of Liege

SUMMARY

This paper describes the functional peculiarities of the pulmonary vascular diseases in domestic animals.

KEY WORDS

Respiratory system - Pulmonary function - Vascular diseases.

1. INTRODUCTION

There is a close relationship between the airways and the pulmonary vasculature. Each system is closely related to the other and a dysfunction of one of the systems may impair the function of the other. Dysfunction in the pulmonary vascular bed is frequently related to changes in the vascular tone.

The vasomotor tone in the pulmonary vessels actually results from a balance between vasoconstriction and vasodilatation. Substances such as autacoids, cytokines and neuropeptides are potent vasomodulators of the pulmonary circulation. For instance, histamine, serotonin, thromboxane, tumor necrosis factor and endothelins are vasoconstrictors while bradykinins, vasoactive intestinal peptide and nitric oxide are vasodilators. Some mediators such as substance P, histamine, serotonin, bradykinin, platelet activating factor, complement, leukotrienes and tumor necrosis factor are also able to modify the vascular permeability.

In the normal lung, some of these substances are inexistent, some are metabolized and inactivated by the vascular endothelium and some are counterbalanced by the action of other factors.

In the diseased lung, the inflammatory response is mediated by some of these vasoactive substances, inducing modifications in the vascular smooth muscle tone. The increased effect of the vasoactive substances is related to (1) an increased production, (2) a decreased inactivation, for instance when the vascular endothelium is damaged, or (3) a decrease of antagonistic vasoactive substances.

The main alterations in the vascular pulmonary diseases are related to (1) an increase of the pressure in the pulmonary artery, i.e. pulmonary hypertension, (2) an increased permeability of the vessel membranes, (3) an obturation of the vessels, i.e. pulmonary embolism, and (4) a rupture of the vascular wall, i.e. pulmonary hemorrhage.

This paper summarizes the influence of vascular dysfunction on the pulmonary function. After a general description of the main functional syndromes, their physiopathological mechanisms and their functional consequences, some species peculiarities are presented.

2. PULMONARY HYPERTENSION

The mean pulmonary artery pressure is maintained between strict physiological limits that are specific for each species. When the mean pulmonary artery pressure exceeds the normal resting values, the patient is said to suffer from pulmonary hypertension. The increase in vascular pressure may in turn induce disorders at the level of the lung ventilation. The ultimate pathophysiologic consequence of pulmonary hypertension is right heart hypertrophy and failure. This so-called "cor pulmonale" refers to right heart disease secondary to primary disease of the lung.

The three fundamental causes of pulmonary hypertension are increases (1) in pulmonary blood flow, (2) in outflow pressure, generally left atrial pressure, and (3) in pulmonary vascular resistance. In the first and the last cases, the pulmonary wedge pressure, representing the left atrial pressure, remain unchanged, while in the second case, this pressure is increased.

2.1. Increase in pulmonary blood flow

Exercise is a physiological factor which induces a sharp increase in pulmonary blood flow. The pulmonary artery and the wedge pressures are increased approximately in the same proportion, while the pulmonary vascular resistance decreases, because of the recruitment and/or dilation of the pulmonary vasculature. Mean pressure increases from 28 to 80 mmHg have been reported in the pulmonary artery of fast running horses (Erickson et al, 1992). Nevertheless, this hypertension is transient and has no deleterious consequences on the respiratory function.

Congenital heart diseases with a left-to-right shunt through interventricular or interatrial septal defects cause an increase in pulmonary blood flow, which in turn induces a rise in pulmonary arterial pressure (Edward, 1988). This phenomenon is rather small because of the ability of the pulmonary capillaries to sustain high blood flow (Reeves et al, 1989). Sometimes, the pulmonary pressures may nevertheless reach systemic levels, causing right-to-left shunts and arterial hypoxemia.

With persistent pulmonary hypertension, a thickening of the pulmonary arterial wall occurs (Edward, 1988), inducing a secondary increase in the vascular pressure.

2.2. Increase in outflow pressure

Increase in left atrial pressure occurs by mitral stenosis, by a left ventricular failure or by an increased preload induced for instance by aortic valve insufficiency. When the pulmonary venous pressure is increased, the pulmonary artery pressure also increases, but to a lesser extent, because the pulmonary vascular resistance decreases. In acute conditions, the principal consequence is the occurrence of pulmonary edema. In contrast, in chronic conditions, a sequence of changes occurs in both the lung parenchyma and vasculature, leading to increased pulmonary vascular resistance, and hence, to an increase in pulmonary artery pressure. The consequent pulmonary hypertension is stipulated as "passive".

In the early stage, the lung is congested and the interstitial spaces are expanded by edema. The basement membranes become thickened. With connective tissue proliferation, the lung becomes heavy and stiff. In later stages, these changes progress into alveolar fibrosis, local collection of macrophages and mast cells, scattered hemorrhages and even patchy ossifications. As the vascular pathology progresses, the vascular lumen is narrowed or even closed, and part of the increase in resistance is due to the reduction of the cross-sectional area of the vessels.

2.3. Increase in pulmonary vascular resistance

The increase in pulmonary vascular resistance is the most common cause of pulmonary hypertension. The resistance may increase following vasoconstrictive, obstructive or obliterative problems.

2.3.1. Vasoconstriction

Hypoxic pulmonary vasoconstriction results from alveolar hypoxia in animals living at high altitude or in patients suffering from respiratory disorders. The stimulation for hypoxic vasoconstriction is related to both the alveolar and the mixed venous oxygen tension. The greater the hypoxia and the larger the fraction of lung involved, the more the response shifts from the homeostatic maintenance promoting blood oxygenation towards the physiopathologic endpoint of generalized pulmonary vasoconstriction with pulmonary hypertension and increased right heart work.

The most typical form of acute or chronic pulmonary hypertension results from hypoxia at high altitude. The hypoxic pulmonary vasoconstriction response is present in the entire lung. In some species, the acute condition results in right heart failure and pulmonary edema, while the chronic condition may change in the pulmonary vasculature. There is however a large variability in the responses among species. Cattle have a vigourous hypoxic constrictor response, causing a right ventricular failure known as brisket disease (Robinson, 1982). Pigs, ponies and goats are slightly less reactive than cattle (Tucker et al, 1975; Bisgard et al, 1975) while dogs, cats and sheep do not develop pulmonary hypertension at altitude (Tucker et al, 1975).

Acute lung injury occurs in some patients suffering from septicemia or endotoxemia.

An experimental study, performed in sheep, demonstrated two main phases following administration of endotoxin (Brigham et al, 1979; Demling et al, 1981). There was an early and transient increase in pulmonary vascular resistance with pulmonary hypertension. This early pulmonary hypertension was due to vasoconstriction but the mechanisms leading to this vasoconstriction remain unclear. Various factors such as the increase of the plasma level of thromboxane (Parratt et al, 1982), the platelet release of serotonin (Demling et al, 1985) and adenosine diphosphate (Minnear et al, 1982), the activation of neutrophils by 12-lipoxygenase metabolites and the platelet-activating factor, the damage of the endothelium induced by the release of arachidonic acid products, oxygen free radicals and proteases (Brigham and Meyrick, 1984) have been suggested to be partly responsible for this primary phase of pulmonary hypertension. After approximately 3 hours, there was an increased vascular permeability with increased lymph flow, and the pulmonary pressure decreased. It was suggested that in this stage the pathophysiological processes were related to endotoxin that activates the complement and the release of tumor necrosis factor, which in turn activate the inflammatory cells to release other mediators and free radicals (Gee et al, 1985; Leeper-Woodford et al, 1991).

This has also been suggested by studies performed on isolated perfused pig lungs (Gustin et al, 1992; Urbain et al, 1992)

2.3.2. Loss of vasculature due to obstructive or obliterative disorders

Pulmonary hypertension can also result from mechanical obstruction or destruction of the vascular bed (Malik, 1983). The occlusion of a vessel generally results from thromboembolism, circulating fat, air or parasites.

Humoral factors released from leukocytes (Harlan, 1985), platelets (Vaage, 1982), plasma, lung endothelium, macrophages and mast cells (Harlan, 1985; Peters et al, 1987) also contribute to vascular injury (Malik, 1985).

Obliterative lesions occur in emphysema, when the capillary bed is partly destroyed. Other pulmonary parenchymal diseases such as scleroderma, interstitial fibrosis and granulomatous disease also increase pulmonary vascular resistance because they destroy blood vessels.

3. PULMONARY EDEMA

Fluid is normally exchanged between the pulmonary circulation and the interstitium, between the interstitium and the pleural space, and between the airway interstitium and epithelial surface. The fluid exchanges are well regulated, so that excessive fluid does not accumulate in the pulmonary interstitium nor in the pleural space. The accumulation of excessive fluid is

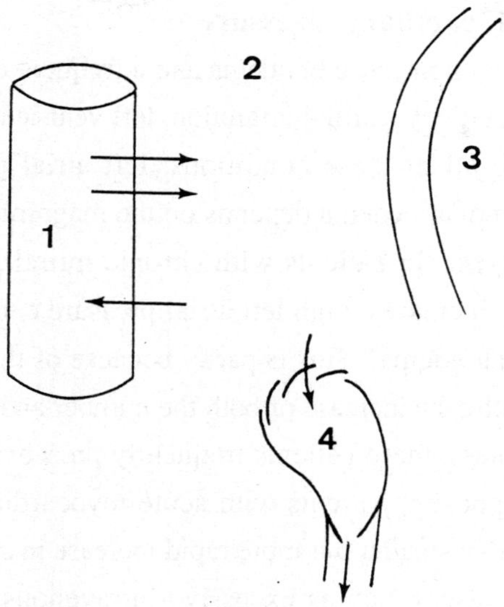

Fig. 12-1. Interrelationship between the pulmonary capillary (1), interstitium (2), alveolus (3) and lymphatic vessel (4). The arrows indicate the fluid movements in physiological conditions.

also prevented by the extensive lymphatic system that drains these areas. In healthy lungs, fluid formation equals fluid removal so that excessive fluid cannot enter the lung interstitium, alveoli or airways. Normally, transcapillary fluid exchange is controlled within very narrow limits, but in pathological conditions fluid may accumulate in the extravascular spaces and tissues of the lung. This phenomenon is called pulmonary edema. It can complicate a variety of heart and lung diseases, altering the gas exchange and the mechanics of breathing. Two stages of pulmonary edema are recognized, but the clinical differentiation may be difficult. The first phase is *interstitial edema*, which is characterized by engorgement of the perivascular and peribronchial interstitial tissues. The second phase is *alveolar edema*, when fluid moves into the alveoli (Fig. 12-1.).

3.1. Etiology

3.1.1. Increased capillary pressure

This is the most common cause of edema and a frequent complication of heart diseases such as acute myocardial infarction, left ventricular failure and mitral valve disease. In all of these conditions, left atrial pressure rises. The occurrence of pulmonary edema depends on the magnitude and on the rate of the pressure changes. In patients with chronic mitral failure in which the pressure gradually increases, high left atrial pressure can be reached without evidence of alveolar edema. This is partly because of the adjustement of the lymphatic drainageby the increase of both the number and the caliber of lymph vessels. Nevertheless, these patients frequently present a marked interstitial edema. On the opposite, patients with acute myocardial failure present an alveolar edema with a smaller but more rapid increase in capillary pressure. Noncardiogenic causes, such as excessive intravenous saline perfusion or acute renal failure, can also induce pulmonary edema. In these conditions, the edema is partly caused by the rise in the hydrostatic pressure, but also by an increase in capillary permeability apparently due to stretching of the endothelium induced by the increase of the capillary pressure.

3.1.2. Increased capillary permeability

Inhaled toxins such as sulfur dioxide or nitrogen oxide, or circulating toxins such as endotoxin, cause pulmonary edema because they increase capillary permeability. Immunologically-mediated processes such as purpura hemorrhagica also increase vascular permeability by complement activation.

3.1.3. Lymphatic insufficiency

This occurs in diseases in which the normal lymphatic drainage is impaired because of obliteration, distortion or compression of lymphatic vessels.

3.1.4. Others

Decreased interstitial pressure, as in pneumothorax or decreased osmotic

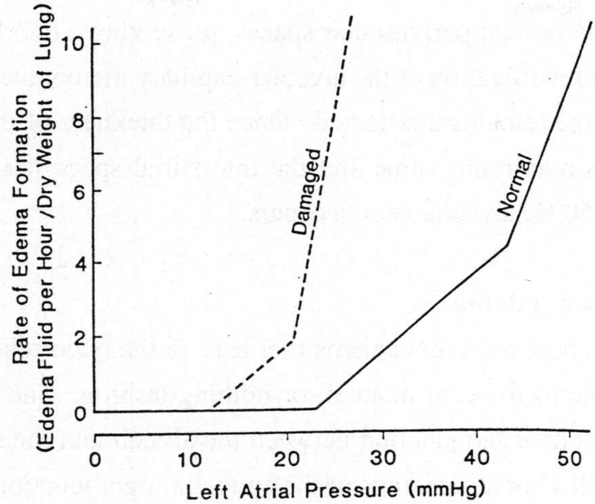

Fig. 12-2. Effect of the integrity of the lung capillary wall on the rate of edema formation (Taylor and Rippe, 1986).

pressure, as in hypoproteinemia, provoke much more rarely the occurrence of pulmonary edema.

3.2. Physiopathology

When left atrial pressure is abnormally high, the rise in capillary pressure rapidly causes fluid accumulation in the pulmonary interstitium. Furthermore, the rate of edema formation is accelerated by an increased concentration of interstitial proteins or a disruption of the alveolar-capillary membrane. Moreover, when the endothelium of the capillary wall is damaged, the fluid begins to accumulate more rapidly in the lung tissue even at a low left atrial pressure (Fig. 12-2.).

3.2.1. Interstitial edema

The occurrence of interstitial edema increases the alveolar-capillary membrane thickness by only 15-20 %. This modest increase is due to an expanded interstitial space. The tissue fluid moves rapidly from the gas exchange sites into the more compliant perivascular spaces, preserving a thin barrier for gas exchange. The modification of the alveolar-capillary membrane is so minimal that gas exchange remains unaffected. Once the thickness of the interstitium has reached its maximum value and the interstitial space has expanded by approximately 50 %, alveolar edema occurs.

3.2.2. Alveolar edema

Little is know about the mechanisms that lead to the occurrence of alveolar edema, but it seems to occur in an all-or-nothing fashion. The leaking site is supposed to be either the junction between the alveoli and the small alveolar ducts (Staub, 1984) or at openings of the epithelial tight junctions (Taylor and Rippe, 1986). These leakage sites are clearly not selective and do not restrict the passage of plasma proteins (Vreim et al, 1976). Once the fluid begins to fill the alveoli, blood oxygenation is affected (Aukland and Nicolaysen, 1981).

3.2.3. Alveolar safety factors

Edema formation is not detectable until left atrial pressure exceeds a certain level. The question of knowing why has led to the concept of tissue edema safety factors, which oppose the formation of pulmonary edema when capillary pressure is elevated (Guyton et al, 1975). The three tissue safety factors are : (1) a decreased filtration pressure because the tissue pressure increases immediately (Misserochi and Negrini, 1989); (2) an increased osmotic value because the protein concentration in the tissue is diluted (Erdmann et al, 1975); (3) a 5 to 10-fold increase in the lymph flow that carries away an important additional amount of fluid (Ishibashi et al, 1990). These safety factors are less efficient when the pulmonary capillary endothelium is damaged. In this case, the inefficiency of the safety factors is due to the fact that the lymphatic vessels are less effective in fluid removal and that the osmotic pressure in the tissues remains high because the capillary wall is permeable to plasma proteins (Gaar et al, 1967). For example, it has been shown that the capillary pressure required to induce edema is decreased from 23 to 12 mmHg for alloxan-treated canine lungs (Drake and Gabel, 1980) and from 23 to 15 mmHg in endotoxin-challenged sheep lungs (Gabel et al, 1984). In this condition, pulmonary edema can result even when the left atrial and the capillary pressures are normal. This phenomenon is called "low pressure edema" or "permeability edema", in opposition to "high pressure edema" which is due to left heart failure.

3.3. Functional effects

When capillary pressure increases, the pulmonary blood vessels are dilated (congestion) and interstitial edema begins to develop. This phenomenon induces a sharp drop in the dynamic lung compliance, while arterial blood gases remain steady in resting conditions. With further accumulation of extravascular lung water, alveolar edema occurs. As the result of surface tension forces, the edematous alveoli shrink in size. The alveolar ventilation and alveolo-arterial diffusion are impaired and arterial partial pressure in oxygen drops dramatically while the alveolo-arterial gradient increases. The arterial partial pressure in carbon dioxide is generally normal because of increased ventilation of the nonedematous alveoli.

The alveolar edema induces a further decrease in lung compliance. This decrease is related to the reduced distensibility of the lung because of the fluid within the interstitium, to the changes in surface properties related to alveolar edema, and to the decrease in lung volume.

During vascular congestion and edema formation, the vascular resistance and consequently the pulmonary arterial pressure rise because cardiac output remains normal. Hypoxic vasoconstriction of the poorly or unventilated areas contributes to this phenomenon. In addition, the perivascular "cuffing" probably also plays a role by compressing extra-alveolar vessels. Lastly, the collapse of the edematous alveoli and the edematous alveolar walls may compress the capillaries.

Airway resistance may be increased in severe cases because the blood vessel engorgement and fluid in the airways reduce their cross-sectional area. Reflex bronchoconstriction following stimulation of irritant receptors in the bronchial wall may also play a role.

The impaired oxygenation can be improved by mechanical ventilation of the patient, by increasing the inspired oxygen concentration and by diuretics.

4. PULMONARY EMBOLISM

4.1. Definition and pathophysiology

One of the functions of the lung is to filter the blood. The frequency of solid particles trapped in the blood vessels is unknown, but it is likely that it is not unusual. Small emboli are probably very common and frequently undiagnosed. In contrast, larger emboli may induce hemorrhage and atelectasis, and even pulmonary infarction, which are potentially fatal.

Most pulmonary emboli arise from venous thrombi formed in the deep veins of the lower extremities. Fat, air and amniotic fluid are also potential thrombi but this occurs more rarely. Factors which favor the formation of venous thrombi are stasis of the blood (local pressure, immobilization, venous obstruction), alterations in the blood coagulation system (change in blood viscosity) and abnormalities of the vascular walls (trauma, inflammation, phlebitis).

4.2. Functional effects

4.2.1. Effect on pulmonary hemodynamics

The most spectacular effect of pulmonary thromboemboli on pulmonary hemodynamics is an increase in pulmonary artery pressure (McIntyre and Sasahara, 1971). The pulmonary circulation normally has a large reserve capacity because many capillaries are unfilled. This reserve is so important that at least half of the pulmonary circulation can be obstructed by an embolus before there is a substantial rise in pulmonary artery pressure. In addition to the purely mechanical effect of the embolus, there is some evidence that active

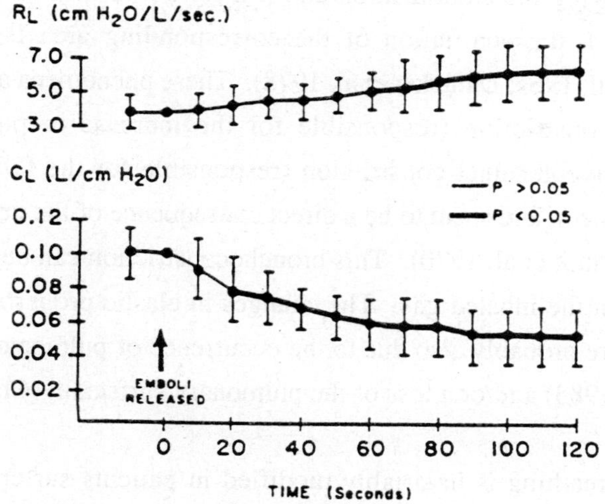

Fig. 12-3. Effect of pulmonary embolization on total pulmonary resistance (R_L) and dynamic lung compliance (C_L) (Thomas et al, 1964)

(hypoxic) vasoconstriction occurs in the remaining perfused area lasting at least for some minutes after embolization. In experimentally embolized dog lungs, a local release of serotonin from platelets associated with the embolus has been put forwards to explain this phenomenon, as well as a vasoconstriction reflex via the sympathetic nervous system (Dantzker et al, 1978).

If the embolus is large, the pulmonary arterial pressure may increase dramatically and right ventriclar failure may result. In few cases, pulmonary edema may occur, probably caused by leakage from those capillaries which are not protected from the raised pulmonary arterial pressure.

4.2.2. Effect on the respiratory and lung mechanics

In experimental animals, the response to thromboemboli is an increase in pulmonary resistance and a fall of both dynamic and static compliance (Fig. 12-3.) (Cahill et al, 1961; Thomas et al, 1964). These changes occur immediatly following the embolization and last for 30-40 min (Clark et al, 1970). Furtheron, the ventilation of the corresponding area is reduced (Severinghaus et al, 1961; Dantzker et al, 1978). These phenomena are due to a local bronchoconstriction (responsible for the increase in pulmonary resistance) and alveolar duct constriction (responsible for the fall of lung dynamic compliance), and seem to be a direct consequence of the decrease in alveolar PCO_2 (Clark et al, 1970). This bronchoconstriction can be reversed by adding CO_2 in the inhaled gas. The changes in elastic properties of the embolized area are probably also due to the occurrence of pulmonary edema (D'Alonzo et al, 1983) and/or a loss of the pulmonary surfactant (Chernick et al, 1966).

The pattern of breathing is invariably modified in patients suffering from pulmonary embolization. The respiration is rapid and shallow as well as dyspneic. Stimulation of pulmonary chemoreflex via the activation of pulmonary C fibers by the release of prostaglandins (Armstrong and Miller, 1980; Roberts et al, 1986) as well as serotonin (Coleridge and Coleridge, 1977), and stimulation of irritant receptors have been implicated in these modifications.

The constrictive response to vascular obstruction is generally weaker than the vascular response to airway obstruction (hypoxic vasoconstriction). However, it also aims to avoid a wastage, by reducing the physiological dead space. In man, this adaptation seems to be short-lasting or even nonexistant because several hours after a pulmonary embolization, the distribution of ventilation does not show a difference between the embolized and the unaffected areas.

4.2.3. Effect on gas exchange

Moderate hypoxemia without carbon dioxide retention is often seen in case of pulmonary embolism (Dantzker and Bower, 1982). Measurements by the multiple inert gas elimination technique have demonstrated that the abnormal gas exchange in patients suffering from embolism results from a combination

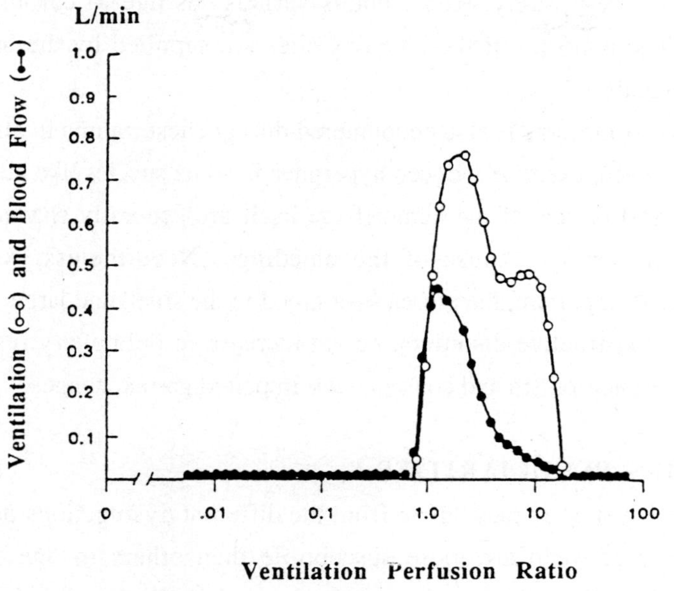

Fig. 12-4. Ventilation perfusion inhomogeneity in a patient suffering from a severe pulmonary embolism (D'Alonzo et al, 1983)

of several mechanisms including ventilation/perfusion inhomogeneity as main reason, and physiological shunts, increase in physiological dead space and diffusion impairment as more minor reasons (Fig. 12-4.) (D'Alonzo et al, 1983; Manier et al, 1985). Lastly, it has been shown that embolized lungs have areas with very high ventilation/perfusion ratio, i.e. sharp reduction of blood flow through the embolized regions, and very low ventilation/perfusion ratio, i.e. blood flow through areas of hemorrhagic atelectasis (Dantzker et al, 1978).

5. PULMONARY HEMORRHAGE

Most of the time, pulmonary hemorrhage is secondary to severe pulmonary lesions and generally originates in highly vascularized tissues such as the wall of a necrotizing bacterial cavity, the site of chronic bronchiectasis, a bronchial adenoma, or, very rarely, from venous varicosities due to chronic mitral stenosis. The majority of the bleeding sites are supplied by the bronchial artery collaterals.

Pulmonary hemorrhage is also encountered during chest trauma in all species and during severe exercise-induced hyperpnea in some species like horses.

The functional effects of the hemorrhage itself are generally shaded by the effect of the primary cause of the bleeding. Nevertheless, when the hemorrhage is important, the presence of blood in the small and larger airways may induce obstructive disorders, i.e. an increase in pulmonary resistance, ventilation asynchronism and consequently impaired gas exchanges.

6. SPECIES PECULIARITIES

Although each species may suffer from the different dysfunctions described above, some of them are more susceptible than others to one of these pathological conditions, according to their morphological and/or functional characteristics.

6.1. Equine species

6.1.1. Exercise-induced pulmonary hemorrhage

6.1.1.1. Definition, prevalence and epidemiology

Exercise-induced pulmonary hemorrhage is not a clinical entity nor a syndrome. It is rather a clinical sign that may be the result of heavy exercise and/or pathological changes and is defined as the presence of blood in the tracheobronchial tree following strenuous exercise. It is mainly described in horses. Endoscopic surveys of the lower airways in racing horses have demonstrated that a large number of horses show exercise-induced pulmonary hemorrhage, with a relatively low percentage presenting epistaxis. Several competitive events may induce the occurrence of exercise-induced pulmonary hemorrhage, especially when horses run at speeds of 14 m/sec or more. Reported incidences are approximately 30 % in Standardbred horses, 60 % in Quarter Horses (Hillidge et al, 1984) and up to 75 % in Thoroughbred horses

(Raphel and Soma, 1982). Repeated endoscopic examinations of horses after exercise reveal an even higher incidence of exercise-induced pulmonary hemorrhage : 95 % of the examined horses bled on at least one occasion (Burrell, 1985). Bleeding may occur soon after the start of training and tends to have an increasing incidence with increasing age (Raphel and Soma, 1982). There is no apparent sex difference in exercise-induced pulmonary hemorrhage susceptibility, and little geographic variation is found in the incidence either within or between countries.

6.1.1.2. Symptomatology

Most of the clinical signs are non-specific. They include blood in the tracheo-bronchial airways, and much less frequently epistaxis, either during or after exercise when the horse is released in its stall and allowed to lower its head. Other signs are more variable and include abnormal respiratory sounds, swallowing while running and labored breathing. As far as its effect on performance is concerned, in some horses there is no influence at all while in others a definite exercise intolerance is observed. Some authors did not find any association between race finishing position and exercise-induced pulmonary hemorrhage (Pascoe et al, 1981; Raphel and Soma, 1982; Sweeney and Soma, 1983). However, other studies showed that racing times are adversely influenced in the races in which horses suffering pulmonary hemorrhage were recognized (Soma et al, 1985).

6.1.1.3. Diagnosis

Several complementary tests are available to assess the diagnosis.

Blood may be detected in the trachea by endoscopic examination of the lower airways performed 60 to 90 minutes after the race (Fig. 12-5.). This blood is still visible 4 to 6 hours later. If exercise-induced pulmonary hemorrhage is strongly suspected and blood is not present in the trachea 60 minutes after exercise, a repeated endoscopic examination is recommended one hour later.

Cytologic examination of broncho-alveolar lavage reveals the presence of

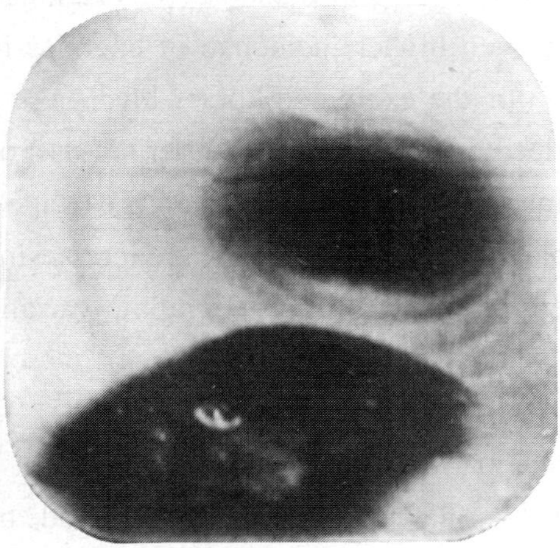

Fig. 12-5. Intratracheal endoscopic view of a "bleeder" after a race.

numerous haemosiderophages, neutrophils and sometimes eosinophils.

Radiographic evaluation of the lungs is of limited usefulness, as the interpretation of the findings is difficult. In horses suffering exercise-induced pulmonary hemorrhage, a discernible increase in interstitial density may be observed in the caudodorsal lobes of the lungs (O'Callaghan and Goulden, 1982; O'Callaghan et al, 1987c).

Ventilation/perfusion ratio scans show a variable reduction of ventilation and a loss of perfusion in the caudodorsal fields, with collateral supply from the bronchial circulation (O'Callaghan et al, 1987d).

6.1.1.4. Necroscopy findings

Because exercise-induced pulmonary hemorrhage is rarely fatal, necroscopic investigations have been generally performed on confirmed "bleeders" and the lesions observed are considered as end-stage findings. Post-mortem examination shows evidence that the caudodorsal lung lobes are the primary

sites of hemorrhage : blue-brown colored areas are generally distributed dorsally and laterally within the dorsal half of the caudal lobe. There is an increase in bronchial arterial vessels due to neovascularisation. The damaged regions receive their vascular supply almost exclusively from the bronchial arterial circulation (O'Callaghan et al, 1987a; 1987b).
The microscopic examination of these regions reveals mainly bronchiolitis and an increase in fibrous connective tissue.

6.1.1.5. Pathogenesis

While the epidemiology and the end-stage pathology are firmly established, there is still little understanding of the factors that predispose horses to exercise-induced pulmonary hemorrhage.
Exercise-induced pulmonary hemorrhage is so frequently encountered irrespective of the breed, the sport discipline, the age or sex of the horse, the regions of the world and the methods of management, that it is highly improbable that it has an unique etiology. Most likely, it is the result of the co-existence of multiple factors, some favouring or predisposing to the condition and others triggering the episode of exercise-induced pulmonary hemorrhage.

6.1.1.5.1. Affected vessels

Micropathological examination of end-stage exercise-induced pulmonary hemorrhage lesions shows destruction of alveolar tissue, extensive proliferation of bronchial blood vessels and greatly increased numbers of anastomoses between the bronchial and pulmonary circulations. The extent of the anastomotic flow depends on the relative pressure in the bronchial and pulmonary vasculature and on the alveolar pressure (Modell et al, 1981). The increase in the pressure gradient between the bronchial and the pulmonary artery could perhaps favour bronchial blood flow into the pulmonary circulation. The pulmonary capillaries could consequently be submitted to the high systemic pressure and rupture. However, it remains to be elucidated

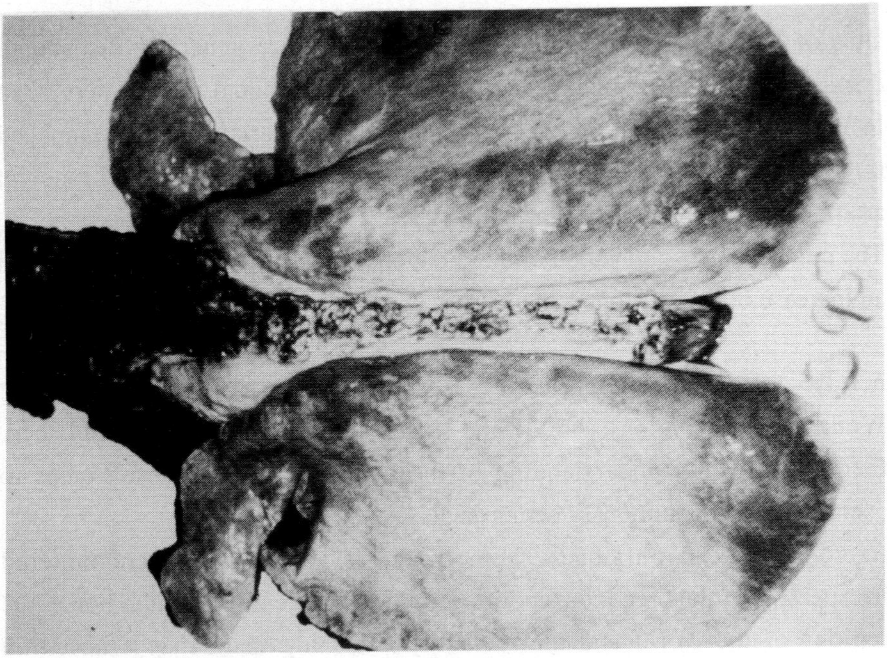

Fig. 12-6. Lungs of a "bleeder" showing dark colored areas in the caudodorsal lobes (O'Callaghan et al, 1987a).

whether the bronchial neovascularisation, which is a response to inflammation and is considered as integral part of pulmonary repair, occurs before or after the very first episode of exercise-induced pulmonary hemorrhage.
Therefore, until now, the exact source of bleeding remains unknown. Rupture of pulmonary or bronchial vessels at the capillary or arterial level may potentially be the source of the blood.

6.1.1.5.2. Coagulation

Although there is evidence of coagulation alteration in any exercising horse, platelet adhesiveness may decrease more in hemorrhage-positive horses than in normal horses, following exercise (Bayly et al, 1983). However, it is questionable whether this modification is sufficient to elicit spontaneous bleeding and why hemorrhages occur only at the level of the lungs.

6.1.1.5.3. Sites of bleeding

Most of the affected areas appear to be distributed in the caudodorsal broncho-pulmonary segments (Fig. 12-6.). There are some anatomical and functional characteristics of these regions which could explain their predispositon to bleeding during exercise.

First, this segment is subtended by the terminal divisions of the principal bronchus. Because of its axial alignment with the principal bronchus, it is likely that this segment would be a predilected site for deposition of inhaled particles. Secondly, because of the more negative intrapleural pressure at this level (Derksen and Robinson, 1980), the alveoli of these regions are fully dilated and consequently weakened. Thirdly, relatively smaller alveoli and thicker septa result in a regional difference in elastic properties and consequently in a greater respiratory asynchronism. Moreover, the regional decrease in the distribution of the pores of Kohn and therefore in the collateral ventilation enhances the inhomogeneity of the distribution of ventilation. Lastly, the caudodorsal region of the lung is the least well perfused by the pulmonary circulation in the resting horse : this could favour the bronchial blood flow to enter into the pulmonary circulation via the anastomoses.

6.1.1.5.4. Obstructive disorders

Chronic obstructive pulmonary disease has been suggested to be the underlying lesion in exercise-induced pulmonary hemorrhage. Using the presence of mucus or muco-purulent material in the trachea to diagnose chronic obstructive pulmonary disease, several studies failed to point out any association between exercise-induced pulmonary hemorrhage and chronic obstructive diseases (Speirs et al, 1982; Burrell, 1985; McNamara et al, 1990). Moreover, exercise-induced pulmonary hemorrhage is universally encountered, while, conversely, chronic obstructive pulmonary disease is absent in some regions of the world.

However, the bronchiolitis found in exercise-induced pulmonary hemorrhage-positive horses could be induced by respiratory disorders other than chronic obstructive pulmonary disease. Few pathogens are known to affect horses with the wide variety of epidemiological conditions under which exercise-induced pulmonary hemorrhage is known to occur. An ubiquitous virus, with high morbidity and low mortality, affecting most of the young horses, such as the EHV1, has been suggested to be this pathogen (O'Callaghan et al, 1987e). Small airway disease is a general feature in confirmed bleeders as proven by thorough imaging and post-mortem studies (O'Callaghan et al, 1987a; 1987b). The inflammatory processes found in the lungs of exercise-induced pulmonary hemorrhage positive horses suggest that local inflammatory lesions causing small airway disease are likely predisposing causes of exercise-induced pulmonary hemorrhage and may precede the hemorrhagic lesions. However, exercise-induced pulmonary hemorrhage could also occur the very first time in healthy horses and lead to secondary inflammatory lesions and small airway disease. Indeed, the instillation of autologous blood in the lung of healthy horses has been shown to induce both physiological and morphological modifications, the latter being similar to those observed in horses suffering exercise-induced pulmonary hemorrhage (Aguilera-Tejero et al, 1991; Tyler et al, 1991).

It has also been suggested that exercise-induced pulmonary hemorrhage could be secondary to upper airway obstruction associated with laryngeal hemiplegia (Cook, 1989).

6.1.1.5.5. Mechanical stress

The occurrence of exercise-induced pulmonary hemorrhage following strenuous exercise and not after prolonged exercise of lower intensity (Sweeney and Soma, 1983) suggests that the syndrome is the result of extreme mechanical forces applied to lung tissues and vessels. During heavy exercise, alveolar pressure is likely to become highly negative (Art et al, 1990), while the intravascular pressure (both pulmonary and bronchial) increases greatly. Consequently, transmural pressure, i.e. the pressure gradient between airways and blood vessels, is expected to reach high values.

Moreover, because of the poor collateral ventilation, the transmural pressure in asynchronous regions is suspected to become sufficiently high to cause capillary rupture.

Pulmonary vascular hypertension has been rejected as a possible cause of exercise-induced pulmonary hemorrhage (Robinson, 1979). The author asserts that pulmonary edema would occur before capillary pressure could increase enough to rupture a vessel. However, both alveolar and pulmonary capillary blood pressures are subjected to continuous cyclic variations induced by respiration and cardiac contraction respectively. Consequently, transmural pressure (between pulmonary circulation and alveoli or between bronchial circulation and alveoli) is expected to present important, irregular and sudden variations which could cause capillary rupture, rather than a continuous high value causing pulmonary edema.

In "bleeders", increased interstitial fibrosis is evident in interlobular and interalveolar septa, as well as around airways and vessels. This probably contributes to a loss of elasticity of the lung tissue in the affected regions. Because of interconnection, this loss of compliance may induce an increasing shear stress at the interface between the normal and affected areas. This decrease in compliance, whether or not it is primary of secondary to exercise-induced pulmonary hemorrhage, will probably favour the occurrence of new episodes of hemorrhage.

6.1.1.5.6. Vessel and tissue fragility

Several factors are likely to decrease the stress resistance of the pulmonary tissues. On the one hand, lung injury and hemorrhage may result from inflammatory processes, mainly due to a local release of toxic products (heparin, oxygen metabolites) by phagocytic cells such as neutrophils or macrophages (Ward and Mulligan, 1991). On the other hand, it has been shown in rabbits that a high lung volume increases stress failure of pulmonary capillaries and may cause disruption of the capillary endothelium, alveolar epithelium, or sometimes all layers of the wall (Fu et al, 1992). If the same is true in the horse, the alveoli of the caudodorsal regions of the lung should also be more fragile, since they are more distended because of gravitational effects. Therefore, the presence of chronic pulmonary inflammatory processes and/or the increase in lung volume during high exercise intensity may be partly responsible for increased blood vessel fragility and therefore for the occurrence of "bleeding".

6.1.2. Hypoxic vasoconstriction in chronic obstructive pulmonary disease

Pulmonary artery hypertension secondary to chronic pulmonary disease is of major importance in human medicine. Chronic bronchiolitis is frequently observed in horses, and pulmonary hypertension due to an hypoxic vasoconstriction may sometimes occur (Dixon, 1978). This could induce a right ventricular hypertrophy and eventually a right heart failure. However, this complication seems to be uncommon in horses (Dixon et al, 1982)

6.2. Bovine species

6.2.1. Brisket disease

Brisket disease is a bovine disease which is also called high altitude disease. It is a typical example of cor pulmonale. The most common clinical signs are tachycardia, jugular venous distension and subcutaneous edema of the brisket. This species peculiarity is due to the fact that cattle have a vigourous hypoxic pulmonary vasoconstrictor response (Robinson, 1982) and, when taken to altitude, develop pulmonary hypertension as a result of increased pulmonary vascular resistance (Fig. 12-7.) (Alexander et al, 1960). The resulting pressure overload on the right ventricle is responsible for the progressive cardiac hypertrophy, dilation and failure (Will et al, 1962).

The severity of the disease depends on the level of alveolar hypoxia, on the speed with which the condition develops and on the individual reactivity to chronic hypoxia. Indeed, some strains of cattle are less sensitive to both acute and chronic hypoxia (Will et al, 1975). Species such as sheep and dog, which

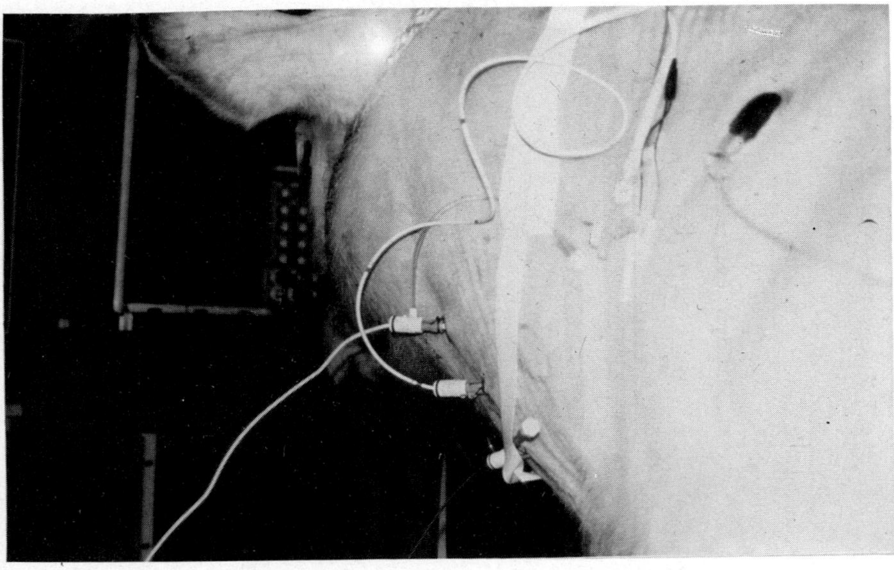

Fig. 12-7. Measurement of the increase in pulmonary vascular resistance during hypoxic pulmonary vasoconstriction in cattle (courtesy of H. Amory).

are hyporeactive to hypoxia, fail to develop right heart failure at high altitude (Harris et al, 1982; Robinson, 1982). It is interesting to note that the degree of right ventricular insufficiency during chronic hypoxia is correlated with the thickness of the intermediate smooth muscle layer of the small pulmonary arteries prior to exposure to hypoxia (Tucker et al, 1975).

Severe hypoxic vasoconstriction, which must be considered as a disadvantage during chronic lung disease (Nuytten et al, 1985), is of critical importance in the minute to minute matching of ventilation and perfusion in the lung, particularly in species, such as cattle and pigs, without collateral ventilation (Sylvester et al, 1980).

6.2.2. Acute endotoxinic pasteurellosis

Intratracheal or intravenous inoculation of high doses of *Pasteurella haemolytica* organisms is responsible for a severe pulmonary vascular disease

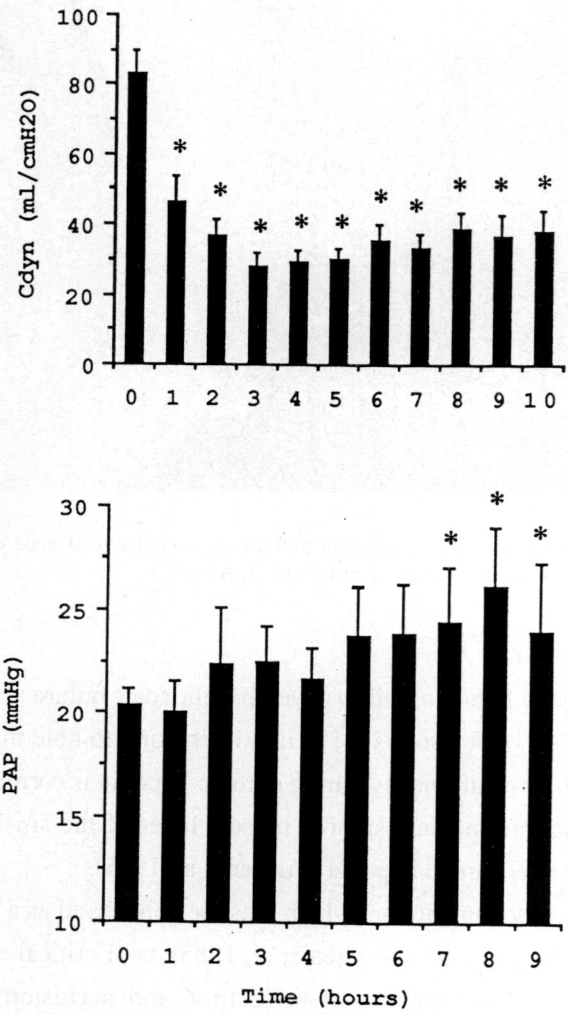

Fig. 12-8. Effect of acute endotoxinic pasteurellosis on dynamic lung compliance (Cdyn) and pulmonary artery pressure (PaP) in newborn calves. T0 : Baseline values; T1 to T10 : 1 to 10 hours post-inoculation; * : Significantly different from baseline (Linden et al, 1993).

in calves. The early changes in the mechanics of breathing consist of a decrease in lung dynamic compliance without change in total pulmonary resistance (Fig. 12-8.). This suggest that respiratory tract injury in acute bovine pasteurellosis is initiated from the parenchyma and does not result from extension of lesions from the conducting airways (Slocombe et al, 1984; 1990; Linden et al, 1993).

The gas exchange impairments observed during this syndrome result first from ventilation-perfusion mismatching in injured lung segments, and later from pulmonary edema. This may result from increased pulmonary vascular permeability due to endothelial damage generated by activated neutrophils and oxygen radical release (Heflin and Brigham, 1981), and from pulmonary hypertension due to left heart failure (Amory et al, 1993).

On the other hand, acute pasteurellosis may attenuate both the physiological pulmonary hypoxic vasoconstrictior response (Alnoor et al, 1986) and the adrenoceptor function in the pulmonary venous compartment (Greenless et al, 1987). These sequels could further impair the gas exchanges.

6.2.3. 3-Methylindole toxicosis

Acute bovine pulmonary edema and emphysema may be caused by the conversion of L-tryptophan ingested in the lush forage to 3-methylindole which is a pneumotoxic compound (Carlson et al, 1975). This leads to the development of acute pulmonary edema, alveolar epithelial hyperplasia and interstitial emphysema (Breeze and Carlson, 1982).

The functional disorders induced by 3-methylindole in the early stage of the disease consist of a large decrease in dynamic lung compliance and arterial oxygen tension and a large increase in minute viscous work and arterial carbon dioxide tension, without change in total pulmonary resistance. These dysfunctions are compatible with severe interstitial and pulmonary edema (Table 12-1.) (Lekeux et al, 1985).

The severity of this syndrome is dependent of the 3-methylindole dosage, the individual susceptibility and the age of the patient (Lekeux et al, 1985).

Table 12-1. Effect of 3-methylindole toxicosis on pulmonary function in calves.

Values	Unit	Baseline	Post-dosage
f	min^{-1}	31 (2)	103 (24)
t_I/t_{TOT}	-	0.47 (0.02)	0.48 (0.04)
V_T	L	1.20 (0.20)	0.88 (0.10)
V_e	$L.min^{-1}$	37 (5)	89 (12)
maxΔPpl	kPa	0.72 (0.08)	2.49 (0.30)
Cdyn	$L.kPa^{-1}$	2.85 (0.46)	0.61 (0.23)
R_L	$kPa.sec.L^{-1}$	0.16 (0.04)	0.16 (0.03)
Wvis	$J.min^{-1}$	13.4 (2.9)	91.0 (23.0)
HR	min^{-1}	78 (4)	100 (12)
pH	-	7.42 (0.01)	7.33 (0.02)
PaO_2	mmHg	100.5 (6.0)	38.25 (7.5)
$PaCO_2$	mmHg	43.5 (3.0)	58.5 (17.25)
$A\text{-}aDO_2$	mmHg	5.25 (1.5)	53.25 (22.5)

Data are expressed as mean ± SD. f : Respiratory frequency; t_I/t_{TOT} : Inspiratory time/total time of the breathing cycle ratio; V_T : Tidal volume; V_e : Minute volume; maxΔPpl : Peak to peak change in pleural pressure; Cdyn : Dynamic lung compliance; R_L : Total pulmonary resistance; Wvis : Minute work of breathing; HR : Heart rate; PaO_2 and $PaCO_2$: Arterial oxygen and carbon dioxide tensions; $A\text{-}aDO_2$: Alveolo-arterial oxygen gradient.

6.3. Canine species

6.3.1. Pulmonary hypertension

With the exception of dirofilariasis, little attention has been devoted to the detection of spontaneous pulmonary hypertension in chronic respiratory disease of cats and dogs.

The presence of *Dirofilaria immitis* in the pulmonary arteries and the right heart, and the shedding of metabolic products and antigens by microfilariae and adult worms are responsible for the wide range of changes observed in the pulmonary vascular bed and lung parenchyma. However, cor pulmonale is seen almost exclusively in severe chronic infections.

The major vaso-occlusive effects are due to chronic endarteritis and endothelial proliferation of the peripheral pulmonary branches (Knight, 1977).

Dirofilariasis causes 4 types of clinical signs : acute venae cavae syndrome, chronic cardio-pulmonary disease, chronic occult cardio-pulmonary disease, and ectopic abnormalities by adult worms developing in systemic arteries (Jackson, 1975). The diagnosis is based upon radiographic findings in dogs (Thrall et al, 1980) as well as in cats (Hawe, 1979), result of Knott's test, serologic findings, cardiac catheterization and angiography (Rawlings et al, 1978; Thrall et al, 1979; Rawlings, 1980).

The major differential diagnosis of secondary and primary cor pulmonale include the Eisenmenger's syndrome and chronic pulmonary thromboembolism. The Eisenmenger's syndrome refers to cyanotic heart diseases with right-to-left shunting due to a blood flow obstruction in the pulmonary vascular bed.

The most common congenital cardiac defect causing systemic to pulmonary shunting is the patent ductus arteriosus (Patterson, 1976; Bonagura, 1989). Females of certain small breeds are at greatest risk for the development of this disorder which is also well recognized in the cat.

Due to the higher aortic than pulmonary blood pressure, blood shunts continuously into the main pulmonary artery. This results in a continuous cardiac murmur, increased pulmonary flow, and increased venous return to the left atrium and ventricle. Left ventricular failure with pulmonary edema develops from volume overload. In a small percentage of cases, the lumen of the patent ductus arteriosus is so large that pulmonary vascular pressure markedly increase.

Many other cardiac congenital defects are recognized and may lead to pulmonary hypertension. In cases of interatrial or interventricular septal defects, blood shunts from the left to the right. However, in conditions such as tricuspid or pulmonic stenosis that increase right atrial or ventricular pressures, right-to-left shunting may develop.

6.3.2. Pulmonary edema

Most pulmonary edemas in dogs and cats are cardiogenic in origin. Left heart failure remains the most common cause of pulmonary edema in the dog and cat. Left heart failure is usually evidenced by dyspnea, pulmonary rales, and exercise intolerance. In most patients with left heart failure, the presence of pulmonary congestion can be confirmed by thoracic radiography. The nature and distribution of lesions on chest X-rays and the concurrent presence of cardiomegaly associated with a systolic murmur usually implicate the failing heart as the cause of pulmonary congestion. When equivocal evidence of left heart failure is present in patients in which pulmonary infiltrates of uncertain etiology are identified, left atrial pressure can be estimated by measurement of pulmonary artery wedge pressure using a Swan-Ganz catheter.

Noncardiogenic edema may be due to a great variety of pathogenetic mechanisms, and are either high-pressure or high-permeability edemas.

Acute respiratory failure with massive pulmonary edema, also called adult respiratory distress syndrome (ARDS), or shock lung syndrome, is the common response of the lung to a great variety of injuries. Pulmonary edema following pancreatitis in the dog is one of the many forms of this syndrome (Lees et al, 1978). In dogs and cats, aspiration of gastric content during anesthesia, unconsciousness or dysphagic troubles, and inhalation of smoke or toxic inhalants are common causes of permeability edema (Farrow, 1975). Pulmonary edema in dogs and cats with terminal uremia is also common. Infectious diseases, including viral, bacterial and parasitic pneumonia, may result in inflammatory lung edema. Hypersensitivity or idiosyncrasy reactions to therapeutic agents, vaccines or other biological products are relatively uncommon when one considers their extensive use. Neurogenic pulmonary edema may occur following seizures, head trauma or electrocution. Hypoglycemia in severely stressed hunting dogs might be the inciting factor for pulmonary edema (Lord et al, 1975)

6.3.3. Pulmonary thromboembolism (PTE)

The best recognized thromboemboli disease syndromes in companion animals are the aortic thromboembolism associated with cardiomyopathy in the cat and pulmonary thromboembolism due to heartworm disease and treatment in the dog.

The clinical clinical signs of this syndrome are not pathognomonic and consist of acute onset of dyspnea, tachypnea and nonspecific signs of cardiopulmonary diseases. Therefore, identification of conditions that predispose to pulmonary thromboembolism is helpful (Baty and Hardie, 1992). Deep venous thrombosis is less prevalent in companion animals than in humans. In animals, this disorder has been associated with hypothyroidism, pancreatitis, nephrotic syndrome, renal amyloidosis, disseminated intravascular coagulation (Cornelissen et al, 1985), antithrombin III deficiency, hyperadrenocorticism (King et al, 1985), and immune-mediated hemolytic anemia (Klein et al, 1989).

Pulmonary thromboembolism is a common clinical disease in dogs but it is frequently underdiagnosed. Postmortem diagnosis is complicated by the rapid dissolution of thrombi, and antemortem diagnosis requires specialized diagnostic techniques. Hypoxemia is a common but inconstant finding, and thoracic radiographs are frequently normal (Fluckiger and Gomez, 1984). Pulmonary scintigraphy is a noninvasive procedure which shows the combination of a normal ventilation scan and an abnormal perfusion scan (Fig. 12-9.) (Clercx et al, 1989). Such ventilation/perfusion mismatch aids in the diagnosis of thromboembolism. Pulmonary arteriography is the "gold standard" for diagnosis but it is an invasive procedure that has potential limitations and complications (Koblik et al, 1989).

6.3.4. Lung hemorrhage

Pulmonary injuries are common consequences of chest trauma, a condition which is frequently encountered in dogs and cats. Lung laceration or contusion are associated with hemorrhage and edema. In lung contusion,

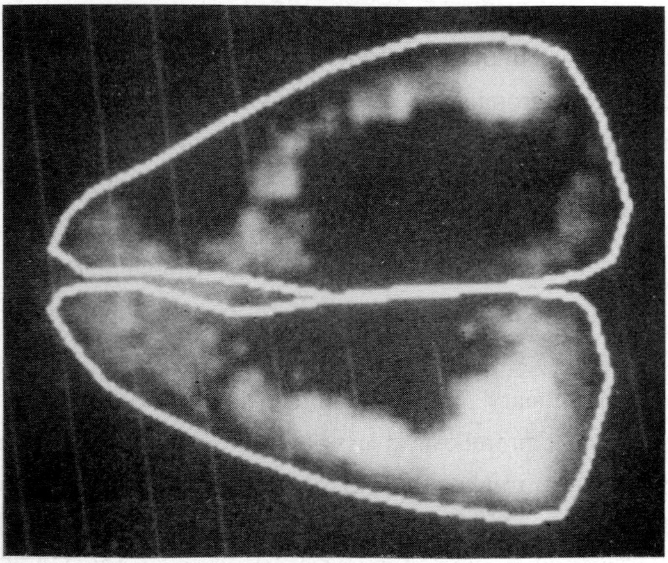

Fig. 12-9. Pulmonary scintigraphic image of a dog suffering from severe pulmonary thromboembolism. White areas are ventilated but unperfused.

intrapulmonary hemorrhage results from the tearing of capillaries and small blood vessels, and leads to alveolar wall disruption, intertitial hemorrhage, aspiration of blood and atelectasis. The severity of the clinical signs depends on the extent of the lung injury, and the type and severity of the concurrent lesions. Localized lung injury without pneumothorax or rib fracture may cause no overt clinical signs. When several lung lobes are involved, dyspnea, coughing, hemoptysis and cyanosis may be observed. Except for hemoptysis and signs of hypovolemia, the clinical signs are nonspecific, and lung contusion needs to be confirmed radiographically (Krahwinkel, 1980).

Blood can accumulate within the pleural cavity. Hemothorax is a particularly serious situation. Exsanguination into the pleural cavity caused by injuries to the great vessels, and the intercostal, tracheobronchial or internal thoracic arteries, is likely to cause death before the animal can be admitted to a clinic. Bleeding from the high-pressure systemic arterial system is more rapidly fatal than bleeding from the low-pressure pulmonary arterial system or the intrathoracic veins. Respiratory signs of restrictive pulmonary disease go along with signs of hypovolemia.

Primary or secondary thrombocytopenia and a large number of primary or secondary coagulopathies can lead to diffuse, nontraumatic pulmonary hemorrhage. The etiologies are very diverse and include thrombocytopenia caused by bone-marrow depression or imune-mediated diseases, and coagulopathies associated with congenital diseases, warfarin toxicity, treatment with cytostatica and anticoagulants. The diagnosis of hemorrhage has to be based on physical findings and laboratory results. The animals show a wide variety of nonspecific signs depending on the underlying primary disease and the degree of bleeding and anemia. Suspicious signs include prolonged bleeding time after venupuncture, subcutaneous, mucosal or submucosal hemorrhage, and dyspnea. Hemoptysis often occurs, but this is not a consistent sign. Radiographically, diffuse nontraumatic hemorrhage is indistinguishable from pulmonary permeability edema, acute interstitial pneumonia, and adult respiratory distress syndrome (Suter, 1981).

7. CONCLUSIONS

Even more than other respiratory dysfunctions, vascular pulmonary diseases present manifest species peculiarities. For instance, exercise-induced pulmonary hemorrhage, brisket disease and pulmonary embolism are quite exclusively observed in horses, cattle and dogs, respectively.

Therefore, these species pecularities must be taken into account when dealing with the diagnosis, the treatment and the prevention of vascular pulmonary diseases.

REFERENCES

AGUILERA-TEJERO E., PASCOE J.R., TYLER W.S., WOLINER M.J. Pulmonary function after instillation of autologous blood in the lungs of horses. In Proceedings :

10th Comparative Respiratory Society Meeting, Urbana, USA, 1991, S-6.

ALEXANDER A.F., WILL D.H., GROVER R.F., REEVES J.T. Pulmonary hypertension and right ventricular hypertrophy in cattle at high altitude. *Am. J. Vet. Res.* 1960, 21, 199-204.

ALNOOR S.A., SLOCOMBE R.F., DERKSEN F.J., ROBINSON N.E. Hemodynamic effects of acute pneumonia experimentally induced in newborn calves inoculated with *Pasteurella haemolytica*. *Am. J. Vet. Res.* 1986, 47, 1382-1386.

AMORY H., LINDEN A., DESMECHT D., LEKEUX P. Evidence of cardiovascular dysfunction during *Pasteurella haemolytica*-induced acute pneumonia in calves. 1993, submitted for publication.

ARMSTRONG D.J., MILLER S.A. Lung irritant and C-fibre response to embolism in thrombocytopenia rabbits. *J. Physiol. London* 1980, 303, 41-42.

ART T., ANDERSON L., WOAKES A.J., ROBERTS C., BUTLER P.J., SNOW D.H., LEKEUX P. Mechanics of breathing during strenuous exercise in thoroughbred horses. *Respir. Physiol.* 1990, 82, 279-294.

AUKLAND K., NICOLAYSEN G. Interstitial fluid volume: local regulation mechanism. *Physiol. Rev.* 1981, 61, 556-643.

BATY C.J., HARDIE E.M. Pulmonary thomboembolism: diagnosis and treatment. In : *Current Veterinary Therapy XI Small Animal Practice*, Kirk, R.W., Bonagura, J.D. (Eds), W.B. Saunders Company, Philadelphia, 1992, pp 137-142.

BAYLY W.M., MEYERS K.M., KECK M.T., HUSTON L.J., GRANT B.D. Effects of furosemide on exercise-induced alterations in haemostasis in thoroughbred horses exhibiting post-exercise epstaxis. In : *Equine Exercise Physiology*, Snow, D.H., Persson, S.G.B., Rose, R.J. (Eds), Granta Editions, Cambridge, 1983, pp 64-70.

BISGARD G.E., ORR J.A., WILL J.A. Hypoxic pulmonary hypertension in the pony. *Am. J. Vet. Res.* 1975, 36, 49-52.

BONAGURA J.D. Congenital heart disease. In : *Ettinger Textbook of Veterinary Internal Medicine*, Ettinger, S.J. (Ed.), W.B. Saunders Company, Philadelphia, 1989, pp 976-1030.

BREEZE R.G., CARLSON J.R. Chemical-induced lung injury in domestic animals. *Adv. Vet. Sci. Comp. Med.* 1982, 26, 201-231.

BRIGHAM K.L., BOWERS R., HAYNES J. Increased sheep lung vascular permeability caused by *Escherichia coli* endotoxemia. *Circ. Res.* 1979, 45, 292-297.

BRIGHAM K.L., MEYRICK B. Interaction of granulocytes with the lungs. *Circ. Res.* 1984, 54, 623-635.

BURRELL M.H. Endoscopic and virological observations on respiratory disease in a group of young thoroughbred horses in training. *Equine Vet. J.* 1985, 17, 99-103.

CAHILL J.M., ATTINGER E.O., BYRNE J.J. Ventilatory responses to embolization of lung. *J. Appl. Physiol.* 1961, 16, 469-472.

CARLSON J.R., DICKINSON E.O., YOKOYAMA M.T., BRADLEY B. Pulmonary edema and emphysema in cattle after intraruminal and intravenous administration of 3-methylindole. *Am. J. Vet. Res.* 1975, 36, 1341-1347.

CHERNICK V., HODSON W.H., GREENFIELD L.J. Effect of chronic pulmonary artery ligation on pulmonary mechanics and surfactant. *J. Appl. Physiol.* 1966, 21, 1315-1320.

CLARK S.W., GRAF P.D., NADEL J.A. *In vivo* visualization of small airway constriction after pulmonary microembolism in cats and dogs. *J. Appl. Physiol.* 1970, 29, 646-650.

CLERCX C., VAN DEN BROM W.E., VAN DEN INGH T.S.G.A.M., de VRIES H.W. Scintigraphical analysis as a diagnostic tool in canine experimental lung embolism. *Lung* 1989, 167, 225-236.

COLERIDGE H.M., COLERIDGE J.C.G. Impulse activity in afferent vagal C-fibers with endings in the intrapulmonary airways of dogs. *Respir. Physiol.* 1977, 29, 125-142.

COOK W.R. Specifications for speed in the racehorse : the Airflow Factors, The Russell Meerdink Company Ltd, Menasha, Wi, 1989.

CORNELISSEN J.M.M., WOLVEKAMP W.T.H.C., STOKHOF A.A., VAN DEN BROM W.E., de VRIES H.W. Primary occlusive pulmonary vascular disease in a dog diagnosed by a lung perfusion scintigram. *J. Am. Anim. Hosp. Assoc.* 1985, 21, 293-297.

D'ALONZO G.E., BOWER J.S., DEHART P., DANTZKER D.R. The mechanisms of abnormal gas exchange in acute massive pulmonary embolism. *Am. Rev. Respir. Dis.* 1983, 128, 170-172.

DANTZKER D.R., WAGNER P.D., TORNABENE V.M., ALAZRAKI N.P., WEST J.B. Gas exchange after pulmonary thromboembolism in dogs. *Circ. Res.* 1978, 42, 92-103.

DANTZKER D.R., BOWER J.S. Alterations in gas exchange following pulmonary thromboembolism. *Chest* 1982, 81, 495-501.

DEMLING R.H., SMITH M., GUNTHER R. The effect of prostacyclin infusion on endotoxin induced lung injury. *Surgery* 1981, 89, 257-263.

DEMLING R.H., WONG C., FOX R., HECHTMAN H., HUVAL W. Relationship of increased lung serotonin levels to endotoxin-induced pulmonary hypertension in sheep; effects of a serotonin antagonist. *Am. Rev. Respir. Dis.* 1985, 132, 1257-1261.

DERKSEN F.J., ROBINSON N.E. Esophageal and intrapleural pressures in the healthy conscious pony. *Am. J. Vet. Res.* 1980, 41, 1756-1761.

DIXON P.M. Pulmonary artery pressures in normal horses and in horses affected with chronic obstructive pulmonary disease. *Equine Vet. J.* 1978, 10, 195-198.

DIXON P.M., NICHOLLS J.M., McPHERSON E.A., LAWSON G.H., THOMSON J.R., PIRIE H.W., BREEZE R.G. Chronic obstructive pulmonary disease. Anatomical cardiac studies. *Equine Vet. J.* 1982, 14, 80-82.

DRAKE R., GABEL J. Effects of histamine and alloxan in canine pulmonary vascular permeability. *Am. J. Physiol.* 1980, 239, H96-H100.

EDWARD W.D. Pathology of pulmonary hypertension. *Cardiovasc. Clin.* 1988, 18, 321-359.

ERDMANN A.J., VAUGHAN T.R., BRIGHAM K.L., WOOLVERTON W.C., STAUB N.C. Effect of increased vascular pressure on lung fluid balance in unanesthetized sheep. *Circ. Res.* 1975, 37, 271-284.

ERICKSON B.K., ERICKSON H.H., COFFMAN J.R. Pulmonary artery and aortic pressure changes during high intensity treadmill exercise in the horse: effect of furosemide and phentolamine. *Equine Vet. J.* 1992, 24, 215-219.

FARROW, C.S. Smoke inhalation in the dog: current concepts of pathophysiology and management. *Vet. Med. Small Anim. Clin.* 1975, 70, 404-414.

FLUCKIGER M.A., GOMEZ J.A. Radiographic findings in dogs with spontaneous thrombosis or emboli. *Vet. Radiol.* 1984, 25, 124-131.

FU Z., COSTELLO M.L., TSUKIMOTO K., PREDILETTO R., ELLIOTT A.R., MATHIEU-COSTELLO M., WEST J.B. High lung volume increases stress failure in pulmonary capillaries. *J. Appl. Physiol.* 1992, 73, 123-133.

GAAR K.A., TAYLOR A.E., OWENS L.J., GUYTON A.C. Effect of capillary pressure and plasma proteins on the development of pulmonary edema. *Am. J. Physiol.* 1967, 213, 79-82.

GABEL J., HARRIS T., DRAKE R. Effect of endotoxin on lung fluid balance in unanesthetized sheep. *J. Appl. Physiol.* 1984, 56, 489-494.

GEE M.H., TAHAMONT M.V., PERKOWSKI S.Z., FLYNN J.T. Arachidonic acid metabolites as mediators of lung injury during intravascular complement activation.

Prog. Biochem. Pharmacol. 1985, 20, 108-119.

GREENLEES K.J., SHEWEN P., YAGER J., EYRE P. Induced pasteurellosis and pulmonary vascular adrenoceptor function in bull calves. *Am. J. Vet. Res.* 1987, 48, 1584-1588.

GUSTIN P., URBAIN B., DELAUNOIS A., ZEIMES K., ANSAY M. Permeability of the endothelium and partitioning of the pulmonary blood flow resistance in isolated perfused pig lungs: effects of breed and age. *Vet. Res. Commun.* 1992, 16, 69-82.

GUYTON A.C., TAYLOR A.E., GRANGER H.J. Circulatory Physiology. II. Dynamics and Control of body Fluids, W.B. Saunders Company, Philadelphia, 1975, pp 149-193.

HARLAN J.M. Leukocyte-endothelial cell interaction. *Blood* 1985, 65, 513-525.

HARRIS P., HEATH D., SAUTH P., WILLIAMS D.R., RAMIREZ A., KRUGER H., JONES D.M. Pulmonary circulation of the llama at high and low altitudes. *Thorax* 1982, 37, 38-45.

HAWE R.S. The diagnosis and treatment of occult dirofilariasis in a cat. *J. Am. Anim. Hosp. Assoc.* 1979, 15, 577-582.

HEFLIN A.C., Jr, BRIGHAM K.L. Prevention by granulocyte depletion of increased vascular permeability of sheep lung following endotoxemia. *J. Clin. Invest.* 1981, 68, 1253-1260.

HILLIDGE C.J., LANE T.J., JOHNSON E.L. Preliminary investigations of EIPH in racing Quarter Horse. *Equine Vet. Sci.* 1984, 4, 21-23.

ISHIBASHI M., REED R.K., TOWNSLEY M.I., PARKER J.C., TAYLOR A.E. Capillary-interstitial barrier properties to albumin in the canine lung. *FASEB J.* 1990, 4, A589.

JACKSON W.F. Physical examination, anamnesis, and chief complaint. In Proceedings : Heartworm Symposium 1974, Morgan, H.C. (Ed.), VM Publishing, Inc, Bonner Springs, Kansas, 1975, P16-18.

KING R.R., MAUDERLY J.L., HAHN F.F., WOLFF R.K., MUGGENBURG B.A., PICKRELL J.A. Pulmonary function studies in a dog with pulmonary thromboembolism associated with Cushing's disease. *J. Am. Anim. Hosp. Assoc.* 1985, 21, 555-562.

KLEIN M.K., DOW S.W., ROSYCHUK R.A.W. Pulmonary thomboembolism associated with immune-mediated hemolytic anemia in dogs: ten cases (1982-1987). *J. Am. Vet. Med. Assoc.* 1989, 195, 246-250.

KNIGHT D.H. Heartworm heart disease. *Adv. Vet. Sci. Comp. Med.* 1977, 21, 107-149.

KOBLIK P.D., HORNOF W., HARNAGEL S.H., FISHER P.E. A comparison of pulmonary angiography, digital subtraction angiography, and 99m Tc-DTCPA/MAA ventilation-perfusion scintigraphy for detection of experimental pulmonary emboli in the dog. *Vet. Radiol.* 1989, 30, 159-168.

KRAHWINKEL D.J. Thoracic trauma. In : *Current Veterinary Therapy VII*, Kirk, R.W. (Ed.), W.B. Saunders Company, Philadelphia, 1980, pp 268-271.

LEEPER-WOODFORD S.K., CAREY P.D., BYRNE K., JENKINS J.K., FISHER B.J., BLOCHER C., SUGERMAN H.J., FOWLER III A.A. Tumor necrosis factor. Alpha and beta subtypes appear in circulation during onset of sepsis-induced lung injury. *Am. Rev. Respir. Dis.* 1991, 143, 1076-1082.

LEES, G.E., SUTER P.F., JOHNSON G.C. Pulmonary edema in a dog with acute pancreatitis and cardiac disease. *J. Am. Vet. Med. Assoc.* 1978, 172, 690-696.

LEKEUX P., HAJER R., VAN DEN INGH T.S.G.A.M., BREUKINK H.J. Pathophysiologic study of 3-methylindole-induced pulmonary toxicosis in immature cattle. *Am. J. Vet. Res.* 1985, 46, 1629-1631.

LINDEN A., DESMECHT D., AMORY H., ROLLIN F., LEKEUX P. An experimental trial of intramuscular metrenperone to induce respiratory improvement during pneumonia

in neonatal calves. *Arch. Int. Physiol. Bioch.* 1993, 101, P9.
LORD P.F., OLSSON S.E., AUDELL L. Acute pulmonary edema and seizures in hunting dogs. *Nord. Vet. Med.* 1975, 27, 112-116.
MALIK A.B. Pulmonary microembolim. *Physiol. Rev.* 1983, 1114-1207.
MALIK A.B. Mechanism of neurogenic pulmonary edema. *Circ. Res.* 1985, 57, 1-8.
MANIER G., CASTAING Y., GUENARD H. Determinants of hypoxemia during the acute phase of pulmonary embolism in humans. *Am. Rev. Respir. Dis.* 1985, 132, 332-338.
McINTYRE K.M., SASAHARA A.A. The hemodynamic response to pulmonary embolism in patients without prior cardiopulmonary disease. *Am. J. Cardiol.* 1971, 28, 288-294.
McNAMARA B., BAUER S., IAFE J. Endoscopic evaluation of exercise-induced pulmonary hemorrhage and chronic obstructive pulmonary disease in association with poor performance in racing standardbreds. *J. Am. Vet. Med. Assoc.* 1990, 196, 443-445.
MINNEAR F.L., MOON D.G., KAPLAN J.E., MALIK A.B. Effect of ADP induced platelet aggregation on lung fluid balance. *Am. J. Physiol.* 1982, 11, H645-H661.
MISSEROCHI G., NEGRINI D. Interstitial pulmonary pressure in anesthetized, paralyzed rabbits with intact pleural space. *Physiologist* 1989, 32, P201.
MODELL H.E., BECK K., BUTLER J. Functional aspects of canine bronchial-pulmonary vascular communications. *J. Appl. Physiol.* 1981, 50, 1045-1051.
NUYTTEN J., MUYLLE E., OYAERT W. Pulmonary haemodynamics in healthy calves and in calves suffering from respiratory disorders. *Zbl. Vet. Med. A* 1985, 32, 81-85.
O'CALLAGHAN M.W., GOULDEN B.E. Radiographic changes in the lungs of horses with exercise-induced epistaxis. *N. Z. Vet. J.* 1982, 30, 117-118.
O'CALLAGHAN M.W., PASCOE J.R., TYLER W.S., MASON D.K. Exercise-induced pulmonary haemorrhage in the horse: results of a detailed clinical, post mortem and imaging study. II. Gross lung pathology. *Equine Vet. J.* 1987a, 19, 389-393.
O'CALLAGHAN M.W., PASCOE J.R., TYLER W.S., MASON D.K. Exercise-induced pulmonary haemorrhage in the horse: results of a detailed clinical, post mortem and imaging study. III. Subgross findings in lungs subjected to latex perfusions of the bronchial and pulmonary arteries. *Equine Vet. J.* 1987b, 19, 394-404.
O'CALLAGHAN M.W., PASCOE J.R., TYLER W.S., MASON D.K. Exercise-induced pulmonary haemorrhage in the horse: results of a detailed clinical, post mortem and imaging study. VI. Radiological/pathological correlations. *Equine Vet. J.* 1987c, 19, 419-422.
O'CALLAGHAN M.W., HORNOF W.J., FISHER P.E., PASCOE J.R. Exercise-induced pulmonary haemorrhage in the horses: results of a detailed clinical, post mortem and imaging study. VII. Ventilation/perfusion scintigraphy in horses with EIPH. *Equine Vet. J.* 1987d, 19, 423-427.
O'CALLAGHAN M.W., HORNOF W.J., FISHER P.E., MASON D.K. Exercise-induced pulmonary haemorrhage in the horses: results of a detailed clinical, post mortem and imaging study. VIII. Conclusions and implications. *Equine Vet. J.* 1987e, 19, 429-434.
PARRATT J., COKER S., HUGHES B. The possible role of prostaglandin and thromboxane in the pulmonary consequences of experimental endotoxic shock and clinical sepsis. In : *Role of Chemical Mediators in the Pathophysiology of acute Illness and Injury*, McConn, R. (Ed.), Raven Press, New York, 1982, pp 195-219.
PASCOE J.R., FERRARO G.L., CANNON J.H., ARTHUR R.M., WHEAT J.D. Exercise-induced pulmonary hemorrhage in racing thoroughbreds: a preliminary study. *Am. J. Vet. Res.* 1981, 42, 703-707.
PATTERSON D.F. Congenital defects of the cardiovascular system of dogs: studies in

comparative cardiology. *Adv. Vet. Sci. Comp. Med.* 1976, 20, 1-37.

PETERS S.P., SCHLEIMER R.P., NACLERIO R.M., McGLASHAN D.W., TOGIAS A.G., PROUD D., FREELAND H.S., FOX C., ADKINSON N.F., LICHTENSTEIN L.M. The pathophysiology of human mast cells. *Am. Rev. Respir. Dis.* 1987, 135, 1196-1200.

RAPHEL C.F., SOMA L.R. Exercise-induced pulmonary hemorrhage in thoroughbreds after racing and breezing. *Am. J. Vet. Res.* 1982, 43, 1123-1127.

RAWLINGS C.A., McCALL J.W., LEWIS R.E. The response of the canine heart and lungs to *Dirofilaria Immitis*. *J. Am. Anim. Hosp. Assoc.* 1978, 14, 17-32.

RAWLINGS C.A. Acute response of pulmonary blood flow and right ventricular function to *Dirofilaria immitis* adults and microfilaria. *Am. J. Vet. Res.* 1980, 41, 244-249.

REEVES J.T., DEMPSEY J.A., GROVER B.M. Pulmonary circulation during exercise. In : *Pulmonary Vascular Physiology and Pathophysiology*, vol 38, Weir, E.K., Reeves, J.T. (Eds), Marcel Dekker, New York, 1989, pp 107-133.

ROBERTS A.M., BHATTACHARYA J., SCHULTZ H.D., COLERIDGE H.M., COLERIDGE J.C.G. Stimulation of pulmonary vagal afferent C fibers by lung edema in dogs. *Circ. Res.* 1986, 58, 512-522.

ROBINSON N.E. Functional abnormalities caused by upper airway obstruction and heaves: their relationship to the etiology of epistaxis. *Vet. Clin. North Am. Large Anim. Pract.* 1979, 1, 17-34.

ROBINSON N.E. Some functional consequences of species differences in lung anatomy. *Adv. Vet. Sci. Comp. Med.* 1982, 26, 1-33.

SEVERINGHAUS J.W., SWENSON E.W., FINLEY T.N., LATEGOLA M.T., WILLIAMS J. Unilateral hypoventilation produced in dogs by occluding one pulmonary artery. *J. Appl. Physiol.* 1961, 16, 53-60.

SLOCOMBE R.F., DERKSEN F.J., ROBINSON N.E. Interactions of cold stress and *Pasteurella haemolytica* in the pathogenesis of pneumonic pasteurellosis in calves: changes in pulmonary function. *Am. J. Vet. Res.* 1984, 45, 1764-1770.

SLOCOMBE R.F., MULKS M., KILLINGSWORTH C.R., DERKSEN F.J., ROBINSON N.E. Effect of *Pasteurella haemolytica*-derived endotoxin on pulmonary structure and function in calves. *Am. J. Vet. Res.* 1990, 51, 433-438.

SOMA L.R., LASTER L., OPPENLANDER F., BARR-ALDERFER V. Effects of furosemide on the racing times of horses with exercise-induced pulmonary hemorrhage. *Am. J. Vet. Res.* 1985, 46, 763-768.

SPEIRS V.C., van VEENENDAAL J.C., HARRISON I.W., SMYTH G.B., ANDERSON G.A., WILSON D.V., GILBO B. Pulmonary haemorrhage in standardbred horses after racing. *Aust. Vet. J.* 1982, 59, 38-40.

STAUB N.C. Pathophysiology of pulmonary edema. In: *Edema*, Staub, N.C., Taylor, A.E. (Eds), Raven Press, New York, 1984, pp 719-786.

SUTER P.F. The radiographic diagnosis of canine and feline heart disease. *Comp. Cont. Educ.* 1981, 3, 441-454.

SWEENEY C.R., SOMA L.R. Exercise induced pulmonary haemorrhage in horses. In : *Equine Exercise Physiology*, Snow, D.H., Persson, S.G.B., Rose, R.J. (Eds), Granta Editions, Cambridge, 1983, pp 51-56.

SYLVESTER J.T., HARABIN A.L., PEAKE M.D., FRANK R.S. Vasodilator and constrictor responses to hypoxia in isolated pig lungs. *J. Appl. Physiol.* 1980, 49, 820-825.

TAYLOR A.E., RIPPE B. Pulmonary edema. In : *Physiology of Membrane Disorders*, Andreoli, T.E., Hoffman, J.F., Fanestal, D.D., Schultz, S.G. (Eds), Plenum Press, New York, 1986, pp 1025-1039.

THOMAS D., STEIN M., TANABE G., REGE V., WESSLER S. Mechanism of bronchoconstriction produced by thromboemboli in dogs. *Am. J. Physiol.* 1964, 206, 1207-1212.

THRALL D.E., BADERTSCHER R.R., McCALL J.W., LEWIS R.E. The pulmonary arterial circulation in dogs experimentally infected with *Dirofilaria immitis*. Its angiographic evaluation. *J. Am. Vet. Rad. Soc.* 1979, 20, 74-78.

THRALL D.E., BADERTSCHER R.R., LEWIS R.E., McCALL J.W., LOSONSKY J.M. Radiographic changes associated with developing dirofilariasis in experimentally infected dogs. *Am. J. Vet. Res.* 1980, 41, 81-90.

TUCKER A., McMURTRY I.F., REEVES J.T., ALEXANDER A.F., WILL D.H., GROVER R.F. Lung vascular smooth muscle as a determinant of pulmonary hypertension at high altitude. *Am. J. Physiol.* 1975, 228, 762-767.

TYLER W.S., PASCOE J.R., AGUILERA-TEJERO E., WOLINER M.J., HINDS D.M., BAKER G.L., JAIN S., KANN M. Morphological effects of autologous blood in airspaces of equine lungs. In Proceedings : 10th Comparative Respiratory Society Meeting, Urbana, USA, 1991, S-7.

URBAIN B., GUSTIN P., ANSAY M. Endotoxin-induced microvascular injury in isolated and perfused pig lungs. *Vet. Res. Commun.* 1992, 16, 453-464.

VAAGE J. Intravascular platelet aggregation and pulmonary injury. *Ann. N Y Acad. Sci.* 1982, 384, 301-318.

VREIM C.E., SNASHALL P., STAUB N.C. Protein composition of lung fluids in anesthetized dogs with acute cardiogenic edema. *Am. J. Physiol.* 1976, 231, 1466-1469.

WARD P.A., MULLIGAN M.S. Lung injury by toxic oxygen metabolites. In Proceedings : 10th Comparative Respiratory Society Meeting, East Lansing, USA, 1991, P1-P5.

WILL D.H., ALEXANDER A.F., REEVES J.T., GROVER R.F. High altitude-induced pulmonary hypertension in normal cattle. *Circ. Res.* 1962, 10, 172-177.

WILL D.H., HICKS J.L., CARD C.S., ALEXANDER A.F. Inherited susceptibility of cattle to high-altitude pulmonary hypertension. *J. Appl. Physiol.* 1975, 38, 491-494.

CHAPTER XIII

FUNCTIONAL EFFECTS OF RESTRICTIVE PULMONARY DISEASES

P. Lekeux[1], C. Clercx[2], T. Art[3]

[1] Laboratory for Functional Investigation
[2] Department of Small Animal Medicine
[3] Equine Sport Medicine Unit
Faculty of Veterinary Medicine
University of Liege

SUMMARY
This paper describes the functional peculiarities of several types of restrictive diseases in domestic animals.

KEY WORDS
Respiratory system - Pulmonary function - Restrictive diseases.

1. INTRODUCTION

The main functional consequences of restrictive lung diseases are a decrease in dynamic lung compliance and a reduction in lung volumes, i.e. vital capacity, residual volume and total lung capacity. Nevertheless, abnormal gas transfer and extensive morphological changes in lung biopsies may occur with normal lung volumes.

The respiratory airflow is generally well preserved, except if the patient suffers from a pulmonary disease with a combination of both restrictive and obstructive patterns.

Three classes of defects lead to a restrictive pattern : (1) alteration in lung parenchyma, (2) intraparenchymal changes and (3) extraparenchymal changes.

2. PARENCHYMAL CHANGES

The parenchymal diseases are generally characterized by cellular infiltrations and progressive pulmonary fibrosis. These alterations in lung tissue may be caused by conditions such as idiopathic pulmonary fibrosis or diffuse carcinomatosis.

In other cases, pulmonary fibrosis may be secondary to severe infectious pulmonary diseases. This fibrosis is generally localised to those pulmonary lobes which have been affected by the acute inflammatory disorders.

2.1. Physiopathology of interstitial lung disorders

In human medicine, at least 130 different syndromes of interstitial lung disease, classified according to their physiopathologic characteristics, have been described (Keogh and Crystal, 1982). Their etiology is unknown, although in some cases an immunological reaction is suspected. These fibrotic lung disorders include disorders of the lower respiratory tract characterized by injury to the lung parenchyma and by replacement of the normal architecture by mesenchymal cells and connective tissue matrix secreted by these cells (Crystal and Ferrans, 1988). The name of interstitial lung disorders reflects the concept that the fibrosis is confined to the interstitium of the alveolar walls.

However, it has been demonstrated that most of the fibrotic disorders are alveolar as well as intersitial. They are injuries of the epithelial surface often associated with (a) the interstitial contents moving through rents into the epithelial basement membrane and (b) mesenchymal cells and their products accumulating in spaces normally occupied by air (Basset et al, 1986). The fundamental process underlying these modifications is relatively simple. The fibrotic lung disorders are chronic inflammatory disorders in which the inflammatory processes in the lower respiratory tract damage the lung and modulate the proliferation of mesenchymal cells that form the basis of the fibrotic scare (Crystal et al, 1981). The pulmonary fibrosis is therefore similar to a normal wound-healing process, but whereas wound-healing is normally localised in space and confined in time, the fibrotic lung disorders generally involve the entire organ and are chronic on-going processes. Several mediators such as peptides and cytokines are involved in this condition (Crystal et al, 1991). Because it is the inflammation that drives the mechanism of fibrosis, the differences between the various fibrotic disorders are explained by the difference between the types of inflammation (Crystal et al, 1981). For instance, the inflammation of some interstitial lung disorders is dominated by alveolar macrophages, whereas in others, the major components of inflammation are neutrophils, lymphocytes, and/or eosinophils (Keogh and Crystal, 1982).

Eosinophilic and immune-mediated diseases are disorders arbitrarily characterized by their inflammatory response as primarily eosinophilic and primary mononuclear (granulomatous), respectively. The condition seems to be characterized by restrictive or obstructive features or a combination of both (Bedrossian et al, 1975). In most instances, no offending agent can be discovered, and immunosuppressant therapy is necessary to control the response. Clinical signs are extremely variable. Coughing is nonresponsive to antibiotic therapy. The cell blood count classically reflects the eosinophilic response. However, peripheral eosinophilia may be absent in spite of marked pulmonary involvement. Radiographs can show a mild interstitial pattern, alveolar densities, and even large masses which can be confused with neoplasias or fungal granulomas. A bronchial component also may be present. Cytologic evaluation is necessary in order to determine whether eosinophilic inflammation predominates. Specimens should be critically evaluated for any source of antigen, such as parasites, bacteria, fungi, and neoplasia. These antigens must then be removed by an appropriate treatment. Corticosteroids are frequently successful in controlling the inflammatory process (Noone, 1986).

2.2. Functional effects of interstitial lung disorders

The functional effects of these disorders depend on the stage of the condition. The pulmonary function may be normal despite the presence of histologically proven disease. As the condition worsens, the respiratory function is impaired. The main features are (a) an increased radial traction on the airway due to increased lung recoil, which promotes the airflow and (b) an increase in thickness of the alveolar-capillary membrane inducing a reduction in the diffusing capacity. In summary, the modifications generally observed include a decrease in the total lung and vital capacity (Line et al, 1978), a fall in dynamic and static lung compliance (Fulmer et al, 1977), an increase in maximal expiratory flow (Tan and Tashkin, 1981), a decrease in diffusing capacity (Fulmer et al, 1977; Line et al, 1978), a widening in the end-tidal/arterial differences for partial pressure in oxygen and carbon dioxide (Barrocas et al, 1971; Popius et al, 1975), an increased deadspace volume/tidal volume ratio (Barrocas et al, 1971; Poppius et al, 1975) and a ventilation/perfusion ratio inequality (Wagner et al, 1976).

Pulmonary arterial hypertension has been also observed in patients suffering from diffuse intersitial fibrosis (Radwan and Daum, 1980).

The respiratory frequency is increased and the tidal volume and inspiratory time are decreased, whereas the expired minute volume and the inspiratory time to total breathing time ratio remain unchanged (Savoy et al, 1981).

In large animals, the functional effects of the interstitial disorders are the same as those described in humans, i.e. decreased arterial partial pressure in oxygen, decreased dynamic compliance, unchanged pulmonary resistance and tachypnea (Derksen et al, 1982; Breeze, 1985).

2.3. Interstitial lung diseases in animals

These conditions are rarely described in large animals. One case of chronic restrictive pulmonary disease has been described in the equine species (Derksen et al, 1982).

Two types of chronic interstitial pneumonia of uncertain etiology have been identified in cattle, i.e. fibrosing alveolitis and bronchiolitis obliterans (Breeze, 1985). The fibrosing alveolitis is characterized by diffuse inflammation of the lung tissue beyond the terminal bronchiole. Approximately 50 % of cases are positive for precipitating antibodies to *Micropolyspora feani*, and it is possible that these cases may represent chronic farmer's lung, whereas the others may be chronic stages of hypersensitivity to unindentified antigens. The etiology of the bronchiolitis obliterans is unknown and could be a sequel of viral infection or hypersensitive pneumonitis (Breeze, 1985). On the other hand, bovine respiratory syncytial virus pneumonia, which induces an obstructive disease during the acute stage of this process, is responsible for the occurrence of a subclinical restrictive disease during the chronic stage (Fig. 13-1.) (Lekeux et al, 1985).

Granulomatous pulmonary diseases described in dogs include eosinophilic granulomatosis (Calvert, 1992), lymphomatoid ganulomatosis, and granulomatosis associated with systemic lupus erythematosus (Posterino et al, 1987).

3. INTRAPARENCHYMAL CHANGES

Intraalveolar accumulation of fluid (as in edema) or cells (as in mycoplasma infection), and lack or immaturity of the surfactant induce also restricitve pulmonary problems.

Intraparenchymal disorders are frequently encountered in dogs and cats and

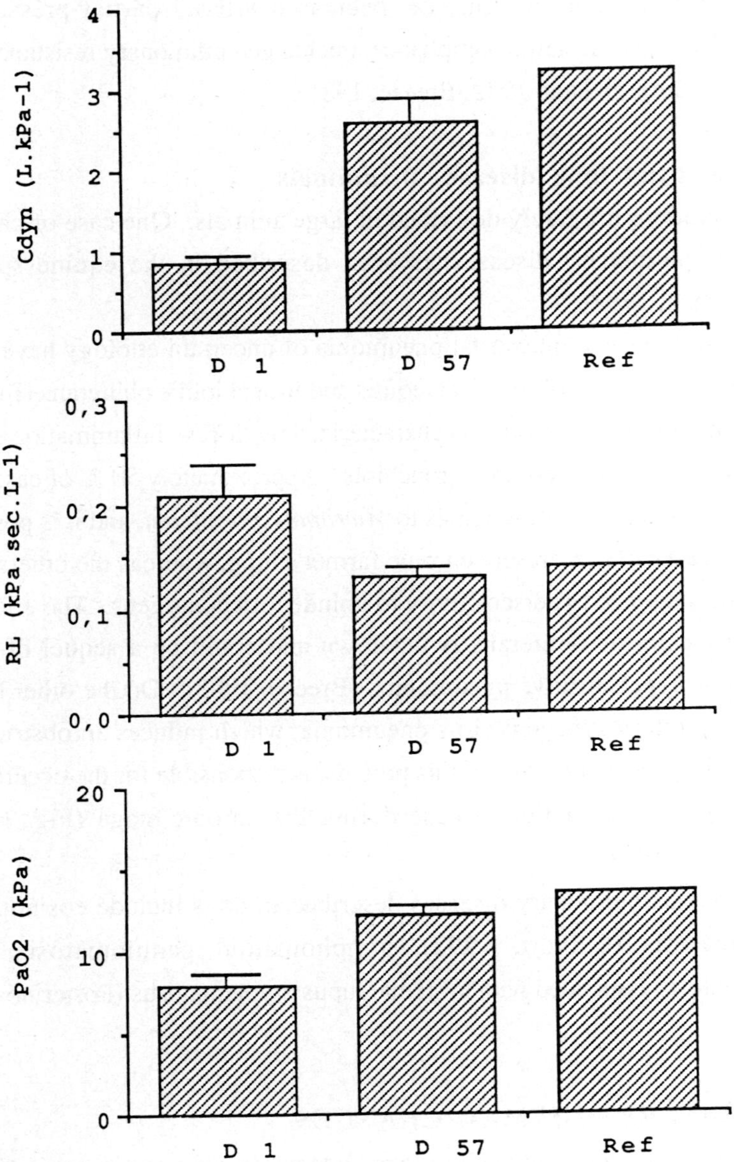

Fig. 13-1. Effect of respiratory syncytial virus infection on dynamic lung compliance (Cdyn), total pulmonary resistance (R_L) and arterial partial pressure in oxygen (PaO_2) in calves.

include non-neoplastic and neoplastic disorders. Affected animals frequently present signs of coughing, dyspnea, or exercise intolerance. Systemic signs may occur concurrently or as the only complaint. Thoracic radiographs are used to localize and characterize the disease process, certain patterns being suggestive of particular diseases. Cytologic or histologic evaluation is often required to obtain a definitive diagnosis; bronchoscopic collections (Hawkins et al, 1992), lung aspirates, or lung biopsies may be necessary (Roudebush et al, 1981; Teske et al, 1991). Less invasive tests, such as antibody titers for infectious diseases or fecal examinations for parasites may be helpful in confirming a specific diagnosis.

3.1. Non-neoplastic diseases

These disorders include viral, bacterial, protozoal, fungal and parasitic diseases and lead to intraparenchymal accumulation of fluid and/or cells.

With uncomplicated viral pneumonia, there is a loss of airway epithelial cells and influx of neutrophils into the airways, infiltration of peribronchial mononuclear cells, thickening and hyperhemia of alveolar septa, exudate with an increase in lymphocytes and neutrophils and fluid in alveoli, interstitial infiltrations with white blood cells and capillary thrombosis (Ada and Jones, 1986). Secondary bacterial infections are common sequels to viral infections.

The biological agents responsible for pulmonary diseases are numerous and generally specific according to the species. For instance, in dogs, canine distemper virus infects epithelial tissue throughout the body. This viral infection is characterized by an interstitial pattern on thoracic radiographs and a lymphopenia. However, the secondary bacterial pneumonia commonly dominates the clinical image (Greene and Appel, 1990). In cats, calicivirus infection can result in an interstitial pneumonia (Hoover and Kahn, 1975). In horses, the most important viruses that cause equine respiratory diseases are *Equine Influenza A/Equine 2* and *Equine Herpesvirus* type 4 (or *Rhinopneumonitis*).

Bacterial pneumonia is a common cause of respiratory disease in dogs, but is unusual in cats. Primary bacterial infection can occur as the result of *Bordetella bronchiseptica* (Bemis and Appel, 1977) and possibly *Streptococcus zooepidemicus*. In horses, the two streptococcal species of primary importance in respiratory diseases are *Streptococcus zooepidemicus* and *Streptococcus equi*.

A wide variety of other bacteria can cause pneumonia, often as secondary invaders (Roudebush, 1990). Possible primary etiologies should not be overlooked (Roudebush, 1992), since bacterial pneumonia is often a sequel of different clinical conditions such as viral, mycoplasmal or fungal respiratory infections, dysphagia, reduced levels of consciousness, severe metabolic disorders, immunosuppressive therapy, therapy with certain drugs like aspirin or digoxin, functional and anatomic disorders like tracheal hypoplasia or primary ciliary dyskinesia, immunodeficiency like phagocytic lymphocyte dysfunction, or intravenous catheterization.

Systemic oral or parenteral antibiotics that are active against the bacterial organism and are administered in high doses for long periods of time, are the principal therapy (McKiernan, 1984).

Other infectious bronchopneumonias in animals include mycobacterial (tuberculosis) (Clercx et al, 1992a; 1992b), protozoal (toxoplasmosis), fungal, parasitic and rickettsial diseases.

3.2. Neoplastic diseases

Lung tissue can be affected by primary pulmonary neoplasia, metastatic neoplasia, lymphosarcoma, and neoplasia invading from adjacent tissues (Mehlhaff and Mooney, 1985).

Surveys of equine neoplasms indicate a very low incidence of thoracic neoplasia in the horse (Sundberg et al, 1977).

In dogs and cats, neoplasia arising primarily from the lung is not very common, especially when compared to metastatic pulmonary neoplasia. The majority of lung neoplasms are carcinomas, which are most frequently adenocarcinomas (Moulton et al, 1981). Intrapulmonary spread of primary

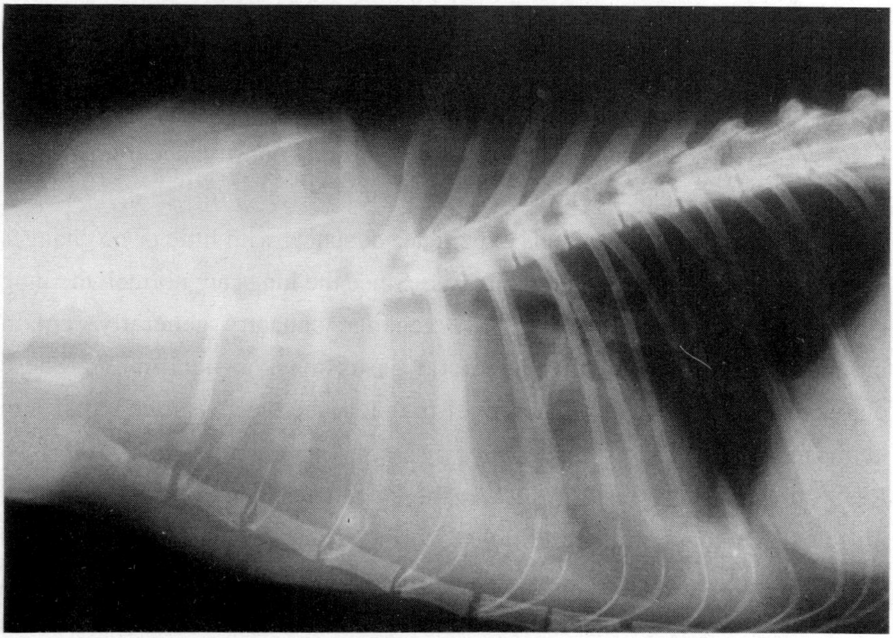

Fig. 13-2. Lateral radiographical view of the thorax of a cat with mediastinal tumor.

lung tumors is common. Clinical signs result from the primary pulmonary tumors and intrathoracic metastases (compression or obstruction of airways, regional ventilation/perfusion inequalities, ...), from extrathoracic metastases and from paraneoplastic conditions. Only few paraneoplastic syndromes have been described in dogs (Madewell and Theilen, 1987). Hypertrophic pulmonary osteopathy is the most frequently reported syndrome in dogs but it is less frequent in cats.

In lymphosarcoma, thoracic radiographs reveal an irregular reticular pattern, often with ill-defined nodular densities (Fig. 13-2.) (Suter, 1984). Intrathoracic lymphadenopathy or pleural effusion can be present.

The lungs are a very common site of metastases. Tumor types with high incidences of pulmonary metastatic lesions include thyroid carcinomas and mammary carcinomas (Suter et al, 1974).

4. EXTRAPARENCHYMAL CHANGES

In these cases, the lung is essentially normal. The restriction may be due to a large variety of conditions such as thoracic tumors, obesity, accumulation of pleural fluid and skeletal deformities

Early in the disease, the patients experience dyspnea, with little or no changes in the standard pulmonary function tests. Since the lungs are normal, the lung compliance and the diffusing gas exchange capacity generally remain unmodified. However, arterial blood gases may be abnormal. These characteristics allow the differential diagnose between parenchymal and extraparenchymal causes of restrictive diseases.

Restriction may also result from weakness or inefficiency of the respiratory muscles due to various conditions such as neural disorders, respiratory muscles fatigue, pneumothorax, diaphragmatic hernia, rib cage fractures, myopathy in young farm animals, tympanism in ruminants, advanced pregnancy and hydrops of the uterus

4.1. Abnormal pleural pressure

Accumulation of fluid (pleural effusion) or air (pneumothorax) in the intrapleural space may be responsible for this restrictive phenomenon. These intrapleural disorders are frequent in dogs and cats.

4.1.1. Functional effects

In these conditions, the absolute pleural pressure is no longer sufficiently negative. During inspiration, the pressure gradient is too weak to induce appropriate volume changes. During expiration, the pleural pressure may become positive, resulting in small airway collapse and/or alveolar atelectasis (Anthonisen, 1977; Nyman et al, 1990). During pneumothorax, active vasoconstriction may occur in the affected lung and a fall in PaO_2 may be observed (Moran et al, 1977).

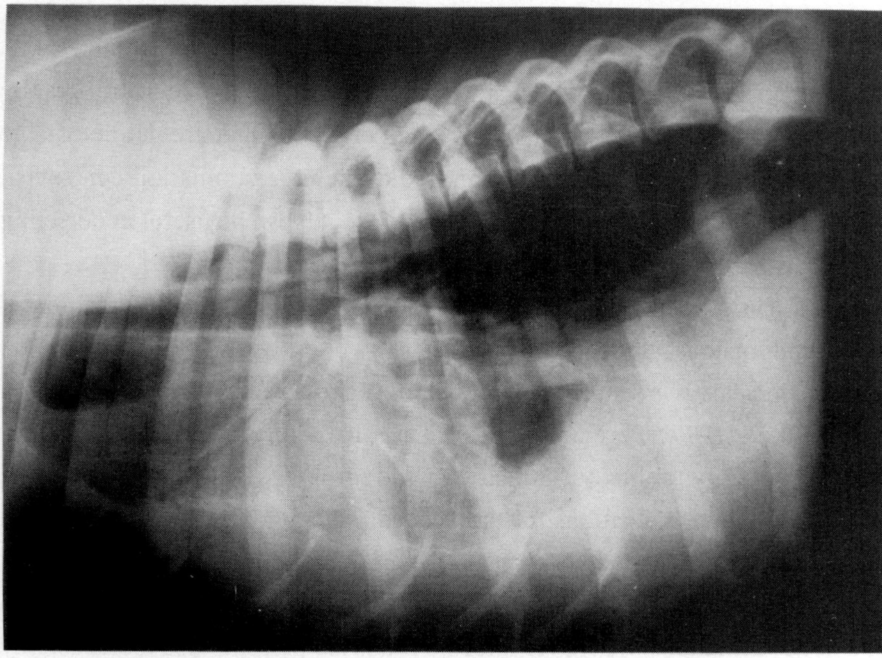

Fig. 13-3. Lateral radiographical view of the thorax of a dog with pleural effusion.

4.1.2. Pleural effusion

Pleural effusion is not a disease by its own, but a complication of severe pulmonary, cardiac, or other diseases. This condition may cause pleuritic pain, reduced movement of the chest and absence of breath sounds, but the pulmonary mechanical parameters often remain unchanged (Brown et al, 1978).

Clinical signs of pleural effusion may occur acutely or develop insidiously (Noone, 1985; Bauer, 1989). The degree of dyspnea does not directly correlate with the volume of pleural fluid. The most common sign is shortness of breath, i.e.tachypnea and shallow respiration. As pleural effusion is only the consequence of various diseases, other symptoms are often observed. Coughing, fever and pleural pain are sometimes present.

Pleural effusions can be detected by thoracic auscultation (characteristic loss or muffling of auscultable breath or cardiac sounds) and percussion (dullness). The diagnosis of pleural effusion must be confirmed by thoracic radiography (Fig. 13-3.), which also demonstrates small effusions that are not detectable on physical examination. Furtheron, radiographic examination can reveal signs of the primary disease. Diagnostic ultrasound can be useful in detecting cardiac diseases, or in locating pockets of pleural fluid.

Pleural fluid can be transudate, modified transudate, exsudate, pyogranulomatous, chylous or hemorrhagic.

Thoracocentesis is essential for establishing a definitive diagnosis (Creighton and Wilkin, 1977; Perman et al, 1979). In addition, removal of fluid improves radiographic visualisation, and provides relief of associated dyspnea. Contra-indications for thoracocentesis are a bleeding disorder and the presence of herniated abdominal content. Therapeutic thoracocentesis is frequently necessary when a large pleural effusion causes lung compression and hypoventilation. Whenever infected fluids are present, tube thoracostomy is mandatory. Pleural biopsy, open biopsy and thoracoscopy are advisable only when thoracocentesis and cytopathological studies have failed to provide a diagnosis.

4.1.3. Pneumothorax

A pneumothorax can either be closed (when air is trapped within the pleural space) or open (when air can escape through the chest wall). When air enters the pleural space, the lung collapses, the rib cage overexpands and the diaphragm is depressed on the affected side. Although the pulmonary function tests show a reduced vital capacity, radiographs are most informative for diagnosing this disorder.

Blunt or penetrating trauma of the thorax or abdomen are the most frequent cause of pneumothorax in dogs and cats. Radiographic findings other than pneumothorax may include rib fractures, subcutaneous emphysema, pneumomediastinum and pulmonary contusions. Pneumothorax can be caused by a number of mechanisms, i.e. direct lung laceration by rib fractures, chest wall disruption, or thoracic compression against a closed glottis. Other causes of pneumothorax include the rupture of pulmonary cysts, bullae or blebs, emphysema, cavitations (infectious or neoplastic), or be iatrogenic (thoracocentesis, biopsies) or spontaneous (Yoshioka, 1982).

Tension pneumothorax is a severe condition that may occur if the lung or pleura acts as an one-way-valve, by which air is allowed to pump into the pleural space by respiratory motions, while its flow back to the airway is prevented. In this case, the intrapleural pressures rise dramatically and become supratmospheric.

4.2. Abnormal thorax

The pulmonary function may be influenced by the thoracic compliance. The latter may be too low (ankylose) or too high, such as in newborn animals. The pulmonary capacity is reduced in the first case. A dramatic increase in the work of breathing and atelectasis result in the second condition.

4.3. Abnormal neuro-muscular function

The diaphragm is the main inspiratory muscle. Therefore, a severe respiratory insufficiency will result from all problems impairing the diaphragmatic work. These problems include diaphragmatic hernia, dysfunction of the phrenic nerve, excessive abdominal pressure as in ruminal tympany in cattle, myopathy, muscle weakness in patients chronically treated by steroids, muscle fatigue as in patients suffering from either acute or chronic respiratory disease. Lastly, pleural pain may also induce voluntary restricted thoracic movements.

4.3.1. Tympany in ruminants

Gastric tympany or bloat is an abnormal distension of the ruminant forestomach compartments with ingesta or gas. Cattle are more susceptible than sheep, but the disease does occur in the same conditions in small ruminants (Guard, 1990).

As the forestomach enlarges, the breathing is impaired because of the important cranial displacement of the diaphragm. Dyspnea is marked and accompanied by mouth breathing, protusion of the tongue, salivation and extension of the neck. The respiratory rate is increased up to 60 /min. Death from asphyxia ultimately results when the distension is extreme enough to compromise the ventilation (Desmecht et al, 1993).

4.3.2. Nutritional myodegeneration

The so called "white muscle disease" is a peracute to subacute myodegenerative disorder of cardiac and/or skeletal muscle. This syndrome occurs in most farm animal species but is most commonly found in young, rapidly growing calves, lambs, kids and foals.

There are two distinct syndromes of nutritional myodegeneration; a cardiac form and a skeletal form. The cardiac form is associated with signs of myocardial decompensation, while the skeletal form is associated with skeletal myasthenia and difficult locomotion. The commonly affected muscles are those of the front and hind limbs and of the neck region. However, in some cases, the diaphragm and the intercostal muscles may also be affected. In these cases, the animals show respiratory distress and evidence of abdominal effort when breathing. Cardiomyopathy often occurs along with the respiratory muscle disorders (Maas et al, 1990).

4.3.3. Syndrome of respiratory muscle weakness or fatigue

Fatigue is defined as the inability of a muscle to maintain a given force. The diaphragm is normally well adapted to resist fatigue. However, some clinical situations in which a combination of adverse factors are present, can lead to diaphragmatic fatigue. The clinical manifestations of inspiratory muscle fatigue include tachypnea, paradoxical abdominal motion, hypercapnia, and, as a preterminal event, bradypnea (Grassino and Macklem, 1984).

From a functional point of view, experimental setting demonstrates a reduced high/low ratio in the power spectrum of the electromyograph and a reduced rate of relaxation, together with a right shift of the force-frequency curve

(Grassino and Macklem, 1984).
Respiratory muscle fatigue has been shown to occur in calves suffering from acute respiratory distress due to experimental pasteurellosis (Desmecht et al, 1992). A bilateral diaphragmatic paralysis of unknown origin has been also described in a pony (Amory et al, 1993).
Lastly, it has been suggested that respiratory muscle fatigue may occur in horses performing exhausting fast exercise and this may be partly responsible for the hypoxemia and hypercapnia observed in this specific condition (Lekeux et al, 1992).

4.3.4. Diaphragmatic dysfunction in pet animals

Obesity (Pickickian syndrome) can affect the pulmonary function in a variety of ways. Intra- and extra-thoracic fat may interfere with expansion of the thoracic cavity and lungs during inspiration, resulting in hypoventilation (Hawkins et al, 1989).
Cranial displacement of the diaphragm may result from obesity, pregnancy, ascites, hepatomegaly and intra-abdominal masses
Herniation of abdominal contents through the diaphragm may occur at any level and may be congenital or acquired (Fig. 13-4.) (Wilson et al, 1986). Traumatic rupture of the diaphragm is usually the result of severe trauma.

5. RESTRICTIVE DISORDERS LEADING TO NEONATE RESPIRATORY DISTRESS SYNDROME

Maturation of the lung involves maturation of the surfactant system, but also a thinning of the alveolar capillary barrier, a decrease in alveolar epithelial permeability and the maturation of chest wall (Jobe, 1983). Although the lack of surfactant is an important factor in the initiation of respiratory distress syndrome, the immaturity of both the lung and chest wall, and the altered permeability characteristics of the lung also play an important role in its expression.

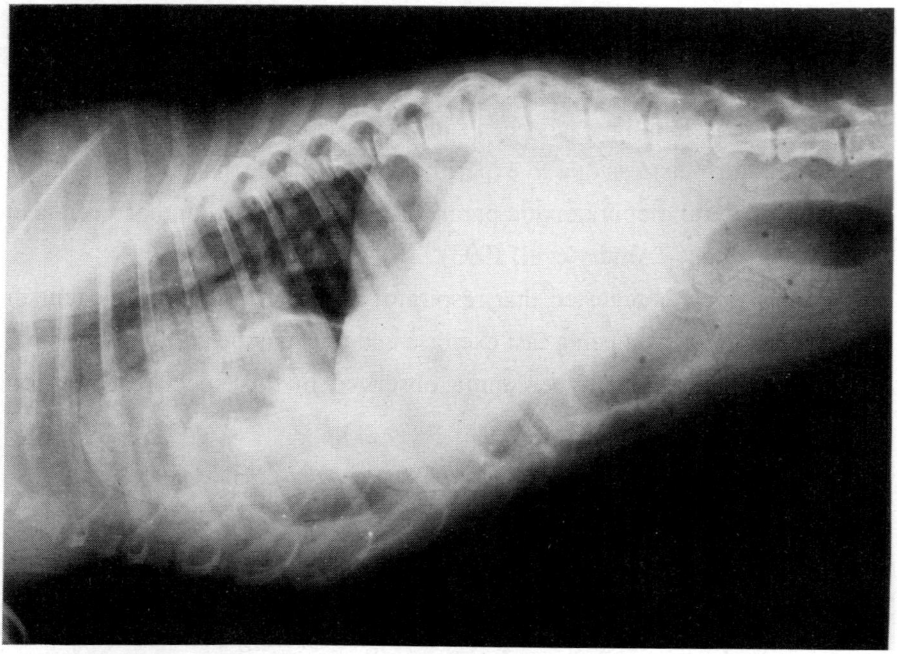

Fig. 13-4. Lateral radiographical view of the thorax of a cat with diaphragmatic hernia.

5.1. Surfactant deficiency

Pulmonary surfactant is a complex material composed mainly of phospholipids and proteins (Rooney, 1985). It has been shown that pulmonary surfactant is required to maintain alveolar stability and to prevent atelectasis. It reduces the work of breathing by increasing lung compliance and enhances alveolar fluid clearance (Clements et al, 1961). It is mainly produced and stored in alveolar epithelial type II cells (King and Clements, 1985). During fetal life, when there is no air-liquid interface within the lung, surfactant is not required. However, an adequate supply of pulmonary surfactant must be present at birth to allow lung stability and prevent atelectasis after the first breath. In the foal, surfactant has been detected as early as 200 days of gestation (Arvidson et al, 1975). Nevertheless, it has been suggested that pulmonary surfactant in the foal is insufficient to maintain

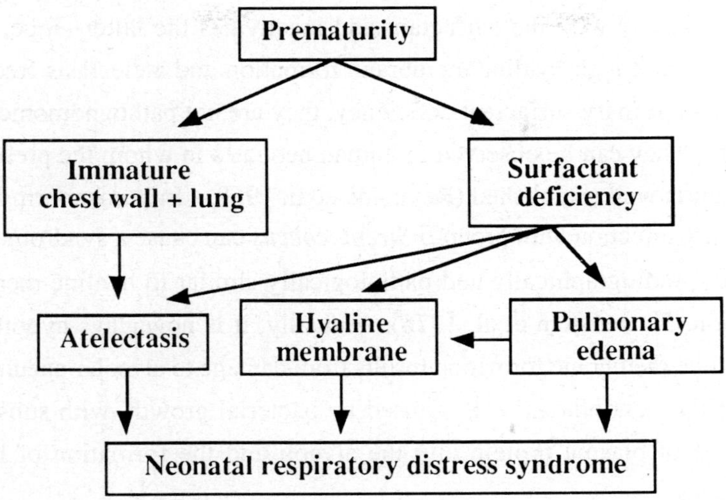

Fig. 13-5. Pathophysiological process of the respiratory distress syndrome in the premature neonate.

lung stability before 300 days of gestation, with large variability among individuals (Pattle et al, 1975). If the production of surfactant is delayed or if the birth is premature, the neonate is likely to suffer from neonatal respiratory distress syndrome (Fig. 13-5.). There is evidence that cortisol, thyroxine, β-adrenergic agonists and other agents stimulate maturation of the surfactant system (Kikkawa and Smith, 1983).

Surfactant system dysfunction may result either from primary (immaturity) or from secondary (due to insults causing surfactant dysfunction) deficiency.

5.2. Altered permeability characteristics and hyaline membrane formation

The neonate respiratory distress syndrome is frequently complicated by hyaline membrane formation, which is caused by aggregation of proteins and cellular debris accumulating in the alveoli as a result of increased alveolar permeability. This protein not only disrupts alveolar architecture but also interact directly with the surfactant and inactivates the latter (Jobe, 1983). Therefore, although hyaline membrane formation and atelectasis frequently complicate primary surfactant deficiency, they are not pathognomonic of this disorder. They can be observed in human neonates in whom the presence of surfactant is well established (Reynolds et al, 1968). In human term infants, pulmonary infection with group *β-Streptococcus* can cause a syndrome that is clinically, radiographically and pathologically similar to hyaline membrane formation (Katzenstein et al, 1976). Actually, it is nowadays hypothetized that hyaline membrane formation results from damage to alveolar pneumocytes and capillary endothelial cells caused by bacterial growth, with subsequent exudation of plasma protein into the alveoli and the formation of hyaline membranes.

5.3. Chest wall immaturity

The highly compliant chest wall of the premature neonate predisposes to a too low end-expiratory lung volume, even in the presence of surfactant. This results in a tendency for airway collapse and atelectasis and necessitates higher pressures to reopen closed airways, increasing the work of breathing. When this condition is further complicated by a deficiency in lung surfactant, the work of breathing will increase accordingly. The respiratory muscles must generate more pressure for inflation of the lungs, and respiratory muscle failure may result.

5.4. Neonate respiratory distress syndrome in large animals

Neonate respiratory distress syndrome has been reported in premature lambs, pigs, calves and foals (Gibson et al, 1976; Slauson, 1979; Eigenmann et al, 1984; Sonea, 1985). The piglets affected by the so called "barker" syndrome present abnormally immature lungs, hyaline membranes, surfactant deficiency and abnormal thyroid glands with clinical sign of hypothyroidism (Gibson et al, 1976). Calves and foals victims of complicated deliveries (cesarean section, dystocia and premature induction of labor) are usually more predisposed to develop respiratory distress syndrom (Koterba and Paradis, 1990).

5.5. Neonate respiratory distress syndrome in small animals

In dogs, age has been shown to influence the phospholipidic composition of the surfactant (Clercx et al, 1989). Besides physiological changes, there is also a pathological condition in which the altered composition of surfactant from neonatal puppies is responsible for a syndrome (fading puppies complex) similar to the acute respiratory distress syndrome in human neonates (Blunden, 1985). The role of surfactant changes in other clinical conditions has not yet been investigated in dogs and cats.

6. CONCLUSIONS

Interstitial pulmonary diseases, i.e. parenchymal restrictive diseases, are uncommon in domestic animals. Intra- and extraparenchymal disorders induce most frequently restrictive diseases, either alone or in combination with obstructive or vascular diseases. The main functional difference between intra- and extraparenchymal disorders is that the latter do not impair the lung mechanisms.

REFERENCES

ADA G.J., JONES P.D. The immune response to influenza infection. *Curr. Topics Microbiol. Immunol.* 1986, 128, 1-54.

AMORY H., LOMBA F., LEKEUX P., COHEN SOLAL A., JAUNIAUX T., DESMECHT D. Bilateral diaphragmatic paralysis of unknown origin in a pony. *J. Am. Vet. Med. Assoc.* 1993, in press.

ANTHONISEN N.R. Regional lung fonction in spontaneous pneumothorax. *Am. Rev. Respir. Dis.* 1977, 115, 873-876.

ARVIDSON G., ASTEDT B., EKELUND L., ROSSDALE P.D. Surfactant studies in the fetal and neonatal foal. *J. Reprod. Fert.* 1975, 23 (suppl.), 663-665.

BARROCAS M., NUCHPRAYOON C.V., CLAUDIO M., KING F.W., DANON J., SHARP J.T. Gas exchange abnormalities in diffuse lung disease. *Am. Rev. Respir. Dis.* 1971, 104, 72-87.

BASSET F., FERRANS V.J., SOLER P., TAKEMURA T., FUDUKA Y., CRYSTAL R.G. Intraluminal fibrosis in interstitial lung disorders. *Am. J. Pathol.* 1986, 122, 433-461.

BAUER T. Mediastinal, pleural, and extrapleural diseases. In : *Textbook of Veterinary Internal Medicine: Diseases of the Dog and Cat*, Ettinger, S.J. (Ed.), WB Saunders Company, Philadelphia, 1989, pp 867-897.

BEDROSSIAN C.W.M., GREENBERG S.D., WILLIAMS L.J. Ultrastructure of the lung in Loeffler's pneumonia. *Am. J. Med.* 1975, 58, 438-443.

BEMIS D.A., APPEL M.J. Aerosol, parenteral, and oral antibiotic treatment of *Bordetella bronchiseptica* infections in dogs. *J. Am. Vet. Med. Assoc.* 1977, 170, 1082-1086.

BLUNDEN A.S. Composition in puppies dying of fading puppy complex. *Res. Vet. Sci.* 1985, 42, 113-118.

BREEZE R.G. Respiratory disease in adult cattle. *Vet. Clin. North Am. Food Anim. Pract.* 1985, 1, 311-346.

BROWN N.E., ZAMEL N., ABERMAN A. Changes in pulmonary mechanics and gas exchange following thoracocentesis. *Chest* 1978, 74, 540-542.

CALVERT C.A. Eosinophilic pulmonary granulomatosis. In : *Current Veterinary Therapy XI Small Animal Practice*, Kirk, R.W., Bonagura, J.D. (Eds), W.B. Saunders Company, Philadelphia, 1992, pp 813-816.

CLEMENTS J.A., HUSTEAD R.F., JOHNSON R.P., GRIBETZ I. Pulmonary surface tension lining and alveolar stability. *J. Appl. Physiol.* 1961, 16, 444-450.

CLERCX C., VENKER-van HAAGEN A.J., den BREEJEN J.N., HAAGSMAN H.P., van den BROM W.E., de VRIES H.W., van GOLDE L.M.G. Effects of age and breed on the phospholipid composition of canine surfactant. *Lung* 1989, 167, 351-357.

CLERCX C., COIGNOUL F., MAINIL J., JAKOVLJEVIC S., HENROTEAUX M., KAECKENBEECK F. Canine tuberculosis: a case report and review of the literature. *J. Am. Anim. Hosp. Assoc.* 1992a, 28, 207-211.

CLERCX C., JAKOVLJEVIC S., HENROTEAUX M., DE GROOTE A., KAECKENBEECK A., COIGNOUL F. Deux cas de tuberculose féline (*Mycobacterium bovis*). *Ann. Méd. Vét.* 1992b, 136, 141-145.

CREIGHTON S.R., WILKIN R.S. Pleural effusion. In : *Current Veterinary Therapy*, Kirk, R.W. (Ed.), WB Saunders Company, Philadelphia, 1977, pp 255-263.

CRYSTAL R.G., GADEK J.E., FERRANS V.J., FULMER J.D., LINE B.R., HUNNINGHAKE G.W. Interstitial lung disease: current concepts of pathogenesis, staging, and therapy. *Am. J. Med.* 1981, 70, 542-568.

CRYSTAL R.G., FERRANS V.J. Reactions of the interstitial space to injury. In : *Pulmonary Diseases and Disorders*, Fishman, A.P. (Ed.), McGraw-Hill, New York, 1988, pp 711-738.

CRYSTAL R.G., FERRANS V.J., BASSET F. Biologic basis of pulmonary fibrosis. In : *The Lung: Scientific Foundations*, Crystal, R.G., West, J.B. (Eds), Raven Press, New York, 1991, pp 2031-2046.

DERKSEN F.J., SLOCOMBE R.F., BROWN C.M., ROOK J., ROBINSON N.E. Chronic restrictive pulmonary disease in a horse. *J. Am. Vet. Med. Assoc.* 1982, 180, 887-889.

DESMECHT D., LINDEN A., AMORY H., LEKEUX P. Effect of experimentally induced acute pneumonia on diaphragmatic strength generation in neonatal calves. *Arch. Int. Physiol. Bioch.* 1992, 100, P4.

DESMECHT D., LINDEN A., LEKEUX P. Respiratory muscle function changes associated with experimental simulation of rumen tympanism in cattle. *Arch. Int. Physiol. Bioch.* 1993, 101, P7.

EIGENMANN U.J.E., SCHOON H.A., JAHN D., GRUNERT E. Neonatal respiratory distress syndrome in the calf. *Vet. Rec.* 1984, 114, 141-144.

FULMER J.D., ROBERTS W.C., VON GAL E.R., CRYSTAL R.G. Small airways in idiopathic pulmonary fibrosis. *J. Clin. Invest.* 1977, 60, 595-610.

GIBSON E.A., BLACKMORE R.J.J., WIJERATNE W.V.S., WRATHALL A.E. The "barker" (neonatal respiratory distress) syndrome in the pig: its occurence in the field. *Vet. Rec.* 1976, 98, 476-479.

GRASSINO A., MACKLEM P.T. Respiratory muscle fatigue and ventilatory failure. *Ann. Rev. Med.* 1984, 35, 625-647.

GREENE G.E., APPEL, M.J. Canine distemper. In : *Infectious Diseases of the Dog and Cat*, Greene, G.E. (Ed.), W.B. Saunders Company, Philadelphia, 1990, pp 226-242.

GUARD C. Bloat or ruminal tympany. In : *Large Animal Internal Medicine*, Smith, B.P. (Ed.), The Mosby Company, Toronto, 1990, pp 789-791.

HAWKINS E.C., ETTINGER S.J., SUTER P.F. Diseases of the lower respiratory tract (lung) and pulmonary edema. In : *Textbook of Veterinary Internal Medicine*, Ettinger, S.J. (Ed.), W.B. Saunders Company, Philadelphia, 1989, pp 846.

HAWKINS E.C. Tracheal wash and bronchoalveolar lavage in the management of respiratory disease. In : *Current Veterinary Therapy XI Small Animal Practice*, Kirk, R.W., Bonagura, J.D. (Eds), W.B. Saunders Company, Philadelphia, 1992, pp 795-800.

HOOVER E.A., KAHN D.E. Experimentally induced feline calicivirus infections: clinical signs and lesions. *J. Am. Vet. Med. Assoc.* 1975, 166, 463-468.

JOBE A. Respiratory distress syndrome - New therapeutic approaches to a complex pathophysiology. *Adv. Pediatr.* 1983, 30, 93-130.

KATZENSTEIN A.L., DAVIS C., BRAUDE A. Pulmonary changes in neonatal sepsis due to group B β-hemolytic *Streptococccus*: relation to hyaline membrane disease. *J. Infect. Dis.* 1976, 133, 430-435.

KEOGH B.A., CRYSTAL, R.G. Alveolitis: the key to the interstitial lung disorders. *Thorax* 1982, 37, 1-10.

KIKKAWA Y., SMITH F. Cellular and biochemical aspects of pulmonary surfactant in health and disease. *Lab. Invest.* 1983, 49, 122-139.

KING R.J., CLEMENTS J.A. Lipid synthesis and surfactant turnover in the lungs. In : *Handbook of Physiology: The Respiratory System*, Vol. 1, Fishman, A.P. (Ed.), American Physiological Society, Bethesda MD, Maryland, 1985, pp 309-336.

KOTERBA A.M., PARADIS M.R. Specific respiratory conditions. In : *Equine Clinical Neonatalogy*, Koterba, A.M., Drummond, W.H., Kosch, P.C. (Eds), Lea & Febiger, Philadelphia, 1990, pp 177-199.

LEKEUX P., VERHOEFF J., HAJER R., BREUKINK H.J. Respiratory syncytial virus pneumonia in Friesian calves: physiological findings. *Res. Vet. Sci.* 1985, 39, 324-327.

LEKEUX P., ART T., DESMECHT D. Effect of exercise on equine alveolar ventilation. In Proceedings : 11th Comparative Respiratory Society Meeting, Urbana, (USA), September 1992, S12.

LINE B.R., FULMER J.D., REYNOLDS H.Y., ROBERTS W.C., JONES A.E., HARRIS E.K., CRYSTAL R.G. Gallium-67 citrate scanning in the staging of idiopathic pulmonary fibrosis: correlation with physiologic and morphologic features and bronchoalveolar lavage. *Am. Rev. Respir. Dis.* 1978, 118, 355-365.

MAAS J., PARISH S.M., HODGSON D.R. Nutritional myodegeneration. In : *Large Animal Internal Medicine*, Smith, B.P. (Ed.), The Mosby Company, Toronto, 1990, pp 1352-1357.

MADEWELL B.R., THEILEN G.H. Tumors of the respiratory tract. In : *Veterinary Cancer Medicine*, Theilen, G.H., Madewell, B.R. (Eds), Lea & Febiger, Philadelphia, 1987, pp 535.

McKIERNAN B.C. Therapeutic strategies involving antimicrobial treatment of the lower respiratory tract in small animals. *J. Am. Vet. Med. Assoc.* 1984, 185, 1155-1158.
MEHLHAFF CJ, MOONEY S. Primary pulmonary neoplasia in the dog and cat. *Vet. Clin. North Am.* 1985, 15, 1061-1067.
MORAN J.F., JONES R.H., WOLFE W.G. Regional pulmonary fonction during experimental unilateral pneumothorax in the awake state. *J. Thorac. Cardiovasc. Surg.* 1977, 74, 396-402.
MOULTON J.E., von TSCHARNER C., SCHNEIDER R. Classification of lung carcinomas in the dogs and cats. *Vet. Pathol.* 1981, 18, 513-528.
NOONE K.E. Pleural effusions and diseases of the pleura. *Vet. Clin. North Am.* 1985, 15, 1069-1084.
NOONE K.E. Pulmonary hypersensitivities. In : *Current Veterinary Therapy IX*, Kirk, R.W. (Ed.), W.B. Saunders Company, Philadelphia, 1986, pp 285.
NYMAN G., FUNKQUIST B., KVART C., FROSTELL C., TOKICS L., STRANDBERG A., LUNDQUIST H., LUNDH B., BRISMAR B., HEDENSTIERNA G. Atelectasis causes gas exchange impairment in the anaesthetised horse. *Equine Vet. J.* 1990, 22, 317-324.
PATTLE R.E., ROSSDALE P.D., SCHOCK C., CREASEY J.M. The development of the lung and its surfactant in the foal and in other species. *J. Reprod. Fert. (suppl.)* 1975, 23, 651-657.
PERMAN V., ALSAKER R.D., RIIS R.C. Cytology of the dog and cat. *Am. Anim. Hosp. Assoc. South Bend. Indiana*, 1979.
POPPIUS H., KORHONEN O., VILJANEN A.A., KREUS K.-E. Arterial to end-tidal CO2 difference in respiratory disease. *Scand. J. Respir. Dis.* 1975, 56, 254-262.
POSTERINO N.C. Canine pulmonary lymphomatoid granulomatosis: 8 cases (1981-1986). *Vet. Can. Soc. News* 1987, 11, 1.
RADWAN L., DAUM S. Evaluation of mixed venous oxygenation on the basis of arterial oxygen tension in chronic lung diseases. *Respiration* 1980, 40, 194-200.
REYNOLDS E.O.R., ROBERTON N.R.C., WIGGLESWORTH J.S. Hyaline membrane disease, respiratory distress and surfactant deficiency. *Pediatrics* 1965, 42, 758-768.
ROONEY S.A. The surfactant system and lung phospholipid biochemistry. *Am. Rev. Respir. Dis.* 1985, 131, 439-460.
ROUDEBUSH P, GREEN R.A., DIGILIO K.M. Percutaneous fine-needle aspiration biopsy of the lung in disseminated pulmonary disease. *J. Am. Anim. Hosp. Assoc.* 1981, 17, 109-116.
ROUDEBUSH P. Bacterial infections of the respiratory system. In : *Infectious Diseases of the Dog and Cat*, Greene, G.E. (Ed.), W.B. Saunders Company, Philadelphia, 1990, pp 114-125.
ROUDEBUSH P. Infectious pneumonia. In : *Current Veterinary Therapy XI Small Animal Practice*, Kirk, R.W., Bonagura, J.D. (Eds), W.B. Saunders Company, Philadelphia, 1992, pp 228-237.
SAVOY J., DHINGRA S., ANTHONISEN N.R. Role of vagal airway reflexes in control of ventilation in pulmonary fibrosis. *Clin. Sci.* 1981, 61, 781-784.
SLAUSON D.O. Naturally occuring hyaline membrane disease syndromes in foals and piglets. *J. Pediatr.* 1979, 95, 889-891.
SONEA I. Respiratory distress syndrome in neonatals foals. *Comp. Cont. Educ. Pract. Vet.* 1985, 7, S462-S469.
SUNDBERG J.P., BURSTEIN T., PAGE E.H., KIRKHAM W.W., ROBINSON F.R. Neoplasms of Equidae. *J. Am. Vet. Med. Assoc.* 1977, 170, 150-152.
SUTER P.F., CARRIG C.B., O'BRIEN T.R., KOLLER D. Radiographic recognition of primary and metastatic pulmonary neoplasms of dogs and cats. *J. Am. Vet. Radiol.*

Soc. 1974, 15, 3-25.
SUTER P.F. Lower airway and pulmonary parenchymal diseases. In : *Thoracic Radiography*, ch. 11, Suter, PF. (Ed.), Wettswil, Switzerland, 1984, pp 517-682.
TAN C.S.H., TASHKIN D.P. Supernormal maximal mid-expiratory flow rates in diffuse interstitial lung disease. *Respiration* 1981, 42, 200-208.
TESKE E., STOKHOF A.A., VAN DEN INGH T.S.G.A.M., WOLVEKAMP W.TH.C., SLAPPENDEL R.J., DE VRIES H.W. Transthoracic needle aspiration biopsy of the lung in dogs with pulmonic diseases. *J. Am. Anim. Hosp. Assoc.* 1991, 27, 289-294.
WAGNER P.D., DANTZKER D.R., DUECK R., de POLO J.-L., WASSERMAN K., WEST J.B. Distribution of ventilation-perfusion ratios in patients with interstitial lung disease. *Chest* 1976, 69 (suppl.), 256-257.
WILSON G.P., HAYES H.M. Diaphragmatic hernia in the dog and cat: a 25-year overview. *Sem. Vet. Med. Surg.* 1986, 1, 318-326.
YOSHIOKA M.M. Management of spontaneous pneumothorax in twelve dogs. *J. Am. Anim. Hosp. Assoc.* 1982, 18, 57-62.

CHAPTER XIV

VENTILATORY FAILURE AND RESPIRATORY MUSCLE FATIGUE

P. Lekeux and D. Desmecht

Laboratory for Functional Investigation
Faculty of Veterinary Medicine
University of Liege

SUMMARY

This paper analyses the concept that respiratory muscles may be unable in somes circumstances or diseases to generate sufficient pressure for an adequate alveolar ventilation in domestic animals.

KEY WORDS

Respiratory system - Pulmonary function - Muscle fatigue.

1. INTRODUCTION

The inspiratory work of breathing required to overcome the resistive, elastic and inertial forces, may considerably increase during some circumstances, i.e. respiratory disease-induced and exercise-induced hyperpnea. It is evident that the integrity of the inspiratory muscles is of primary importance. Indeed, respiratory muscle fatigue may result in alveolar hypoventilation and life threatening hypercapnic ventilatory failure.

The main purpose of this report is to analyse the concept that the respiratory muscles may fail in the same way as locomotor muscles or the cardiac muscle. Respiratory muscle failure is reported to be common in a variety of conditions in human beings (Pittinger and Adamson, 1972; Doekel et al, 1976; Thurlbeck, 1978; Driver and Lebrun, 1980; Bassili and Deitel, 1981; Knochel, 1981; Aubier et al, 1985; Laroche et al, 1988) but has not yet been reported in domestic animals.

Investigations of the diaphragmatic function in large animals models, during mimicked naturally occurring conditions such as pneumonia, gastric tympanism or hypocalcemia, have recently been conducted (Desmecht et al, 1992a). This could result in a better understanding of the inspiratory muscle physiopathology. Whether respiratory muscle fatigue could result in poor athletic performance is now open to question since exercise-induced hypoxemia in horses was shown to be significantly correlated to the exponential evolution of their mechanical work of breathing (Art et al, 1990).

2. RESPIRATORY MUSCLE FUNCTION AND FATIGUE

During respiratory muscle contraction, there is a chain of events which may be divided into three groups : (a) the processes for delivering sufficient electrical activation from the central nervous system to the muscle, (b) the metabolic and enzymatic processes providing energy for the contractile mechanisms, and (c) the excitation-contraction coupling processes (Roussos and Macklem, 1986). Fatigue of these muscles is usually defined as their inability to continue to generate sufficient pressure for an adequate alveolar ventilation. The site of fatigue may theoretically be located at any link of the processes involved in muscle contraction.

3. FACTORS PREDISPOSING TO RESPIRATORY MUSCLE FATIGUE

Factors which can lead to fatigue can be divided into two groups.

The first group of predisposing factors concerns the energy demand of the inspiratory muscles which is conditioned by the work of breathing, the muscle strength and the efficiency. The work of breathing depends on the minute ventilation, the resistance, the compliance and the inertance of the respiratory system. The muscle strength is influenced by the lung volume (Yan et al, 1992) and by the integrity of the neuromuscular system. Finally, respiratory muscle efficiency is affected by increased load, decreased fiber length or isometric contraction.

The second group of predisposing factors concerns the energy supply of the inspiratory muscles which is conditioned by the muscle blood flow (cardiac output, distribution of perfusion, intensity of contraction), the oxygen content of arterial blood (oxygen saturation, hemoglobin concentration), the blood substrate concentration (glucose, free fatty acids), the ability to extract sources of energy and the energy reserves of the muscles (Roussos and Macklem, 1986)

4. DETECTION OF RESPIRATORY MUSCLE FATIGUE

Diaphragmatic fatigue can be detected in various ways (Dureuil and Aubier, 1988).

The assessment of diaphragmatic fatigue is more difficult than for other skeletal muscles because it is impossible to measure directly the tension generated. However, the mechanical transformation of tension into pressure can be evaluateded. Fortunately, the trans-diaphragmatic pressure (Pdi), defined as the difference between the gastric pressure and the esophageal pressure, closely reflects the tension produced by the contracting diaphragm

(Kim et al, 1976). Therefore, this parameter is used to assess diaphragmatic mechanical performance.

There are typical clinical manifestations of inspiratory muscle fatigue. They consist of (1) a paradoxical inward abdominal motion during inspiration ("abdominal paradox") and (2) an alternation between abdominal and rib cage breathing ("respiratory alternans") (Cohen et al, 1982). Respiratory inductive plethysmography is an objective technique to demonstrate these thoraco-abdominal motions. This technique has been used simultaneously with Pdi measurements to diagnose diaphragmatic paralysis in the horse (Figs 14-1. and 14-2.) (Amory et al, 1993).

Diaphragmatic performances can also be evaluated by the measurement of the maximal Pdi a subject can generate during standardized inspiratory maneuvers (the so-called "Mueller maneuvers"). This technique is based on the assumption that a lower diaphragmatic contractility will be associated with lower maximal pressures. However, this parameter depends on the subject's ability and motivation to cooperate and can not be used in animals. Furthermore, the comparison of the peak Pdi achieved at two different times is only possible if the abdominal compliance, the muscle length and the muscle geometry remain unchanged. For all these reasons Pdimax measurement is not a good tool for research in animals.

Spectral analysis of diaphragmatic spontaneous electrical activity is of great interest since the modification of spectral parameters (shift in centroïd frequency and high-to-low ratio) is a precocious indicator of fatigue (Gross et al, 1979). This technique is only reliable when the skin is thin enough to allow the recording of spontaneous diaphragmatic electromyograms via surface electrodes. In the bovine species however, it requires a thoracotomy to insert electrodes into the muscle itself (Close et al, 1991). The signal obtained is not stable over long periods, can only be compared with itself and, up to now, cannot be related to any physiological event. These disadvantages preclude its wide use in research. However, this technique can be useful in clinical conditions such as the follow-up of patients disconnected from

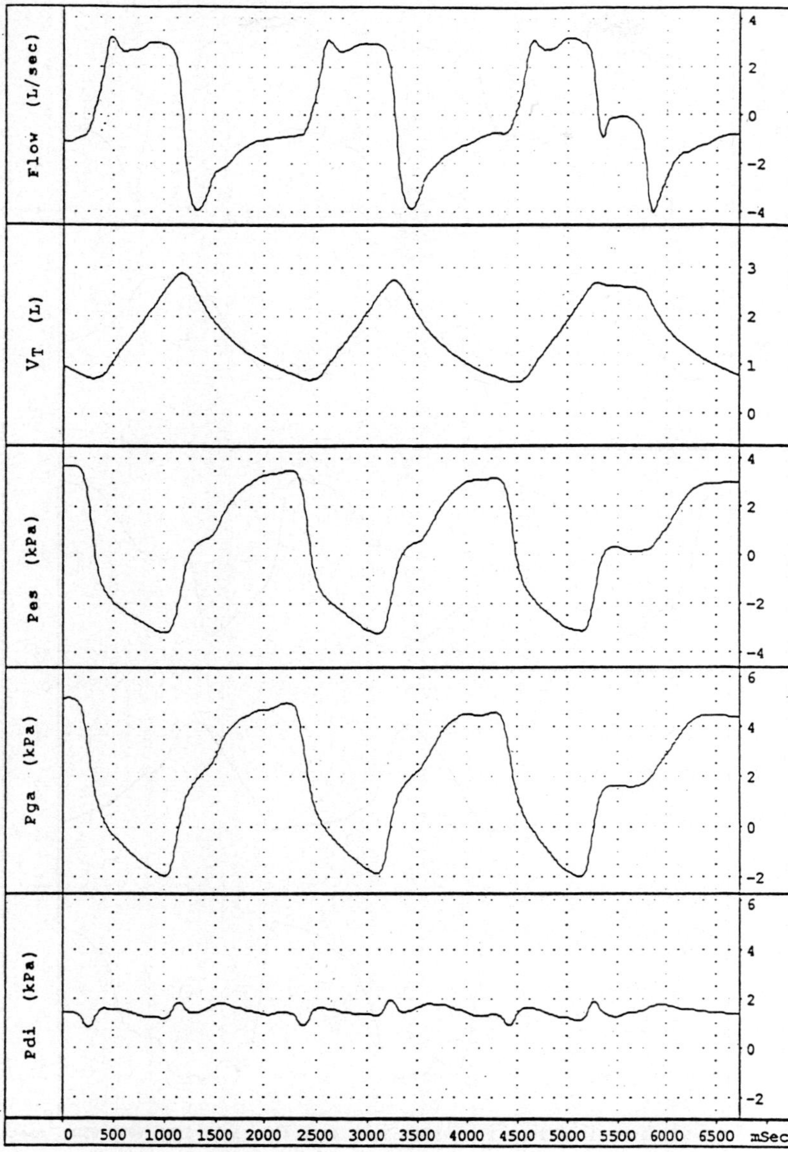

Fig. 14-1. Typical flow, tidal volume (V_T), esophageal (Pes), gastric (Pga) and transdiaphragmatic (Pdi) pressures tracings in the pony studied. Note the close parallelism between Pga and Pes during the whole respiratory cycle, the marked decrease in Pga during inspiration, and the nearly flat Pdi.

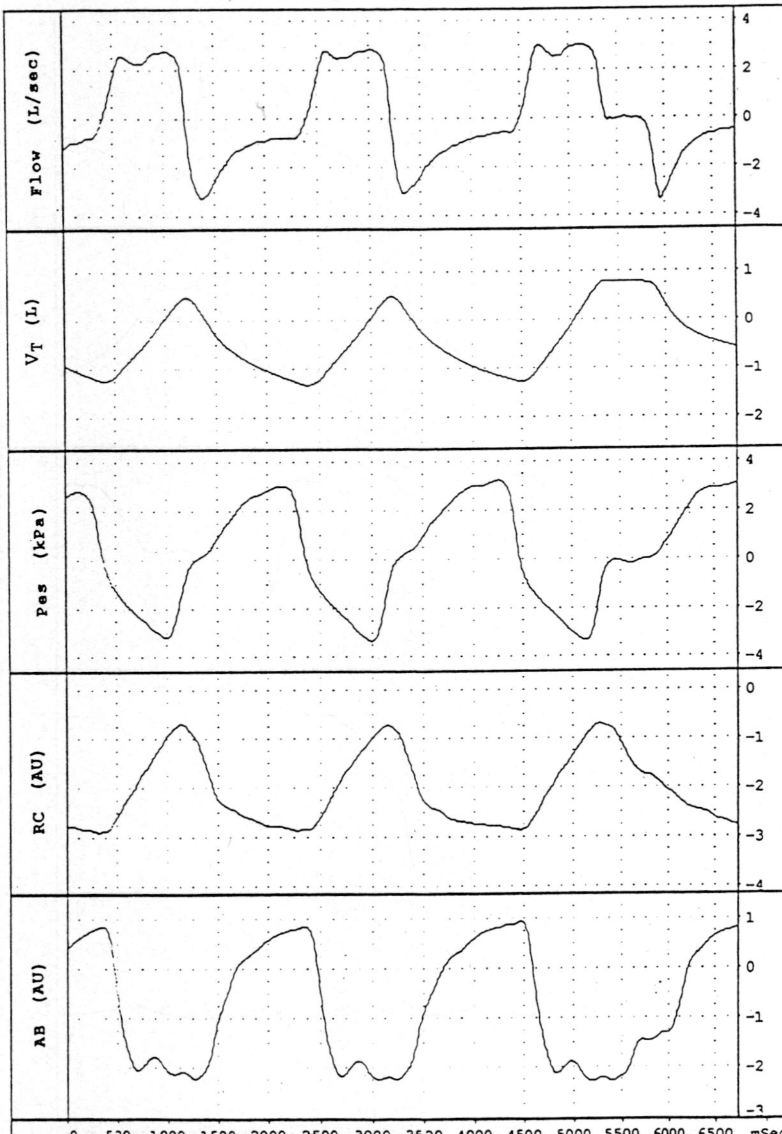

Fig. 14-2. Typical flow, tidal volume (V_T), esophageal (Pes), rib cage motion (RC) and abdominal motion (AB) tracings in the pony studied. A downward deflection on the RC and AB tracings indicate an inward motion of the compartment's wall. Note the inward displacement of the abdomen during inspiration. AU : Arbitrary units.

artificial ventilators (Cohen et al, 1982).

Changes in diaphragmatic contractility are accompanied by changes in muscle relaxation time (Edwards, 1978), as fatigued muscles relax more slowly than fresh muscles. This change in diaphragmatic relaxation time, which appears before the decrease in muscular tension, can be quantified by measuring the maximum Pdi relaxation rate or the time constant of the latter mono-exponential phase of relaxation (Esau et al, 1983; Mal et al, 1987). When this time constant is greater than 75 ms, diaphragmatic dysfunction may be suspected.

The last method to evaluate the diaphragmatic function consists in constructing its pressure-frequency curve, i.e. the pressures the diaphragm can generate in response to supramaximal stimulations of the phrenic nerves at increasing frequencies. This technique is difficult to use in human beings because of discomfort and because of the risks of causing phrenic lesions by inserting stimulating needles or skin burns by using transcutaneous high voltage stimulations. In laboratory animals, this technique requires a thoracotomy in order to catch the phrenic nerves, precluding safe extrapolation of the results obtained in intact subjects. Recently, the feasability, technical, methodological and standardization requirements of this technique have been established in intact and awake subjects of the bovine and equine species (Desmecht et al, 1990; 1993a). It requires the simultaneous recording of evoked diaphragmatic compound action potentials (Fig. 14-3.) by using surface electrodes (Fig. 14-4.) and of evoked transdiaphagmatic pressure changes by using esophageal and gastric balloons (Fig. 14-5.).

5. RESPIRATORY MUSCLE FATIGUE IN DISEASED ANIMALS

5.1. Dog

Impaired blood flow to the respiratory muscles has been associated with muscle fatigue and ventilatory failure in the canine species (Aubier et al, 1981a). However, other studies showed that the blood supply to these

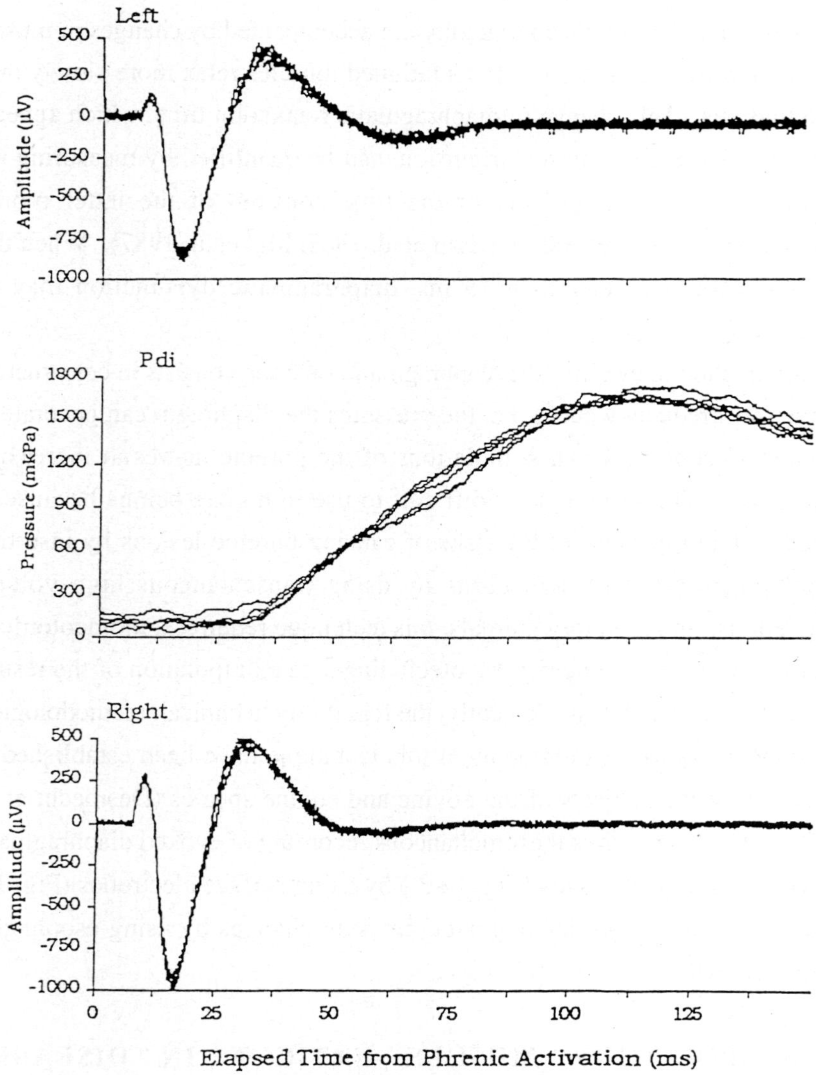

Fig. 14-3. Typical experimental data for monitoring phrenic activation and precontraction diaphragmatic length in cattle. Five superimposed compound hemidiaphragmatic action potentials (CDAP) picked on the right and left chest and the corresponding twitches in transdiaphragmatic pressure (Pdi) after bilateral supramaximal phrenic nerves stimulation at 1 Hz are displayed. Note the repeatability of CDAPs' amplitudes and Pdi values at the time of stimulation.

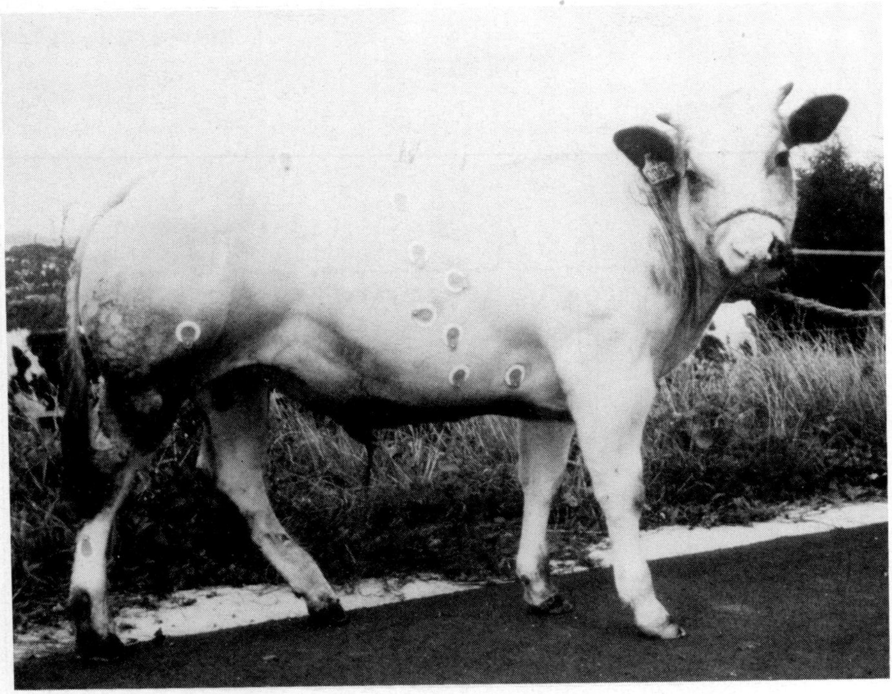

Fig. 14-4. Electrode position arbitrarily chosen for recording of body surface diaphragmatic compound action potential.

muscles is not a limiting factor in dogs breathing through heavy inspiratory loads (Rochester et al, 1976).

5.2. Cattle

5.2.1. Experimental model

A reliable method giving diaphragmatic function parameters in intact, unsedated and spontaneously breathing calves has been recently developed Desmecht et al, 1991). This method is of considerable interest because it gives the opportunity to conduct experiments in intact and unsedated animals so that the conclusions drawn may be extrapolated with minimal risk to

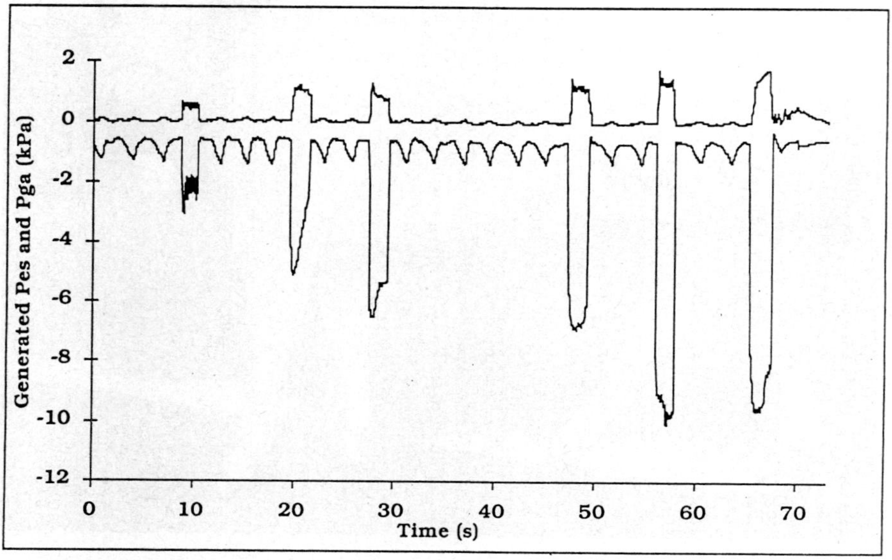

Fig. 14-5. Display of esophageal (Pes) and gastric (Pga) pressure responses to successive bilateral supramaximal phrenic nerves stimulations at frequencies between 10 and 100 Hz (80 V, 2-s trains of 0.2-ms square-wave pulses) in cattle.

naturally occurring conditions.

The measurement of the force generated by a muscle in response to electrical stimulations of its nerve provides an objective technique for assessing its contractility. In the case of the model presented, it requires the simultaneous achievement of three techniques : (1) the measurement of the force output, i.e. the transdiaphragmatic pressure (Pdi) which is measured by subtracting esophageal pressure from gastric pressure, each measured via conventional balloon-tubing-transducer units, (2) the strict control of the neural input by transjugular activation of the phrenic nerves and (3) the monitoring of the evoked electrophysiological response of the diaphragm by electromyography (EMG) in order to be sure that the stimulation remains supramaximal.

The phrenic nerves are stimulated through the wall of the jugular veins, using a catheter equipped with 2 platinum electrodes at its distal end. Square-wave pulses are initiated immediately after introducing the catheter into the vein. The catheter is then slowly and progressively inserted backward until diaphragmatic twitches appear on the Pdi and EMG tracings. The stimulus voltage is then increased until no further increase in twitch occurs. The nerves are then stimulated at different frequencies in order to obtain pressure-frequency curves. The evoked potentials emanating from the left and right hemidiaphragms are captured using a specific pair of electrodes glued on the skin of the chest.

As for any muscle, even if the stimulus voltage is supramaximal, the contractions must be identical on a mechanical point of view. This requires isometric contractions, identical degree and velocity of shortening and same fiber length at the moment of the stimulation. In order to fulfill these conditions, the stimulations are automatically triggered at end-expiratory lung volume (by using the flow signal) against a tightly occluded airway. All conditions of reliability being properly controlled, the force-frequency curves of the diaphragm can be constructed in intact and unsedated calves, giving intra-day, between day and between individuals reproducible measurements of diaphragmatic strength at different frequencies of stimulation. This model has been implemented in three experimental conditions each mimicking a naturally occurring disease in cattle. Interestingly, each of these conditions also corresponds to a peculiar challenge for the diaphragm.

5.2.2. Respiratory muscle fatigue associated with pneumonia

Pneumonia is a condition in which the diaphragmatic quotient energy demand/energy supply is increased. The capacity of the diaphragm to generate pressure is considerably decreased in this circumstance (Desmecht et al, 1992b). As previously mentioned, the pressure generated by the diaphragm for a given stimulation is affected by its fibers length which is determined by the lung volume. Conceivably, the observed changes in Pdi could have been secondary to changes in the end-expiratory lung volume. However, there was a significant decrease of end-expiratory lung volume measured by the helium dilution technique. This indicates that, during pneumonia, the expiratory muscles put the diaphragm on a more efficacious point of its length-tension relationship when the spontaneous inspiration - or phrenic stimulation - begins. That means that Pdi was surely not underestimated. So, Pdi decreased with developing pneumonia for all the frequencies of stimulation. This phenomenon cannot be related to changes in the mechanical behavior of the diaphragm and may thus be called fatigue.

Many pathways from the brain down to the contractile elements are involved in the contraction process of a muscle. However, the present approach of stimulating the muscle directly through its nerve obviously excludes the central steps. Moreover, the observation that the loss of force is not parallelled by a decline in electrical activity of the diaphragm suggests that the decrease in the Pdi-frequency characteristics could be mainly due to an impairment of the excitation-contraction coupling processes. The metabolic processes providing energy for muscle contraction are greatly dependent on muscle perfusion and oxygen availability. During pneumonia, the work of the diaphragm is multiplied by a factor 10 whilst oxygen supply is decreased, due to gas exchange problems (Desmecht et al, 1992b). Both factors may lead to anaerobic metabolism. This study cannot offer a definitive explanation of diaphragmatic failure during pneumonia and further work is needed to fully understand the mechanisms responsible for the impairment of diaphragmatic contraction during pneumonia. This study, however, shows unequivoquely that the precipitating factor leading to death in animals, and perhaps humans as well, suffering from pneumonia may simply be the failure of the inspiratory muscles.

5.2.3. Respiratory muscle fatigue associated with gastric tympanism

Gastric hyperinflation is a condition in which the length and geometry of the diaphragm are completely modified. Moreover, it has been demonstrated that increased intragastric pressure has deleterious effects upon the central circulation and ventilation resulting in arterial hypoxemia and hypercapnia. Presumably, these blood gas changes were the result of mechanical loading on the respiratory apparatus. Accordingly, the effect of an experimental insufflation of the stomach from 0 to 50 cmH_2O on the diaphragmatic strength generation was studied in healthy unsedated young Friesian bulls (Desmecht et al, 1993b). The results of such experiment show that there is a progressive decrease of end-expiratory lung volume as gastric pressure increases. This indicates that experimental insufflation or naturally occurring tympanism displaces the diaphragm forward. The diaphragm is lengthened and put on a more efficacious point of its length-tension curve at the start of spontaneous inspiration or phrenic stimulation. Diaphragmatic force generation increases proportionally with the forward displacement of the diaphragm.

However, whereas diaphragmatic force output increased at stomach pressures of 10 and 20 cm of water, further increase in stomach pressure resulted in progressive decrease of Pdi. According to these results, it seems that an additional factor should be considered to explain the biphasic evolution of Pdi. The initial increase in force corroborates the hypothesis that the diaphragm contracts from progressively longer initial lengths as it is pushed forward.

Consequently, its force output increases according to the relationship of active tension to muscle length characteristic of a skeletal muscle. With respect to the further decrease in force output, the impact of gastric pressure on the shape of the diaphragm should receive attention. Indeed, as a result of higher gastric pressures, the radii of the diaphragmatic curvature may increase and account for a reduction in maximal Pdi. This can be predicted from the Laplace principle according to which, at constant tension, the radii of diaphragmatic curvature and Pdi are inversely related.
In conclusion, at high abdominal pressures, geometric considerations may outweigh length-tension behaviour in explaining the diaphragmatic function in cattle.

6. RESPIRATORY MUSCLE FATIGUE DURING EXERCISE

Inspiratory muscle fatigue has been documented during loaded breathing and acute respiratory failure during various experimental protocols. However, its role in exercise limitation in healthy patients is still undetermined. Up to now, much of the experimental evidence required to determine whether or not the inspiratory muscles can impose limits to exercise performance is not available. This chapter is therefore in part speculative although some experimental clues accumulate.

6.1. Humans

Most healthy human athletes are not hypoxemic nor hypercapnic during maximal exercise, which suggests the lack of significant respiratory muscle fatigue under these circonstances. However, highly trained endurance athletes may show gas exchange impairment during heavy exercise (Dempsey et al, 1984). This could be explained by the observation that these athletes commonly reach mechanical limitations of expiratory flow rate and inspiratory muscle pressure generation at maximal exercise (Johnson and Ferro, 1992), which could result in nonsustainable hyperpnea (Aaron et al, 1992).

6.2. Ponies

Studies on the mechanics of breathing in ponies during moderate exercise have showed that total pulmonary resistance, resistive work of breathing, and pulmonary inertance may constrain further increase in ventilation during maximal exertion (Art and Lekeux, 1989). It is thus possible that during maximal exertion, respiratory muscles need a significant portion of the total body oxygen utilization, and therefore compete with locomotor muscles for available cardiac output. However, neither respiratory acidosis nor hypoxemia have been detected in ponies performing strenuous exercise, indicating that hyperpnea probably meets adequately oxygen demands (Parks and Manohar, 1984). Moreover, to ascertain whether the diaphragm of ponies, like limb muscles, engages in lactate and amonia production during high-intensity exercise, highly invasive experiments were carried out on healthy trained ponies in which phrenic venous catheters had been implanted. Despite the fact that diaphragmatic venous oxygen tension decreased, lactate and amonia concentrations in the diaphragmatics veins did not exceed corresponding arterial values (Manohar et al, 1988; Manohar and Hassan, 1991). These data thus reveal that in intensively exercising ponies, the diaphragmatic energy needs are met by aerobic metabolism. However, there is no further vasodilator reserve in respiratory muscles of maximally exercising ponies (Manohar, 1986), suggesting that these animals reach their maximal aerobic capacity during these conditions.

6.3. Horses

The equine physiology may not parallel that of ponies as the latter have not been selected for their athletic performances. Contrary to ponies, significant changes in arterial gases, i.e. hypoxemia and hypercapnia, were recorded in healthy horses (Bayly et al, 1989; Art et al, 1990). Interestingly, these changes were found to be significantly correlated with the work of breathing. Indeed, in the equine species, total pulmonary resistance increases dramatically with increased ventilation and, therefore, with the intensity of exercise (Art et al, 1990). It was traditionnally tought that in horses, like in humans, the capacity of the respiratory system to increase ventilation was not impeded and that physiological adjustments, such as bronchodilatation and enlargement of the laryngeal cross-sectional area, decrease the airflow resistance. However, inspiratory and expiratory peak flows as high as 66 and 78 L per second, respectively, should clearly overcome any physiological attempt to decrease resistance to flow, whereby frictions and turbulances become of major importance. This phenomenon is likely to be more important in horses than in men, probably because the former are unable to avoid nasal resistance by switching from nasal to oronasal breathing. The large increase in resistance opposed to airflow is undoubtedly the main contributor to the exponential rise in the respiratory work when minute ventilation increases (Art and Lekeux, 1989). When related to the oxygen consumption, the work of breathing is found to reach a substantial percentage of total oxygen uptake. It could therefore be expected that there is a critical level of ventilation above which any further oxygen uptake would be entirely consumed by the respiratory muscles. The increase of the work of breathing to the oxygen consumption ratio with exercise as well as the fact that the arterial hypoxemia and hypercapnia occur earlier in horses than in man suggest that critical ventilation may be reached in horses at a proportionately lower exercise intensity than in man. Moreover, it can be suggested that the volume acceleration at such inspiratory efforts is limited by the metabolic force speed requirements. Indeed, the transformation of chemical energy into mechanical energy has a limiting rate and consequently less tension can be maintained at high velocities of contraction. Therefore, it can be hypothesized that a limiting factor for further increase in minute ventilation may not only be a critical energetic threshold but also the force-velocity characteristics of the respiratory muscles. Moreover, it has been shown in humans breathing against inspiratory resistances that diaphragmatic fatigue occurs when an effort of greater than 50-70 % of maximal transdiaphragmatic force has to be sustained (Roussos and Macklem, 1986). Since pleural pressure changes as high as

8.5 kPa occur during strenuous exercise in horses, the critical fraction of maximal Pdi can also be reached in this species.

7. THERAPEUTIC CONSIDERATIONS

Independently of any etiologic treatment, improvement or prevention of respiratory muscle fatigue may be obtained by increasing the energy supply/demand ratio. Energy supply may be increased by increasing the inspiratory muscle blood flow and the arterial oxygen tension. Energy demand may be decreased by treating both the bronchoconstriction and the pulmonary edema. On the other hand, a respiratory muscle rest via a change in the pattern of breathing or via artificial ventilation may be useful in severe or chronic cases of fatigue (Rochester et al, 1977).

Another way to improve the respiratory muscle fatigue is to improve the muscle contractility pharmacologically. Force and endurance of the human diaphragm seem to be increased by aminophyllin (Aubier et al, 1981b) and β_2-agonists (Nava et al, 1992) but not by theophyllin (Decramer and Janssens, 1989). Domestic animals remain to be investigated in this area.

8. CONCLUSIONS

It has been suggest that respiratory muscle fatigue occurs in domestic animals and can lead to alveolar hypoventilation and ventilatory failure. The inspiratory muscles may fail in the same way and for much the same reasons as the locomotor muscles or even the heart. A method based on standardized phrenic nerve stimulation in calves revealed that the diaphragm fails as a pressure generator during pneumonia and gastric tympanism, due to reduced oxygen and/or glycogen availability or altered geometry, respectively. The same method implemented in the context of hypocalcemia showed that the diaphragm probably needs extracellular calcium for proper functioning and thus behaves more like the heart than like a locomotor muscle.

On the other hand, healthy horses performing intense exercise are found to develop arterial hypoxemia and hypercapnia which are correlated with an exponential-like evolution of the work of breathing. This, along with the amplitude of transpulmonary pressure changes and volume accelerations required by intense exercise, raise questions about the limits of the inspiratory muscles and their possible involvement in equine athletic performance. This however remains to be demonstrated.

REFERENCES

AARON E.A., SEOW K.C., JOHNSON B.D., DEMPSEY J.A. Oxygen cost of exercise hyperpnea: implications for performance. *J. Appl. Physiol.* 1992, 72, 1818-1825.

AMORY H., LOMBA F., LEKEUX P., COHEN SOLAL A., JAUNIAUX T., DESMECHT D. Bilateral diaphragmatic paralysis of unknown origin in a pony. *J. Am. Vet. Med. Assoc.* 1993, in press.

ART T., LEKEUX P. Work of breathing in exercising ponies. *Res. Vet. Sci.* 1989, 46, 49-53.

ART T., ANDERSON L., WOAKES A.J., ROBERTS C., BUTLER P.J., SNOW D.H., LEKEUX P. Mechanics of breathing during strenuous exercise in thoroughbred horses. *Respir. Physiol.* 1990, 82, 279-294.

AUBIER M., TRIPPENBACH T., ROUSSOS Ch. Respiratory muscle fatigue during cardiogenic shock. *J. Appl. Physiol.* 1981a, 51, 499-508.

AUBIER M., DE TROYER A., SAMPSON M., MACKLEM P.T., ROUSSOS C. Aminophylline improves diaphragmatic contractility. *N. Engl. J. Med.* 1981b, 305, 249-252.

AUBIER M., MURCIANO D., LECOCGUIC Y., VIIRES N., JACQUENS Y., SQUARA P., PARIENTE R. Effect of hypophosphatemia on diaphragmatic contractility in patients with acute respiratory failure. *N. Engl. J. Med.* 1985, 313, 420-424.

BASSILI H.R., DEITEL M. Effect of nutritional support on weaning patients off mechanical ventilators. *J. Parenter. Ent. Nutr.* 1981, 5, 161-163.

BAYLY W.M., HODGSON D.R., SCHULZ D.A., DEMPSEY J.A., GOLLNICK P.D. Exercise-induced hypercapnia in the horse. *J. Appl. Physiol.* 1989, 67, 1958-1966.

CLOSE R., DESMECHT D., LEKEUX P. Spectral parameters in diaphragmatic electromyograms : an analysis of stability in one healthy calf. In Proceedings : 10th Comparative Respiratory Society Meeting, East Lansing, (USA), 1991, P-11.

COHEN C.A., ZAGELBAUM G., GROSS D., ROUSSOS CH., MACKLEM P.T. Clinical manifestations of inspiratory muscle fatigue. *Am. J. Med.* 1982, 73, 308-316.

DECRAMER M., JANSSENS S. Theophylline and the respiratory muscles: where are we ? *Eur. Respir. J.* 1989, 2, 399-401.

DEMPSEY JA, HANSON PG, HENDERSON KS. Exercise-induced arterial hypoxaemia in healthy human subjects at sealevel. *J. Physiol. Lond.* 1984, 355, 161-175.

DESMECHT D., ROLLIN F., LINDEN A., LEKEUX P. Assessment of diaphragmatic strength by phrenic nerve stimulation in awake calves. In Proceedings : 9th Comparative Respiratory Society Meeting, Orlando, (USA), 1990, pp A-43.

DESMECHT D., ROLLIN F., LINDEN A., LEKEUX P. Feasibility, reliability and reproducibility of transdiaphragmatic pressure-frequency curve measurements in unanaesthetized calves. *Arch. Int. Physiol. Bioch. Biophys.* 1991, 99, P27.

DESMECHT D., LEKEUX P. Respiratory muscle fatigue in large animals. In Proceedings : IXth International Congress of Electromyography and Clinical Neurophysiology, Jerusalem, Israël, June 1992a, P347.

DESMECHT D., LINDEN A., AMORY H., LEKEUX P. Effect of experimentally induced acute pneumonia on diaphragmatic strength generation in neonatal calves. *Arch. Int. Physiol. Bioch.* 1992b, 100, P4.

DESMECHT D., LINDEN A., GABRIEL A., LOMBA F., LEKEUX P. A first approach to quantify diaphragmatic mechanical performance in intact and awake equines. 3d Congress of the World Equine Veterinary Association, Geneva, December 1993a.

DESMECHT D., LINDEN A., LEKEUX P. Respiratory muscle function changes associated with experimental simulation of rumen tympanism in cattle. *Arch. Int. Physiol. Bioch.* 1993b, 101, P7.

DOEKEL R.C., ZWILLICH C.W., SCOGGIN C.H., KRYGER M., WEIL J.V. Clinical semistarvation: depression of hypoxic ventilatory response. *N. Engl. J. Med.* 1976, 295, 358-361.

DRIVER A.G., LEBRUN M. Iatrogenic malnutrition in patients receiving ventilatory support. *J. Am. Vet. Med. Assoc.* 1980, 244, 2195-2196.

DUREUIL B., AUBIER M. Assessment of diaphragmatic function in the intensive care unit. *Intensive Care Med.* 1988, 14, 83-85.

EDWARDS R.H.T. Physiological analysis of skeletal muscle weakness and fatigue. *Clin. Sci. Mol. Med.* 1978, 54, 463-470.

ESAU S.A., BELLEMARE F., GRASSINO A., PERMUTT S., ROUSSOS C., PARDY R.L. Changes in relaxation rate with diaphragmatic fatigue in humans. *J. Appl. Physiol.* 1983, 54, 1353-1360.

GROSS D., GRASSINO A., ROSS W.D.R., MACKLEM P.T. Electromyogram pattern of diaphragmatic fatigue. *J. Appl. Physiol.* 1979, 46, 1-7.

JOHNSON A., FERRO T.J. TNF-α augments pulmonary vasoconstriction via the inhibition of nitrovasodilator activity. *J. Appl. Physiol.* 1992, 73, 2483-2492.

KIM M.J., DRUZ W.S., DANON J., MACHNACH W., SHARP J.T. Mechanics of the canine diaphragm. *J. Appl. Physiol.* 1976, 41, 369-374.

KNOCHEL J.P. Hypophosphatemia. *West J. Med.* 1981, 134, 15-26.

LAROCHE C.M., CAIRNS T., MOXHAM J., GREEN M. Hypothyroidism presenting with respiratory muscle weakness. *Am. Rev. Respir. Dis.* 1988, 138, 472-474.

MAL H., AUBIER M., PAMELA F., MURCIANO D. Evaluation of the transdiaphragmatic pressure (Pdi) relaxation rate in COPD patients during respiratory failure. *Bull. Eur. Physiopathol. Respir.* 1987, 23 (suppl. 12), P359.

MANOHAR M. Vasodilator reserve in respiratory muscles during maximal exertion in ponies. *J. Appl. Physiol.* 1986, 60, 1571-1577.

MANOHAR M., GOETZ T.E., HOLSTE L.C., NGANWA D. Diaphragmatic O_2 and lactate extraction during submaximal and maximal exertion in ponies. *J. Appl. Physiol.* 1988, 64, 1203-1209.

MANOHAR M., HASSAN A.S. Diaphragmatic energetics during prolonged exhaustive exercise. *Am. Rev. Respir. Dis.* 1991, 144, 415-418.

NAVA S., CROTTI P., GURRIERI G., FRACCHIA C., RAMPULLA C. Effect of a β_2-agonist (broxaterol) on respiratory muscle strength and endurance in patients with COPD with irreversible airway obstruction. *Chest* 1992, 101, 133-140.

PARKS C.M., MANOHAR M. Blood-gas tensions and acid-base status in ponies during treadmill exercise. *Am. J. Vet. Res.* 1984, 45, 15-19.

PITTINGER C., ADAMSON R. Antibiotic blockade of neuromuscular function. *Annu. Rev. Pharmacol.* 1972, 120, 169-184.

ROCHESTER D.F., BETTINI G. Diaphragmatic blood flow and energy expenditure in the

dog. Effects of inspiratory airflow resistance and hypercapnea. *J. Clin. Invest.* 1976, 57, 661-672.
ROCHESTER D.F., BRAUN N.M.T., LARNE S. Diaphragmatic energy expenditure in chronic respiratory failure: the effect of assisted ventilation with body respirators. *Am. J. Med.* 1977, 63, 223.
ROUSSOS C., MACKLEM P.T. Inspiratory muscle fatigue. In : *Handbook of Physiology*, Section 3, The Respiratory System, Volume III, Mechanics of Breathing, Part 2, Fishman, A.P., Fisher, A.B. (Eds), American Physiological Society, Bethesda, 1986, pp 511-527.
THURLBECK W.M. Diaphragm and body weight in emphysema. *Thorax* 1978, 33, 483-487.
YAN S., SIMILOWSKI T., GAUTHIER A.P., MACKLEM P.T., BELLEMARE F. Effect of fatigue on diaphragmatic function at different lung volumes. *J. Appl. Physiol.* 1992, 72, 1064-1067.

CHAPTER XV

TREATMENT OF PULMONARY DYSFUNCTIONS

P. Lekeux[1], B. Genicot[1] and P. Gustin[2]

[1] Laboratory for Functional Investigation
[2] Laboratory for Pharmacology and Toxicology
Faculty of Veterinary Medicine
University of Liege

SUMMARY

This paper describes the potential strategies which could be used in the near future in order to treat the pulmonary dysfunctions in domestic animals.

KEY WORDS

Respiratory system - Pulmonary function - Pulmonary dysfunction - Therapy.

1. INTRODUCTION

Despite the use of preventive and therapeutic agents, respiratory disorders in domestic animals occur at an increasing frequency. This could be due to several factors such as an increase of the population density, an increase of the virulence of some pathogens, an increase of air pollution, etc ...

Another explanation could be that, in the past, respiratory disorders have been analysed only at a pathological but not at a functional level. In the light of new information on animal pulmonary function in health and diseases, it appears that, before the occurrence of irreversible lung damages, there are some reversible dysfunctions at the level of pulmonary ventilation, perfusion or gas diffusion. An early and appropriate correction of these dysfunctions seems to be of critical importance in order to decrease the rate of irreversible lung damages and mortality.

On the other hand, the availability of new, powerful and specific antagonists for many mediators involved in the respiratory physiopathology also contributes to a better understanding and maybe to a better control of these pulmonary dysfunctions.

The purpose of this paper is to review the potential strategies which could improve the treatment of respiratory disorders. Possible preventive treatments will not be discussed in this review.

2. EFFICIENCY FACTORS OF THE RESPIRATORY THERAPY

As for the treatment of other dysfunctions, several factors may play a role in obtaining maximal efficiency, minimal toxicity and minimal residues problems.

An accurate diagnosis of the dysfunctions and injuries is necessary before selecting the most appropriate therapeutic strategy. For instance, a bronchodilator will have little effect if the major cause of an obstructive disorder is edema or hypersecretion in the airways. On the other hand, the presence of diffuse irreversible damages will limit the potential effect of the treatment.

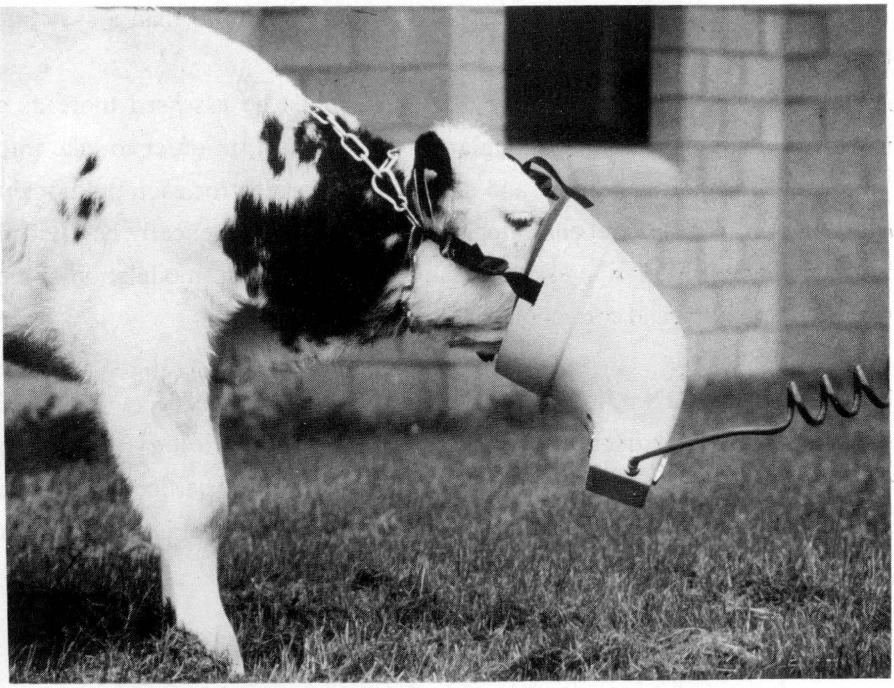

Fig. 15-1. Aerosol therapy as a way to increase the efficiency/toxicity ratio of the treatment.

The fact that several mediators are involved in most of the pulmonary dysfunctions suggests that the blockade of one single mediator should have little effect in the control of physiopathologic processes, and that the use of a "cocktail" of antagonists should be more efficient. However, most of these mediators work in cascade and an early blockade of one basic agonist may contribute to the control of the entire physiopathologic process. Therefore, a detailed understanding of the mechanisms leading to inflammation is important to open new therapeutic methods. Furthermore, the high specificity of the some antagonists may lead to decrease some side effects.

The way of administration of a drug is also of critical importance in the treatment of respiratory disorders. For instance, a local treatment by aerosol therapy may show a much higher efficiency/toxicity ratio than a systemic treatment (Fig. 15-1.).

Finally, the control of respiratory disorders must be assessed more as a modulable strategy than as a single standardized act, in order to take into account the individual, breed and species peculiarities for each pulmonary dysfunction. This global and integrate strategy can theoretically be divided into three targets, i.e. suppression of the etiological agents, modulation of the lung inflammation and correction of the mechanical disorders.

3. SUPPRESSION OF THE ETIOLOGICAL AGENTS

Most respiratory diseases have a multifactorial etiology in which microorganisms play a primary or secondary role. This is particularly true in production animals in which the control of pathogens is crucial in the treatment efficiency.

3.1. Antiviral therapy

Antiviral therapies are rare in veterinary medicine, mainly because of the severe adverse effects of the available drugs (Brochier et al, 1984).

The antiviral agent Ribavirin is effective both in vitro and in vivo against respiratory syncytial virus and influenza A and B virus (Hodes et al, 1975; Breese Hall et al, 1983; Gilbert et al, 1992). In the cat, this antiviral agent may contend a calicivirus infection (Povey, 1978). In calves, parenteral administration of Ribavirin does not decrease the shedding of the bovine respiratory syncytial virus (Mohanty et al, 1981). Inhalation of this drug could increase its efficiency and innocuity (Knight and Gilbert, 1990).

3.2. Antibacterial therapy

Many antibacterial compounds have been shown to be highly active in vitro and in vivo against pulmonary pathogens involved in respiratory diseases (Yancey et al, 1987; Lekeux and Art, 1988; Gourlay et al, 1989; Gustin et al, 1990; Picavet et al, 1991).

In avian (Van Alstine and Hofstad, 1984; Dyer and Van Alstine, 1987), canine (Bemis and Appel, 1977) and bovine (Deprez et al, unpublished data) species, aerosolization of antibacterial compounds has been successfully tested during experimentally-induced respiratory infections.
The in vivo efficacy of all these antibacterial drugs is not only determined by their in vitro activity but also by their pharmacokinetic properties.

3.3. Anthelmintical and antifungal therapy

Anthelmintics have been widely assessed against lung parasites (Turk and Klei, 1984; Lyons et al, 1985a; 1985b; Pouplard et al, 1986; Vandermyde et al, 1987). The effective control of parasite-induced pneumonia depends on both anthelmintic dosage and management factors (Bailey, 1992).
Fungal airway diseases are not rare in domestic animals (Ruoff, 1988), and they are often exarcerbated by long-lasting antibacterial therapy. Aerosolization of iodine compounds is indicated for the control of these fungal pneumonias (Art et al, unpublished data).

3.4. Desensitization

In horses, some inhaled mold spores may reach the deepest areas of the lung and trigger an allergic reaction that is responsible for the signs associated with Chronic Obstructive Pulmonary Disease (COPD). In such cases, several measures relative to environmental factors, bedding materials and forage may be adopted to reduce airborne pollutants (Clarke, 1992). In horses suffering from this obstructive disease, attempts of desensitization have been performed (Evans et al, 1992). Such attempts start with skin testing to identify the offending antigen. Once the antigen is identified, allergens with adjuvant are administered subcutaneously at increasing concentrations. However, because the skin of many clinically normal horses responds vigorously to a large number of antigens, interpretation of skin tests is difficult. Nevertheless, in some horses, immunotherapy may be effective in the treatment of COPD (Beech and Merryman, 1986).

Furthermore, dietary management may help to control some respiratory disorders. In cattle that are abruptly exposed to lush pasture, monensin and supplemental hay reduce ruminal 3-methylindole formation and the subsequent respiratory disorders (Potchoiba et al, 1992). Nutritional and dietary interrelationships with respiratory diseases are also mentioned in feedlot cattle (Johnson, 1991).

3.5. Surgical therapy

Surgical approaches may be adopted to treat tumoral or proliferative processes and some dysfunctions such as dorsal displacement of the soft palate (Ducharme, 1992) or laryngeal hemiplegia (Goble, 1992). Prosthetic laryngoplasty in naturally occurring hemiplegia (Marks et al, 1970) and nerve muscle pedicle graft in experimentally-induced hemiplegia (Fulton et al, 1991) were shown to improve upper airway flow mechanics and restore physiological resistance to airflow in exercising horses (Derksen et al, 1986).

4. MODULATION OF THE LUNG INFLAMMATION

Without any modulation, mediators from the inflammatory processes will bind and act through specific receptors of the target cells.
Consequently, the aim of the modulation of lung inflammation is to block the production and/or the effects of the mediators which interact negatively with the gas exchange processes in the lungs.

4.1. Inhibition of the activation of the inflammatory cells

This inhibition aims to contend substances which are able to stimulate the production of key-mediators involved in the inflammatory cascade. The inhibition of lipopolysaccharides (LPS) is justified in this context. Indeed, LPS are able to activate neutrophils and to induce the production of autacoides, oxygen radical and proteases. This type of treatment will include anti-LPS antibodies (Ziegler et al, 1991), LPS-receptor blockade (Lei and Morrisson, 1988; Morrisson et al, 1990) and inhibition of the activator signal

transmission in the target cell (Scheltze et al, 1991).
Other drugs such as cromolyn sodium are known for their stabilizing properties of mast cells.

4.2. Inhibition of autacoids

The pathways to the production of autacoids should be inhibited when these substances generated during the inflammatory process interact negatively with the defense system of the organism (Bottoms and Adams, 1992).

4.2.1. Complement

Anaphylatoxins (C3a and C5a), which are low-molecular-weight peptides cleaved from the complement system (Garrison and Rall, 1992), are able to enhance the capillary permeability, to stimulate the release of substances from mast cells, to chemotactically attract and induce the release of substances from neutrophilic granulocytes, eosinophil granulocytes and monocytes, and to stimulate the contraction of smooth muscle fibres and the production of leukotrienes (Cotran et al, 1989). These mechanisms have been incriminated during some bovine respiratory diseases (Kimman et al, 1989).
Modulation of the proinflammatory properties of the complement could be obtained by the use of monoclonal antibodies or specific antagonists such as SC-41930 (Fretland et al, 1991).

4.2.2. Histamine

Histamine, which is produced during the acute respiratory distress syndrome (Ogunbiyi et al, 1988), is able to induce a contraction of bovine respiratory smooth muscle (Gustin et al, 1988a). However, the importance of anti-H_1 substances seems to be trivial in the therapeutic schedules of animal respiratory diseases (Gustin et al, 1988b).

4.2.3. 5-Hydroxytryptamine

The administration of exogenous 5-hydroxytryptamine (or serotonin) in

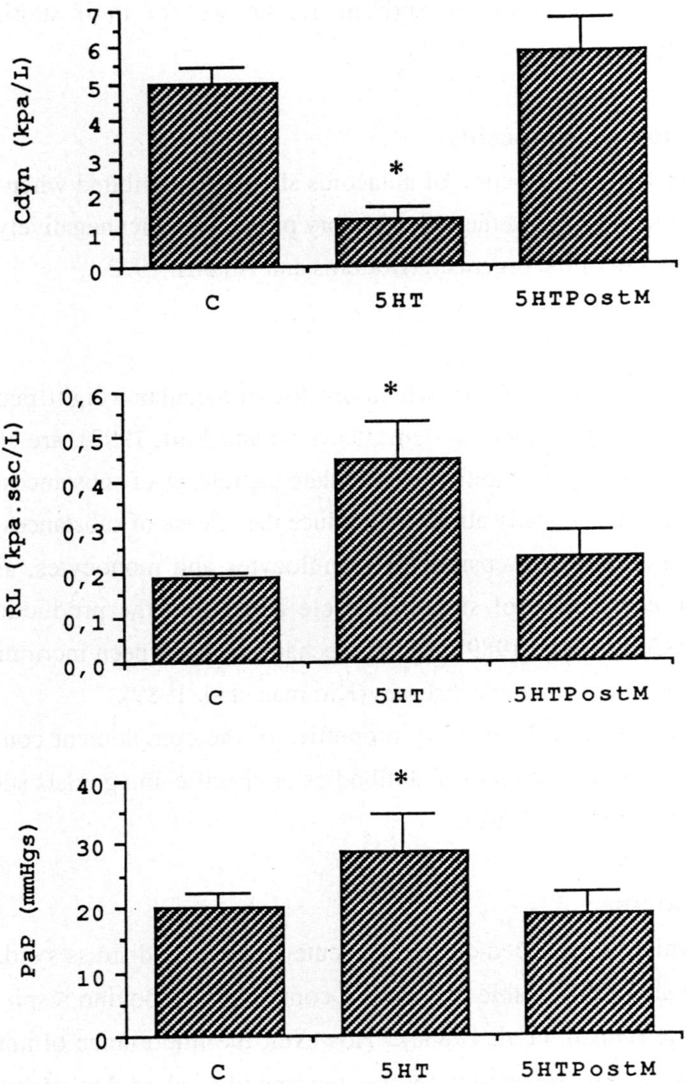

Fig. 15-2. Effect on of blockade of the 5-HT_2 receptors on the 5-HT-induced changes on dynamic lung compliance (Cdyn), total pulmonary resistance (R_L) and pulmonary artery pressure (PaP). C : Control values.

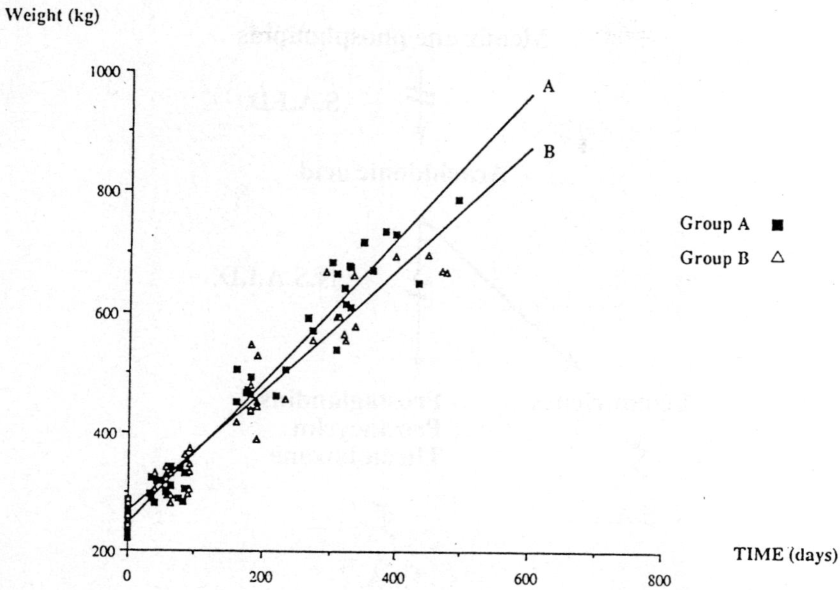

Fig. 15-3. Weight gains during the whole fattening period in calves which were treated for Shipping Fever either with a 5-HT_2 blocker (Group A) or with placebo (Group B), both groups receiving an identical antibacterial therapy (Genicot et al, 1993c).

healthy unsedated calves induces a reversible bronchoconstriction and pulmonary vasoconstriction (Desmecht et al, 1992) which can be prevented by a 5-HT_2-receptor blockade (Fig. 15-2.) (Linden et al, 1993). In double-muscled calves, such a 5-HT_2-receptor blockade has been proved to be effective during both early and late stage of a naturally occurring Acute Respiratory Distress Syndrome (Genicot et al, 1993a; 1993b). Furthermore, economic, clinical and functional consequences of this blockade have been assessed during Shipping Fever pneumonia (Fig. 15-3.) (Genicot et al, 1993c).

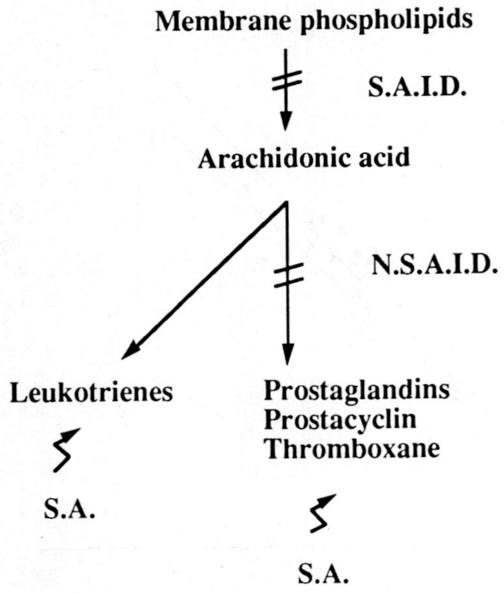

Fig. 15-4. Global or partial inhibition of the production of eicosanoids by steroidal antiinflammatory drugs (S.A.I.D.), non steroidal antiinflammatory drugs (N.S.A.I.D.) or specific antagonists (S.A.).

4.2.4. Eicosanoids

The production of eicosanoids, which are formed from certain polyunsaturated fatty acids (principally, arachidonic acid), increases in response to diverse stimuli (Campbell, 1992). Some of these compounds are involved in pulmonary dysfunctions and their inhibition could be useful in the treatment of respiratory diseases (Fig. 15-4.).

4.2.4.1. Global inhibition of the arachidonate metabolites

The global inhibition of arachidonate metabolites may be obtained by antiinflammatory steroids. The working mechanism of these products has been intensively studied (Snyder et Uranue, 1982; Beutler et al, 1988; Flower, 1988; Lee et al, 1988; Schule et al, 1988; Persico, 1991). However, antiinflammatory steroids may lead to important side-effects such as an inhibition of the hypothalamic-pituitary-adrenal axis, depression of the immune system and osteoporosis. The inhaled route is considered to be much safer than the oral supply of steroid (Lorentzson et al, 1990). Consequently, corticosteroids such as beclomethasone dipropionate, bethamethasone valerate, budesonide, triamcinolone acetonide and flunisolide have been synthetized. They combine the characteristics of enhanced topical antiinflammatory potency with little systemic activity (Phillipps, 1990; Toogood, 1990). During an experimental porcine septicemia, nebulized beclomethasone dipropionate improved pulmonary function and outcome (Walther et al, 1991).

On the other hand, modulation of the membrane fatty acid composition by dietary manipulation (for instance by dietary supplement with α-linoleic acid) may be adopted in order to decrease the production of proinflammatory mediators for instance in response to endotoxin. Such nutritional investigations were successfully carried out in rats (Cook et al, 1981), dogs (Lloyd, 1989) and horses (Henry et al, 1990; 1991; Morris et al, 1991).

4.2.4.2. Inhibition of the cyclooxygenase pathway

Nonsteroidal antiinflammatory drugs (NSAIDs) inhibit the enzymatic production of prostaglandins via the cyclooxygenase pathway (Vane, 1971; Insel, 1992). Other mechanisms of action have also been proposed, i.e. capture of free radicals, decoupling of the oxydative phosphorylation, inhibition of kinin release, inhibition of proteoglycans degradation, inhibition of leucocyte migration, inhibition of neutrophil adhesion reactions, etc ... (Abramson, 1991; Leeper-Woodford et al, 1991; Wu et al, 1991; Malmberg and Yaksh, 1992; Twomey and Dale, 1992; Delannoy et al, 1993).

These antiinflammatory properties probably explain the efficacy of NSAIDs during some acute respiratory diseases (Snapper et al, 1983; Selman et al, 1984; Drazen, 1986; Genicot et al, 1993a). On the other hand, the lack of benefical effects of NSAIDs during other respiratory syndromes may be explained by the fact that NSAIDs not only inhibit the production of prostaglandin (PG) $F_{2\alpha}$ and thromboxanes, which have negative pulmonary effects, but they also inhibit the production of PGI_2 and PGE_2, which are beneficial for the pulmonary function (Drazen, 1986). Furthermore, NSAIDs do not inhibit other proinflammatory mediators nor the lipoxygenase pathway. Consequently, given that the amount of available arachidonic acid is increased through the inhibition of the cyclooxygenase pathway, NSAIDs may enhance the production of leukotrienes (Lees and Higgins, 1985) which may negatively act on the pulmonary function (Hoffstein et al, 1990).

4.2.4.3. Specific inhibition of thromboxane

Thromboxane A_2 (TXA_2) promotes platelet aggregation and vasoconstriction (Campbell, 1992). Drugs such as dazoxiben, that inhibit thromboxane synthetase preferentially (Patrignani et al, 1984), have antithrombotic effects in vivo. Such inhibitors are more selective than salicylates. They inhibit the production of TXA_2 without interfering with PGI_2 production (Campbell, 1992). Thromboxane inhibitors were assessed to reduce vascular thrombi (Gensini, 1992). In endotoxic horses, a selective thromboxane synthetase inhibitor did not lead to any clinical improvement (Moore et al, 1990).

4.2.4.4. Specific inhibition of leukotrienes

Among leukotrienes issued from the lipoxygenase pathway, leukotriene C_4 (LTC_4), LTD_4 and LTE_4 take part in the pulmonary inflammatory process and pulmonary dysfunction observed during respiratory diseases (Barnes and Dixon, 1984; Hoffstein et al, 1990; Tagari et al, 1990). The use of specific blockers seems to decrease the intensity of these phenomena (Coggeshall et al, 1988; Hoffstein et al, 1990).

In cats, LTD_4/LTE_4 blockers enhanced the survival rate and prevented the acute pulmonary effects observed in endotoxinic shocks (Pacciti et al, 1987) although other investigations failed to point out any advantage of such a blockade (Olson et al, 1988; 1990b; Ahnfelt-Ronne, 1991).

4.2.5. Platelet activating factor (PAF)

Pathological functions of PAF have been widely investigated (Braquet et al, 1987; Henderson, 1991; Lantz et al, 1991; Chung, 1992). During acute respiratory distress syndrome, PAF seems to be responsible for several pulmonary dysfunctions (Hwang et al, 1985; Christman et al, 1988).

Many compounds have been described that selectively inhibit the actions of PAF in vivo and in vitro (Braquet et al, 1987; Saunders and Handley, 1987). Furthermore, PAF-blockers are also able to modulate the 5- and 12-lipoxygenase pathway (Braquet et al, 1987; Olson et al, 1990a). The development of PAF antagonists is still in its early stages, and their clinical utility has not yet been established (Campbell, 1992). Some reports seem to forward beneficial effects on the pulmonary function (Hwang et al, 1985; Shen et al, 1985; Imai et al, 1988) although this is refuted by others (Chung, 1992).

4.3. Modulation of neurogenic inflammation

The neuropeptides involved in the neurogenic inflammation, i.e. substance P, neurokinin A and calcitonin gene-related peptide (Barnes et al, 1991; Desmecht et al, 1991), could be inhibited by three different mechanisms, i.e. (1) inhibition of the activation of the C-fibers by local anesthesia (Wolfe, 1988), cromolyn sodium (Dixon et al, 1979), nedocromil sodium (Jackson et al, 1989) and nebulized furosemide (Ventresca et al, 1990), (2) inhibition of the sensory neuropeptide release by opioids (Belvisi et al, 1988), γ-amino butyric acid (Barnes, 1989) and α_2-agonist (Delaunois et al, 1993), and (3) inhibition of sensory neuropeptide effects by specific tachykinin receptor blockade (Snider et al, 1991).

Many other neuropeptides are involved in lung inflammation (Barnes et al, 1991). However, the usefulness of their inhibition by specific antagonists or antibodies during pulmonary diseases remains to be proven.

4.4. Modulation of pro-inflammatory cytokines

The inhibition of pro-inflammatory cytokines may be performed through an inhibition of their synthesis, an inhibition of their soluble form or an inhibition of their action on the target cell (Delannoy et al, 1993).

A modulation of the cytokine synthesis may be achieved through an inhibition of the gene transcription (Granelli-Piperno et al, 1990), a translation controlled by means of complementary anti-sense nucleotides (Burch and Mahan, 1991), an inhibition of the cytokine release (Rubartelli and Sitia, 1991), or an inhibition of promediator transformation (Dinarello and Thompson, 1991; Dinarello, 1992) (Fig. 15-5.).

Inhibition of soluble cytokine may be achieved through the use of anti-cytokine antibodies. In this field, anti-tumor necrosis factor antibodies were able to reduce the mortality from endotoxinic shock (Tracey et al, 1987; Sheehan et al, 1989). The soluble cytokine may also be blocked by exogenous soluble receptors (Lesslauer et al, 1991; Fisher et al, 1992) or by binding proteins (James, 1990).

Recombinant interleukin-1-receptor antagonist (IL1RA), which specifically binds type I and II receptors (Eisenberg et al, 1990), has been successfully assessed during pulmonary inflammation processes (Ulich et al, 1991) and during various septic shocks (Fisher et al, 1992).

4.5. Inhibition of cytolytic inflammatory products

4.5.1. Antiproteases

Proteases such as elastase and thrombin are responsible for pulmonary inflammatory injuries (Schraufstatter et al, 1984).

In vitro results suggest that antiproteinases protect lung endothelial cells from endotoxin injury (Tumen et al, 1988).

In sheep, a single dose of aerosolized secretory leukoprotease inhibitor (rSLPI) results after 3 hours in a four-fold decrease of the antineutrophil elastase capacity in epithelial lining fluid. This effect has a half-life of 12 hours. This demonstrates that it is feasable to use aerosolized rSLPI to

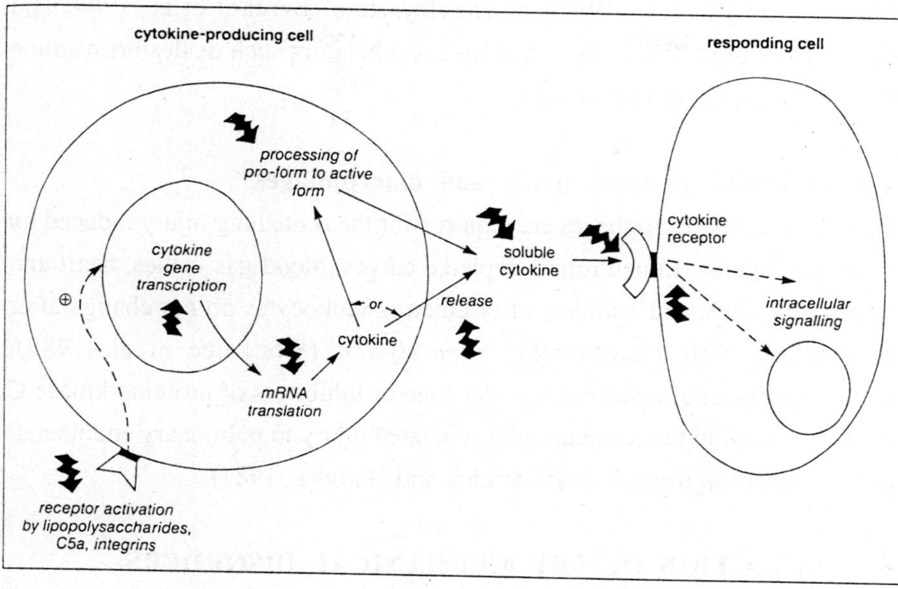

Fig. 15-5. Potential ways to inhibit the synthesis or action of cytokines (Henderson and Blake, 1992).

directly increase the antiprotease capacity of the lung, particularly on the pulmonary epithelial surface (Vogelmeier et al, 1990).

4.5.2. Oxygen radical scavengers

Free radicals derived from oxygen during respiratory disorders are able to induce severe pulmonary injuries (Travis, 1987; Southorn and Powis, 1988). In dogs, inorganic particles phagocytized by lung tissues cause alveolar macrophages to generate reactive oxygen compounds extra- and intracellularly (Beck-Speier et al, 1993).

Inhibition of these compounds may be obtained by enzymatic antioxydants such as catalase, superoxyde dismutase and gluthation peroxydase (McCord et al, 1982; Maunder et al, 1988; Seekamp et al, 1988), by non enzymatic antioxydants such as vitamin A, C and E, taurine (McMillan and Boyd, 1982;

Macklin and Bendich, 1987), N-acetylcysteine (Bernard et al, 1984) and dimethylthiourea (Fox, 1984), and by iron chelators such as desferioxamine (Halliwell and Gutteridge, 1986).

4.6. Inhibition of neutrophils and macrophages

Neutrophils and macrophages are required for the acute lung injury induced by many pathogens. In neutrophil-depleted calves, blood gas values, heart and respiratory rates, and numbers of circulating leukocytes do not change after inoculation with *Pasteurella haemolytica* (Slocombe et al, 1985). Consequently, substances such as dapsone or inhibitors of proteine-kinase C could be useful to reduce neutrophil-mediated injury to pulmonary endothelial cells (Martin and Kachel, 1985; Struhar and Harbeck, 1987).

5. CORRECTION OF THE MECHANICAL DISORDERS

Impairment of pulmonary ventilation, perfusion and gas diffusion may be due to mechanical disorders generated by dysfunction at the level of lung smooth muscle, secretory glands, ciliated cells and ventilatory muscles.

5.1. Bronchodilation

5.1.1. β_2-Agonists

Clenbuterol, salbutamol, fenoterol and terbutaline may be considered as current β_2-agonists, whereas salmeterol and formoterol belong to a new class of β_2-agonists which are characterized by their exceptionally long duration of action.

Clenbuterol has been clinically assessed in equine (Sasse and Hajer, 1977) and bovine (Fig. 15-6.) (Genicot et al, 1992) respiratory disorders. This drug seems to be more potent when administered by aerosol (Scott et al, 1991) than by oral or parenteral administration (Derksen et al, 1987).

Salmeterol, formoterol and broxaterol have potential clinical advantages over current β_2-agonists (Brittain, 1990; Löfdahl and Chung, 1991). Indeed, in guinea pig trachea and human bronchial smooth muscle, salmeterol

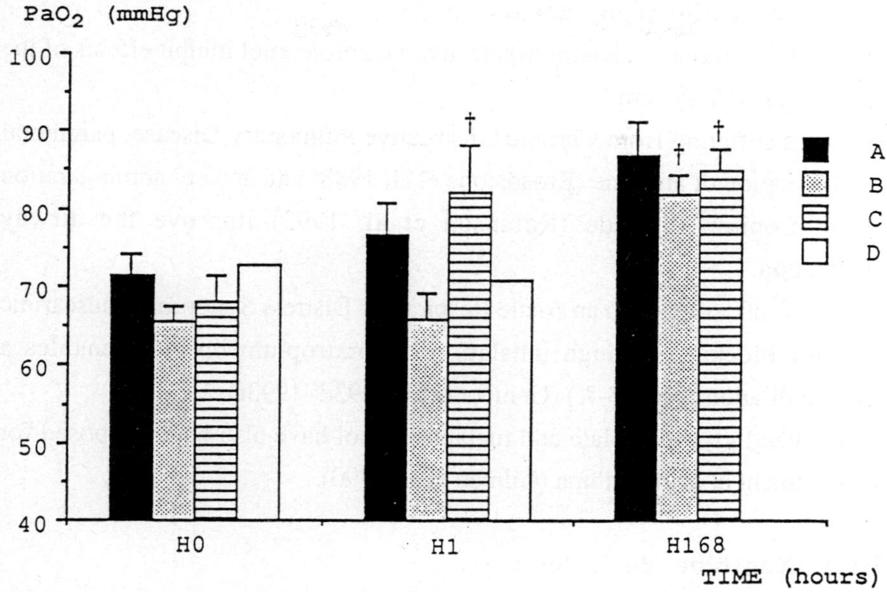

Fig. 15-6. Effect of clenbuterol hydrochlorid (Group A), ipratropium bromide (Group B), both drugs simultaneously (Group C) and saline (NaCl 0.9 %) (Group D) inhalation on arterial oxygen tension during acute respiratory distress syndrome in cattle. † : Significantly ($P < 0.05$) different from initial values collected in the group (Genicot et al, 1993e).

hydroxynaphtoate is more potent than isoprenaline, salbutamol and clenbuterol. Furthermore, salmeterol induces persistent bronchodilation, sustained suppression of mediator release, and long-lasting inhibition of edema formation. In vitro and in vivo, salmeterol inhibits the constriction of airway smooth muscle for up to 7 hours (Johnson, 1990). Formoterol is approximately 35 times more potent than salbutamol to inhibit both microvascular leakage and airflow obstruction induced by histamine aerosol in the guinea pig (Tokuyama et al, 1991).

5.1.2. Anticholinergic agents

Ipratropium bromide, glycopyrrolate and metaproterenol inhibit effects of the parasympathetic system.

In horses suffering from Chronic Obstructive Pulmonary Disease, parenteral administration of atropine (Broadstone et al, 1988) and aerosol administration of ipratropium bromide (Robinson et al, 1993) improve the airway obstruction.

In calves sufferring from an Acute Respiratory Distress Syndrome, muscarinic receptor blockade through inhalation of ipratropium bromide enables a bronchodilation (Fig. 15-7.) (Genicot et al, 1993d; 1993f).

Aerosolized glycopyrrolate and metaproterenol have also been proposed for the treatment of acute asthma (Gilman et al, 1990).

5.1.3. Xanthine derivates

Methylxanthines, and mainly theophylline, are phosphodiesterase inhibitors and work by preventing metabolism of cyclic AMP by phosphodiesterase. They are able to relax the airway smooth muscle, during both experimental and clinical bronchoconstriction (Errecalde et al, 1985; McKiernan et al, 1990). However, the dosage of theophylline must be very precise because the range between the effective and toxic dose is narrow (McKiernan et al, 1990).

5.1.4. Miscellaneous

Other substances such as cromolyn sodium (Soma et al, 1987; Svendsen and Jorgensen, 1991), calcium channel blockers (Ahmed et al, 1988) and potassium channel openers (Chapman et al, 1991; Paciorek et al, 1991) are potent bronchodilators but need to be further investigated during animal respiratory diseases.

5.2. Vasodilation

Inhibition of vasoconstriction can reduce the pulmonary hypertension and the subsequent increase in lung capillary filtration, which is partly responsible for

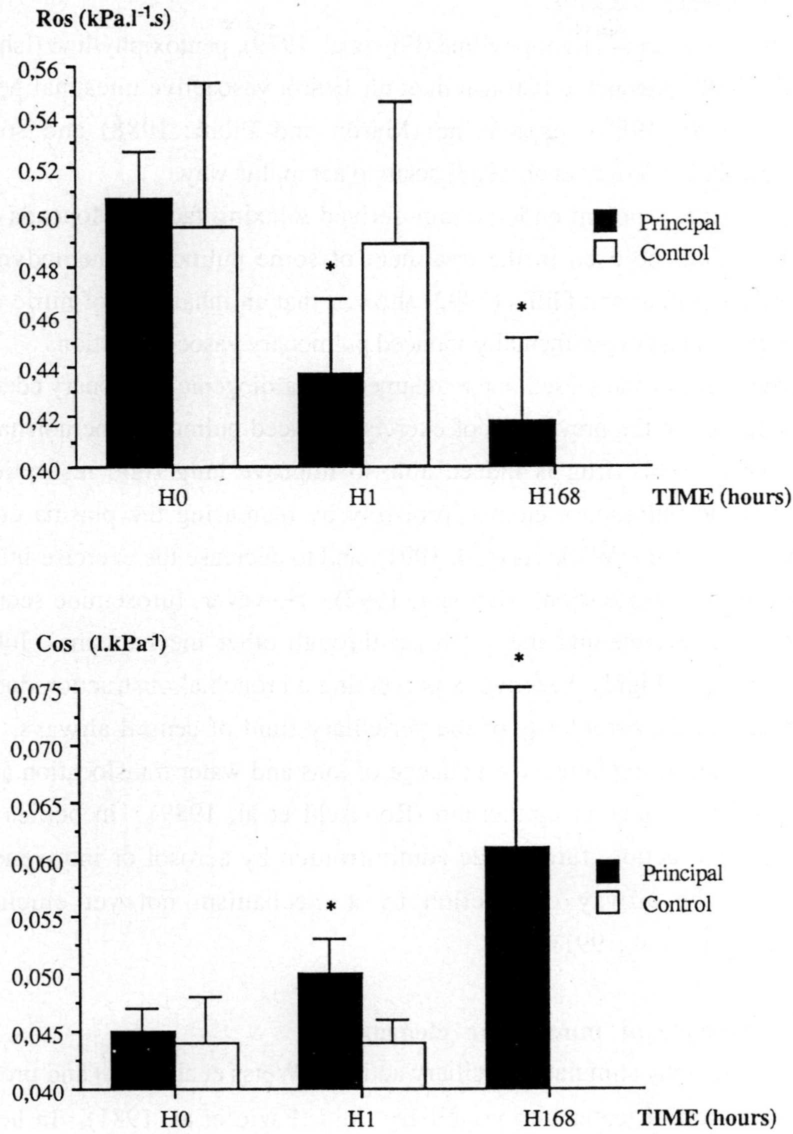

Fig. 15-7. Effect of inhalation of an anticholinergic agent on oscillatory lung resistance (Ros) and oscillatory lung compliance (Cos) in cattle suffering from acute respiratory distress syndrome (Genicot et al, 1993f).

the occurrence of edema.

Substances such as aminophylline (Foy et al, 1979), pentoxiphylline (Ishizaka et al, 1988), adenosine (Cronstein et al, 1986), vasoactive intestinal peptide (Foda et al, 1988), papaverine (Maron and Pilati, 1988) and sodium nitroprusside (Wright et al, 1988) seem to act in this way.

Nitric oxide, a potent endothelium-derived relaxing factor (Moncada et al, 1991), could be used in the treatment of some pulmonary hemodynamic disorders. Rimar and Gillis (1992) showed that an inhalation of nitric oxide may contend an experimentally-induced pulmonary vasoconstriction.

Furosemide is widely used in the treatment of cardiogenic pulmonary edema in the dog and in the prevention of exercise-induced pulmonary hemorrhage in the horse. This drug is indeed able to improve lung fluid resorption in hydrostatic pulmonary edema, probably by increasing the plasma colloid osmotic pressure (Wickerts et al, 1991), and to decrease the exercise-induced pulmonary hypertension (Manohar, 1992). However, furosemide seems to have other effects and may also act through other mechanisms. Inhaled furosemide is highly effective in preventing a bronchial obstruction due to a decrease in the osmolarity of the periciliary fluid of central airways. This effect could be explained by a change of ions and water translocation across the tracheo-bronchial epithelium (Robuschi et al, 1989). In ponies with airway obstruction, furosemide administration by aerosol or intravenously reverses the airway obstruction by a mechanism not yet elucidated (Broadstone et al, 1991).

5.3. Increase of mucociliar clearance

β-Agonists may stimulate the ciliary activity (Weiss et al, 1981) and promote the secretion of water into periciliary fluid (Fazio et al, 1981). In horses, clenbuterol increases the mean speed of tracheal mucociliar clearance both in healthy (Kiely et al, 1985) and horses with Chronic Obstructive Pulmonary Disease (Turgut and Sasse, 1989). In cattle, clenbuterol has been associated with antibacterial drugs in order to improve the mucociliar clearance (Davies and Webster, 1989).

Xanthine derivates may also have beneficial mucokinetic effects in dogs (Wanner, 1981).

Bromhexine has been shown to increase mucociliar clearance in both healthy and diseased cattle (Davies and Webster, 1987). In horses, its efficiency after systemic administration is controversial (Pearce et al, 1978; De Backer et al, 1980).

Mucolytics, such as acetylcysteine, and hypertonic saline aerosol increase the rate of mucokinesis (Pavia, 1984; Dixon, 1992).

Hyperperfusion, i.e. intravenous infusion of 30 litres of saline in 3 hours for three days, has also been suggested to act as a bronchomucotropic agent in the horse (Costa and Deegen, 1986).

5.4. Decrease of the diaphragmatic fatigue

In dogs submitted to a diaphragm fatigue induced by low-frequency electrophenic stimulation, broxaterol (a new β_2-agonist) promotes recovery in a dose-dependent way. On the opposite, theophylline does not improve the force output of fatigued canine diaphragm (Derom et al, 1992). After administration of terbutaline sulfate, feline diaphragmatic contractility shows a greater increase than after administration of aminophylline. Results obtained from the combination of aminophylline and terbutaline sulfate suggest a non-synergistic effect of both drugs on feline diaphragmatic contractility (Nassar et al, 1991).

5.5. Surfactant

In the lung of preterm lambs treated with ovine surfactant, a significant improvement of gas mixing efficiency and alveolar ventilation was recorded (Sandberg et al, 1991). In this species, an improvement of the lung function may be obtained at a very low surfactant dose (Lewis et al, 1991). Furthermore, different surfactant preparations have recently been assessed in surfactant-deficient preterm lambs (Cummings et al, 1992).

After surfactant administration, the immediate improvement in oxygenation is related to increased lung volumes due to increased distention rather than to recruitment of functional alveoli (Goldsmith et al, 1991). After an intratracheal instillation of bovine surfactant (SF-RI 1) in premature lambs, Gortner et al (1990) observed an improvement of the total lung-thorax compliance, and a decrease of $PaCO_2$. Actually, artificial surfactant may be considered as an acceptable substitute for surfactants of biological origin (Levine et al, 1991).

5.6. Oxygen therapy

When arterial oxygen tension is dramatically decreased, for instance in neonates with severe respiratory disorders, the enrichment of the oxygen fraction in inspired air may improve the gas exchange if the alveolar ventilation is sufficient.

When using such a technique, one has to keep in mind the oxygen toxicity occurring as soon as oxygen concentration in inhaled air is too high. In sheep, lung mechanics and airway reactivity were investigated during development of oxygen toxicity (Fukushima et al, 1990).

Since alveolar hypoxia induces hypoxic pulmonary vasoconstriction in some species, oxygen therapy is also a potential treatment for several hemodynamic disorders (Hall and Wood, 1991). However, such a treatment must be applied continuously and has to be removed with a gradual decrease of the inspired oxygen concentration, in order to avoid an acute recurrent hypoxic vasoconstriction (Koterba, 1991).

5.7. Mechanical ventilation

In cases of persistent hypercapnia due to severe alveolar hypoventilation, mechanical ventilatory support may be the only way for improving the gas exchanges.

Continuous positive pressure ventilation and intermittent mandatory ventilation have been recommended in neonates during respiratory distress syndrome

(Coons et al, 1990).

Several nonconventional ventilatory techniques such as high frequency ventilation, high frequency oscillation and high frequency body surface oscillation have been developed in order to optimize the improvement of gas exchange and to minimize the risk of pulmonary barotrauma (Slutsky, 1991).

6. CONCLUSIONS

The control of the pulmonary dysfunctions generated by respiratory diseases is of crucial importance for the health, the performance and the production of domestic animals. Much progress has been made in the understanding of pulmonary physiology, physiopathology and pharmacology, which is susceptible to bring new hope for a better treatment of respiratory disorders. However, much research remains to be done before an optimal therapeutic strategy for each respiratory syndrome in the various animal species can be proposed.

REFERENCES

ABRAMSON S.B. Therapy with and mechanisms of nonsteroidal antiinflammatory drugs. *Curr. Opin. Rheumatol.* 1991, 3, 336-340.

AHMED T., D'BROT J., WASSERMAN M., MUCCITELLI R., ROBINSON M., TUCKER S., MARCHETTE B. Effect of verapamil on pulmonary and eicosanoid responses to endotoxin in awake sheep. *J. Appl. Physiol.* 1988, 64, 1700-1708.

AHNFELT-RONNE I. Rationals for drug development in inflammation: eicosanoids and oxygen-derived free radicals. *Dan. Med. Bull.* 1991, 38, 291-303.

BAILEY M. Lung parasites. In : *Current Therapy in Equine Medicine 3*, Robinson, N.E. (Ed.), W.B. Saunders Company, Philadelphia, 1992, pp 332-334.

BARNES P.J., DIXON C.M.S. The effects of inhaled vasoactive intestinal peptide on bronchial reactivity to histamine in humans. *Am. Rev. Respir. Dis.* 1984, 130, 162-166.

BARNES P.J. Airway neuropeptides: roles in fine tuning and in disease. *NIPS* 1989, 4, 116-120.

BARNES P.J., BARANIUK J.N., BELVISI M.G. Neuropeptides in the respiratory tract. Part II. *Am. Rev. Respir. Dis.* 1991, 144, 1391-1399.

BECK-SPEIER I., DAYAL N., HEILMANN P., KREYLING W.G., LENZ A.G., LEUSCHEL L., MAIER K., MEYER B., MIASKOWSKI U., MÖLLER W. Oxygen radical production of canine alveolar macrophages by inorganic particulate materials. In : *Journal of Aerosol Medicine: Deposition, Clearance, and Effects in the Lung,*

Smaldone, G.C. (Ed.), Mary Ann Liebert, Inc Publishers, New York, 1993d, 6 (Suppl.), p 31.

BEECH J., MERRYMAN G.S. Immunotherapy for equine respiratory disease. *Equine Vet. Sci.* 1986, 6, 6-10.

BELVISI M.G., CHUNG K.F., JACKSON D.M., BARNES P.J. Opioid modulation of non-cholinergic neutral bronchoconstriction in guinea pig in vivo. *Br. J. Pharmacol.* 1988, 95, 413-418.

BEMIS D.A., APPEL N.J. Aerosol, parenteral, and oral antibiotic treatment of *Bordetella bronchiseptica* infections in dogs. *J. Am. Vet. Med. Assoc.* 1977, 170, 1082-1086.

BERNARD G.R., LUCHT W.D., NIEDERMEYER M.E., SNAPPER J.R., OGLETREE M.L., BRIGHAM K.L. Effect of N-acetylcysteine on the pulmonary response to endotoxin in the awake sheep and upon *in vitro* granulocyte function. *J. Clin. Invest.* 1984, 73, 1772-1784.

BEUTLER B., THOMPSON P., KEYES J., HAGERTY K., CRAWFORD D. Assay of a ribonuclease that preferentially hydrolyses mRNA containing cytokine derived UA - Rich instability sequences. *Biochem. Biophys. Res. Commun.* 1988, 152, 973-980.

BOTTOMS G.D., ADAMS R. Involvement of prostaglandins and leukotrienes in the pathogenesis of endotoxemia and sepsis. *J. Am. Vet. Med. Assoc.* 1992, 200, 1842-1848.

BRAQUET P., TOUQUI L., SHEN T.Y., VARGAFTIG B.B. Perspectives in platelet-activating factor research. *Pharmacol. Rev.* 1987, 39, 97-145.

BREESE HALL C., McBRIDE J.T., WALSH E.E., BELL D.M., GALA C.L., HILDRETH S., TEN EYCK L.G., HALL W.J. Aerosolized ribavirin treatment of infants with respiratory syncytial viral infection. *N. Engl. J. Med.* 1983, 308, 1443-1447.

BRITTAIN R.T. Approaches to a long-acting, selective β_2-adrenoceptor stimulant. *Lung* 1990, 168, 111-114.

BROADSTONE R.V., SCOTT J.S., DERKSEN F.J., ROBINSON N.E. Effects of atropine in ponies with recurrent airway obstruction. *J. Appl. Physiol.* 1988, 65, 2720-2725.

BROADSTONE R.V., ROBINSON N.E., GRAY P.R., WOODS P.S., DERKSEN F.J. Effects of furosemide on ponies with recurrent airway obstruction. *Pulm. Pharmacol.* 1991, 4, 203-208.

BROCHIER B., THIRY E., WERENNE J., SCHWERS A., VINDEVOGEL H., PASTORET P.-P. Thérapeutique étiologique des maladies d'origine virale. *Ann. Rech. Vét.* 1984, 15, 35-54.

BURCH R.M., MAHAN L.C. Oligonucleotides antisense to the interleukin-1 receptor mRNA block the effects of interleukin-1 in cultured murine and human fibroblastes and in mice. *J. Clin. Invest.* 1991, 88, 1190-1196.

CAMPBELL W.B. Lipid-derived autacoids: eicosanoids and platelet-activating factor. In : *The Pharmacological Basis of Therapeutics,* Goodman Gilman, A., Rall, T.W., Nies, A.S., Taylor, P. (Eds), Pergamon press, New York, 1992, pp 600-617.

CHAPMAN I.D., MAZZONI L., MORLEY J. Actions of SDZ PCO 400 and cromakalim on airway smooth muscle in vivo. *Agents Actions* 1991, 34, 53-62.

CHRISTMAN B.W., LEFFERTS P.L., KING G.A., SNAPPER J.R. Role of circulating platelets and granulocytes in PAF-induced pulmonary dysfunction in awake sheep. *J. Appl. Physiol.* 1988, 64, 2033-2041.

CHUNG K.F. Platelet-activating factor in inflammation and pulmonary disorder. *Clin. Sci.* 1992, 83, 127-138.

CLARKE A.F. Chronic Obstructive Pulmonary Disease. In : *Current Therapy in Equine Medicine 3*, Robinson, N.E. (Ed.), W.B. Saunders Company, Philadelphia, 1992,

pp 329-332.
COGGESHALL J.W., CHRISTMAN B.W, LEFFERTS P.L., SERAFIN W.E., BLAIR I.A., BUTTERFIELD M.J., SNAPPER J.R. Effect of inhibition of 5-lipoxygenase metabolism of arachidonic acid on response to endotoxemia in sheep. *J. Appl. Physiol.* 1988, 65, 1351-1359.
COOK J.A., WISE W.C., KNAPP D.R., HALUSHKA P.V. Sensitization of essential fatty acid-deficient rats to endotoxin by arachidonate pre-treatment: role of thromboxane A_2. *Circ. Shock* 1981, 8, 69-76.
COONS T.J., KOSCH P.C., CUDD T.A. Respiratory care. In : *Equine Clinical Neonatology*, Koterba, A.M., Drummond, W.H., Kosch, P.C. (Eds), Lea & Febiger, Philadelphia, 1990, pp 200-239.
COSTA P., DEEGEN E. Lung Function and Pulmonary Diseases in the Horse, Deegen, E., Beadle, R. (Eds), Hippiatrika-Verlagsgesellschraft, Calw, Germany, 1986, pp 38.
COTRAN R.S., KUMAR V., ROBBINS S.L. Robbins pathologic basis of disease. In : 4th Editions W.B. Saunders Compagny, Philadelphia, 1989, pp 39-86.
CRONSTEIN B.N., LEVIN R.I., BELANOFF J., WEISSMANN G., HIRSCHHORN R. Adenosine: an endogenous inhibitor of neutrophil-mediated injury to endothelial cells. *J. Clin. Invest.* 1986, 78, 760-770.
CUMMINGS J.J., HOLM B.A., HUDAK M.L., HUDAK B.B., FERGUSON W.H., EGAN E.A. A controlled clinical comparison of four different surfactant preparations in surfactant-deficient preterm lambs. *Am. Rev. Respir. Dis.* 1992, 145, 999-1004.
DAVIES C.P., WEBSTER A.J. Deposition and clearance of monodisperse aerosols in the calf lung: Effects of particle size and a mucolytic agent (bromhexine). *Can. J. Vet. Res.* 1987, 51, 306-311.
DAVIES C.P., WEBSTER A.J. The effects a β_2-agonist (clenbuterol) and antibacterial drugs (trimethoprim sulphadiazine; oxytetracycline) on calves mucociliary clearance. *J. Vet. Pharmacol. Ther.* 1989, 12, 217-224.
DE BACKER P., VANDECASTEELE-THEINPONT L.M.R., JONCKHEERE J.A.A., BELPAIRE F.M., DEBACKERE M., DE LEENHEER A.P. Bioavailability of bromhexine in the horse. *Zbl. Vet. Med. A* 1980, 27, 740-745.
DELANNOY I., MIOSSEC P., LEKEUX P. Potentialités de modulation de la réaction inflammatoire. *Ann. Méd. Vét.* 1993, 137, 163-194.
DELAUNOIS A., GUSTIN P., ANSAY M. Role of neuropeptides in acetylcholine-induced pulmonary edema. *J. Pharmacol. Exp. Therap.*, 1993, in press.
DERKSEN F.J., STICK J.A., SCOTT E.A., ROBINSON N.E., SLOCOMBE R.F. Effect of laryngeal hemiplegia and laryngoplasty on airway flow mechanics in exercising horses. *Am. J. Vet. Res.* 1986, 47, 16-20.
DERKSEN F.J., SCOTT J.S., SLOCOMBE R.F., ROBINSON N.E. Effect of clenbuterol on histamine-induced airway obstruction in ponies. *Am. J. Vet. Res.* 1987, 48, 423-426.
DEROM E., JANSSENS S., GURRIERI G., TJANDRAMAGA T.B., DECRAMER M. Effects of broxaterol and theophylline on fatigued canine diaphragm in vivo. A randomized, controlled study. *Am. Rev. Respir. Dis.* 1992, 146, 22-25.
DESMECHT D., GUSTIN P., LEKEUX P., ANSAY M. Le système nerveux peptidergique du poumon: physiologie, physiopathologie et perspectives thérapeutiques. *Ann. Méd. Vét.* 1991, 135, 15-31.
DESMECHT D., LINDEN A., ROLLIN F., AMORY H., LEKEUX P. Effect of intravenous and aerosol administration of 5-hydroxytryptamine on pulmonary function values in healthy calves. *Am. J. Vet. Res.* 1992, 53, 315-320.
DINARELLO C.A., THOMPSON R.C. Blocking IL1: interleukin-1 receptor antagonist in vivo and in vitro. *Immunol. Today* 1991, 12, 404-410.

DINARELLO C.A. Anti-cytokine strategies. *Eur. cytokine Netw.* 1992, 3, 7-17.

DIXON M., JACKSON D.M., RICHARDS I.M. The effects of sodium cromoglycate on lung irritant receptors and left ventricular receptors in anesthetized dogs. *Br. J. Pharmacol.* 1979, 67, 569-574.

DIXON P.M. Respiratory mucociliary clearance in the horse in health and disease, and its pharmaceutical modification. *Vet. Rec.* 1992, 131, 229-235.

DRAZEN J.M. Chemical mediators of immediate hypersensibility reactions. In : *Handbook of Physiology*, Section 3, Vol III, Fishman, A.P., Macklem, P.T., Mead, J., Geiger, S.R. (Eds), American Physiological Society, Bethesda, USA, 1986, pp 711-718.

DUCHARME N.G. Dynamic pharyngeal collapse. In : *Current Therapy in Equine Medicine 3*, Robinson, N.E. (Ed.), W.B. Saunders Company, Philadelphia, 1992, pp 283-285.

DYER D.C., VAN ALSTINE W.G. Antibiotic aerosolization: tissue and plasma oxytetracycline concentrations in parakees. *Avian Dis.* 1987, 31, 677-679.

EISENBERG S.P., EVANS R.J., AREND W.P., VERDERBER E., BREWER M.T., HANNUME C.H., THOMPSON R.C. Primary structure and functional expression from complementary DNA of a human interleukin-1 receptor antagonist. *Nature* 1990, 343, 341-346.

ERRECALDE J.O., BUTTON C., MULDERS M.S.G. Some dynamic and toxic effects of theophylline in horses. *J. Vet. Pharmacol. Ther.* 1985, 8, 320-327.

EVANS A.G., PARADIS M.R., O'CALLAGHAN M. Intradermal testing of horses with chronic obstructive pulmonary disease and recurrent urticaria. *Am. J. Vet. Res.* 1992, 53, 203-208.

FAZIO F., LAFORTUNA C. Effect of inhaled salbutamol on mucociliary clearance in patients with chronic bronchitis. *Chest* 1981, 80, 827-830.

FISHER E., POUTSIAKA D.D., Van ZEE K.J., MARANO M.A., KENNEY J.S., DINARELLO C.A., LOWRY S.F., MOLDAWER L.L. Interleukin-1 receptor antagonist circulates in experimental inflammation and in human disease. *Blood* 1992, 79, 2196-2200.

FLOWER R.J. Licocortin and the mechanism of action of the glucocorticoids. *Br. J. Pharmacol.* 1988, 87, 57-62.

FODA H.D., IWANAGA T., LIU L.W., SAID S.I. Vasoactive intestinal peptide protects against HCl-induced pulmonary edema in rats. *Ann. N Y Acad. Sci.* 1988, 527, 633-636.

FOX R.B. Prevention of granulocyte-mediated oxidant lung injury in rats by a hydroxyl radical scavenger, dimethylthiourea. *J. Clin. Invest.* 1984, 74, 1456-1564.

FOY T., MARRION J., BRIGHAM K.L., HARRIS T.R. Isoproterenol and aminophylline reduce lung capillary filtration during high permeability. *J. Appl. Physiol.* 1979, 58, 34-44.

FRETLAND D.J., WIDOMSKI D.L., ANGLIN C.P., LEVIN S., GAGINELLA T.S. Modulation of the chemotactic properties of complement fragments C5a and C3 by the anti-inflammatory agent, SC-41930. *Agents Actions* 1991, 34, 5-7.

FUKUSHIMA M., KING L.S, KANG K.H., BANERJEE M., NEWMAN J.H. Lung mechanics and airway reactivity in sheep during development of oxygen toxicity. *J. Appl. Physiol.* 1990, 69, 1779-1785.

FULTON I.C., DERKSEN F.J., STICK. J.A., ROBINSON N.E., WALSHAN R. Treatment of left laryngeal hemiplegia using a nerve muscle pedicle graft. In : *Equine Exercise Physiology*, Persson, S.G.B., Lindholm, A., Jeffcott, L.B. (Eds), ICEEP Publications, Davis, California, 1991, 3, pp 443-448.

GARRISON J.C., RALL T.W. Autacoids; drug therapy of inflammation. In : *The*

Pharmacological Basis of Therapeutics, Goodman Gilman, A., Rall, T.W., Nies, A.S., Taylor, P. (Eds), Pergamon press, New York, 1992, pp 574-599.

GENICOT B., CLOSE R., MOULIGNEAU F., LEKEUX P. Clinical and pulmonary function changes induced by aerosoltherapy during bovine acute respiratory distress syndrome. In Proceedings : XVIIth World Buiatrics Congress, 1992, 3, pp 236-241.

GENICOT B., MOULIGNEAU F., LINDSEY J.K., LAMBERT P., CLOSE R., LEKEUX P. Efficiency of 5-hydroxytryptamine receptor blockade as therapeutic measure during acute respiratory distress syndrome in double-muscled cattle. *J. Vet. Med. A* 1993a, 40, 185-193.

GENICOT B., MOULIGNEAU F., LINDSEY J.K., LAMBERT P., CLOSE R., LEKEUX P. Induction of a serotonin-S_2 receptor blockade during early or late stage of acute respiratory distress syndrome in double-muscled calves: a comparative study. *J. Vet. Med. A* 1993b, 40, 241-248.

GENICOT B., MOULIGNEAU F., ROLLIN F., LINDSEY J.K., CLOSE R., LEKEUX P. Economic, clinical and functional consequences of a treatment using metrenperone during an outbreak of shipping fever in cattle. *Vet. Rec.* 1993c, 132, 245-247.

GENICOT B., MOULIGNEAU F., CLOSE R., LEKEUX P. Are bovine muscarinic receptors activated during respiratory distress syndrome ? In : *Journal of Aerosol Medicine: Deposition, Clearance, and Effects in the Lung*, Smaldone, G.C. (Ed.), Mary Ann Liebert, Inc Publishers, New York, 1993d, 6 (Suppl.), p 80.

GENICOT B.C., CLOSE R.P., LINDSEY J.K., LEKEUX P.M. Clinical and pulmonary function changes induced by three regimens of bronchodilating agents during bovine respiratory distress syndrome. 1993e, submitted for publication.

GENICOT B., MOULIGNEAU F., CLOSE R., LEKEUX P. Functional effects of a muscarinic receptor blockade during acute respiratory distress syndrome in double-muscled calves. *Vet. Rec.* 1993f, in press.

GENSINI G.F. Rationale for a clinical experience with the use of thromboxane A_2 antagonist. In : *Thrombosis*, Neri Serneri, G.G., Gensini, G.F., Abbate, R., Prisco, D. (Eds), Scientific Press, Florence, 1992.

GILBERT B.E., WYDE P.R., AMBROSE M.W., WILSON S.Z., KNIGHT V. Further studies with short duration ribavirin aerosol for the treatment of influenza virus infection in mice and respiratory syncytial virus infection in cotton rats. *Antiviral Res.* 1992, 17, 33-42.

GILMAN N.J., MEYER L., CARTER J., SLOVIS C. Comparison of aerosolized glycopyrrolate and metaproterenol in acute asthma. *Chest* 1990, 98, 1095-1098.

GOBLE D.O. Upper respiratory problems of the draft horse. In : *Current Therapy in Equine Medicine 3*, Robinson, N.E. (Ed.), W.B. Saunders Company, Philadelphia, 1992, pp 92-95.

GOLDSMITH L.S., GREENSPAN J.S., RUBENSTEIN S.D., WOLFSON M.R., SHAFFER T.H. Immediate improvement in lung volume after exogenous surfactant: alveolar recruitment versus increased distention. *J. Pediatr.* 1991, 119, 424-428.

GORTNER L., POHLANDT F., DISSE B., WELLER E. Effects of bovine surfactant in premature calves after intratracheal application. *Eur. J. Pediatr.* 1990, 149, 280-283.

GOURLAY R.N., THOMAS L.H., WYLD S.G. Effect of a new macrolide antibiotic (tilmicosin) on pneumonia experimentally induced in calves by *Mycoplasma bovis* and *Pasteurella haemolytica*. *Res. Vet. Sci.* 1989, 47, 84-89.

GRANELLI-PIPERNO A., NOLAN P., INABA K., STEIMANN R.M. The effect of immunosuppresive agents on the induction of nuclear factors that bind to sites on the interleukin 2 promoter. *J. Exp. Med.* 1990, 172, 1869-1872.

GUSTIN P., DHEM A., LEKEUX P., LOMBA F., LANDSER F.J., VAN DE WOESTIJNE K. Investigation of the effects of histamine inhalation on the

tracheobronchial tree of calves by the forced oscillation technique. *J. Vet. Pharmacol. Therap*. 1988a, 11, 374-380.
GUSTIN P., LOMBA F., LEKEUX P. Pharmacologie des médiateurs de l'hypersensibilité de type 1 chez les bovins. *Ann. Méd. Vét*. 1988b, 132, 549-563.
GUSTIN P., LANDSER F.J., LOMBA F., LEKEUX P. Assessment of respiratory diseases and therapeutics by the forced oscillation technique in feedlot cattle. *Res. Vet. Sci*. 1990, 49, 319-322.
HALL J., WOOD L.D.H. Oxygen Therapy. In : *The Lung: Scientific Foundations*, Crystal, R.G., West, J.B. (Eds), Raven Press, New York, 1991, pp 2143-2153.
HALLIWELL B., GUTTERIDGE J.M. Iron and free radical reactions: two aspects of antioxidant protection. *Trends Biochem. Sci*. 1986, 11, 372-375.
HENDERSON A.R. Eicosanoids and platelet-activating factor in allergic respiratory diseases. *Am. Rev. Respir. Dis*. 1991, 143, S86-S90.
HENDERSON B., BLAKE S. Therapeutical potential of cytokine manipulation. *Trends Pharm. Sc*, 1992, 13, 145-152.
HENRY M.M., MOORE J.N., FELDMAN E.B., FISCHER J.K., RUSSEL B. Effect of dietary alpha-linolenic acid on equine monocyte procoagulant activity and eicosanoid synthesis. *Circ. Schock* 1990, 32, 173-188.
HENRY M.M., MOORE J.N., FISCHER J.K. Influence of an W-3 fatty acid-enriched ration on in vivo responses of horses to endotoxin. *Am. J. Vet. Res*. 1991, 52, 523-527.
HODES D.S., SCHNITZER T.J., KALICA A.R., CAMARGO E., CHANOCK R.M. Inhibition of respiratory syncycial parainfluenza 3 and measles viruses by 2 deoxy-D-glucose. *Virology* 1975, 63, 201-208.
HOFFSTEIN S.T., MALO P.E., BUGELSKI P., WHEELDON E.B. Leukotriene D_4 (LTD_4) induces mucus secretion from goblet cells in the guinea pig respiratory epithelium. *Exp. Lung Res*. 1990, 16, 711-725.
HWANG S.B., LAM M.H., BIFTU T., BEATTIE T.R., SHEN T.Y. Trans-2, 5-bis-tetrahydrofuran. An orally active specific and competitive receptor antagonist of platelet activating factor. *J. Biol. Chem*. 1985, 260, 15639-15645.
IMAI T., VERCELLOTTI G.M., MOLDOW C.F., JACOB H.S., WEIR E.K. Pulmonary-hypertension and edema induced by platelet-activating factor in isolated, perfused rat lungs are blocked by BN52021. *J. Lab. Clin. Med*. 1988, 111, 211-217.
INSEL P.A. Analgesic-antipyretics and antiinflammatory agents: drugs employed in the treatment of rheumatoid arthritis and gout. In : *The Pharmacological Basis of Therapeutics*, Goodman Gilman, A., Rall, T.W., Nies, A.S., Taylor, P. (Eds), Pergamon press, New York, 1992, pp 638-681.
ISHIZAKA A., WU Z., STEPHENS K.E., HARADA H., HOGUE R.S., O'HANLEY P.T., RAFFIN T.A. Attenuation of acute lung injury in septic guinea pigs by pentoxifylline. *Am. Rev. Respir. Dis*. 1988, 138, 376-382.
JACKSON D.M., NORRIS A.A., EADY R.P. Nedocromil sodium and sensory nerves in the dog lung. *Pulm. Pharmacol*. 1989, 2, 179-184.
JAMES K. Interactions between cytokines and 2-macroglobulin. *Immunology Today*. 1990, 11, 163-166.
JOHNSON B. Nutritional and dietary interrelationships with diseases of feedlot cattle. *Vet. Clin. North Am. Food Anim. Pract*. 1991, 7, 133-142.
JOHNSON M. The pharmacology of salmeterol. *Lung* 1990, 168 (Suppl), 115-119.
KIELY R.G., JENKINS W.L., MARTENS R.J. Mucociliary transport rate in the horse and its modification with various pharmacologic agents. In Proceedings : 4th Veterinary Respiratory Symposium, Anaheim, California, 1985, p 7.
KIMMAN T.G., TERPSTRA G.K., DAHA M.R., WESTENBRINK F. Pathogenesis of

naturally acquired bovine respiratory syncytial virus infection in calves: evidence for the involvement of complement and mast cell mediators. *Am. J. Vet. Res.* 1989, 50, 694-700.

KNIGHT V., GILBERT B.E. Aerosol treatment of respiratory viral disease. *Lung* 1990, 168 (Suppl.), 406-413.

KOTERBA A.M. Disorders of the neonatal foal. In : *Equine Respiratory Disorders*, Beech, J. (Ed.), Lea & Febiger, Philadelphia, 1991, pp 403-429.

LANTZ R.C. KELLER G.E., BURRELL R. The role of platelet activating factor in the pulmonary response to inhaled bacterial endotoxin. *Am. Rev. Respir. Dis.* 1991, 144, 167-172.

LEE J.C., GRISWOLD D.E., VOTTA B., HANNA. N. Inhibition of monocyte IL1 production by the anti-inflammatory compound, SK & F 86002. *Int. J. Pharmacol.* 1988, 10, 835-843.

LEEPER-WOODFORD S.K., CAREY P.D., BYRNE K., FISCHER B.J., BLOCHER C., SUGERMAN H.J., FOWLER A.A., Ibuprofen attenuates plasma tumor necrosis factor activity during sepsis-induced acute lung injury. *J. Appl. Physiol.* 1991, 71, 915-923.

LEES P., HIGGINS A.J. Clinical pharmacology and therapeutic uses of non steroidal antiinflammatory drugs in the horse. *Equine Vet. J.* 1985, 17, 83-96.

LEI M.G., MORRISSON D.C. Specific endotoxic LPS-binding proteins on murine splenocytes. II Membrane localization and binding characteristics. *J. Immunol.* 1988, 141, 1006-1011.

LEKEUX P., ART T. Effect of enrofloxacin therapy on Shipping Fever pneumonia in feedlot cattle. *Vet. Rec.* 1988, 123, 205-207.

LESSLAUER W., TABUCHI H., GENTZ M., BROCKHAUS M., SCHLAEGER E.J., GRAU G., PIQUET H., POINTAIRE P., VASSALI P., LOETSCHER H.R. Recombinant soluble TNF receptor proteins inhibit LPS-induced lethality in mice. *Cytokine* 1991, 3, P497.

LEVINE D., EDWARDS D.K., MERRITT T.A. Synthetic vs human surfactants in the treatment of respiratory distress syndrome: radiographic findings. *Am. J. Roentgenol.* 1991, 157, 371-374.

LEWIS J.F., IKEGAMI M., JOBE A.H., TABOR B. Aerosolized surfactant treatment of preterm lambs. *J. Appl. Physiol.* 1991, 70, 869-876.

LINDEN A., DESMECHT D., AMORY H., ROLLIN F., MICHAUX C., LEKEUX P. Pulmonary response to intravenous administration of 5-hydroxyptamine after type-2 receptor blockade in healthy calves. *Am. J. Vet. Res.* 1993, 54, 168-174.

LLOYD D.H. Essential fatty acids and skin disease. *J. Small Anim. Pract.* 1989, 30, 207-212.

LÖFDAHL C.G., CHUNG K.F. Long-acting β_2-adrenoceptor agonists: a new perspective in the treatment of asthma. *Eur. Respir. J.* 1991, 4, 218-226.

LORENTZSON S., BOE J., ERIKSSON G., PERSSON G. Use of inhaled corticosteroids in patients with mild asthma. *Thorax* 1990, 45, 733-735.

LYONS E.T., DRUDGE J.H., TOLLIVER S.C. Ivermectin: treating for naturally occurring infections of lungworms and stomach worms in equids. *Vet. Med.* 1985a, 80, 58-64.

LYONS E.T., TOLLIVER S.C., DRUDGE J.H., SWERCZEK T.W., CROWE M.W. Lungworms: prevalence in live equids in Kentucky. *Am. J. Vet. Res.* 1985b, 46, 921-923.

MACKLIN L.J., BENDICH A. Free radical tissue damage: protective role of antioxidant nutrients. *FASEB J.* 1987, 1, 441-445.

MALMBERG A.B., YAKSH T.L. Hyperalgesia mediated by spinal glutamate or substance P receptor blocked by spinal cyclo-oxygenase inhibition. *Science* 1992, 257,

1276-1279.
MANOHAR M. Furosemide attenuates the exercise-induced rise in pulmonary artery wedge pressure in horses. *Physiologist* 1992, 35, 231.
MARKS D., MACKAY-SMITH M.P., CUSHING L.S., LESLIE A. Observations on laryngeal hemiplegia in the horse and treatment by abductor muscle prosthesis. *Equine Vet. J.* 1970, 2, 158-166.
MARON M.B., PILATI C.F. Effect of papaverine on pulmonary vascular permeability to proteins. *J. Appl. Physiol.* 1988, 65, 1367-1371.
MARTIN G.S., KACHEL D.L. Reduction of neutrophil-mediated injury to pulmonary endothelial cells by dapsone. *Am. Rev. Respir. Dis.* 1985, 131, 544-547.
MAUNDER R.J., WINN R.K., GLEISNER J.M., HILDEBRANDT J., HARLAN J.M. Effect of intravenous catalase on the pulmonary vascular response to endotoxemia in goats. *J. Appl. Physiol.* 1988, 64, 697-704.
McCORD J.M., WONG K., STOKES S.H., PETRONE W.F., ENGLISH D.K. A mechanism for the anti-inflammatory activity of superoxide dismutase. In : *Pathology of Oxygen*, Autor, A.P. (Ed.), Academic Press, New York, 1982, pp 75-83.
McKIERNAN B.C., KORITZ G.D., SCOTT J.S., BERNEY C., ROBINSON N.E. Plasma theophylline concentration and lung function in ponies with recurrent obstructive lung disease. *Equine Vet. J.* 1990, 22, 194-197.
McMILLAN D.D., BOYD G.N. The role of antioxidants and diet in the prevention or treatment of oxygen-induced lung microvascular injury. *Ann. N Y Acad. Sci.* 1982, 384, 535-543.
MOHANTY S., ROCKEMANN D., DAVIDSON J., TRIPATHY R., INGLING A. Chemotherapeutic effect of 2-deoxy-D-glucose against respiratory syncycial virus infection in calves. *Am. J. Vet. Res.* 1981, 42, 336-338.
MONCADA S., PALMER R.M., HIGGS E.A. Nitric oxide: physiology, pathophysiology. *Pharmacol. Rev.* 1991, 43, 109-142.
MOORE K.W., VIEIRA P., FIORENTINO D.F., TROUNSTINE M.L., KLAN T.A., MOSMANN T.R. Homology of cytokine synthesis inhibitory factor (IL-10) to the Esptein-Barr virus gene BCRFI. *Science* 1990, 248, 1230-1234.
MORRIS D.D., HENRY M.M., MOORE J.N., FISCHER J.K. Effect of dietary α-linolenic acid on endotoxin-induced production of tumor necrosis factor by peritoneal macrophages in horses. *Am. J. Vet. Res.* 1991, 52, 528-532.
MORRISSON D.C., SILVERSTEIN R., BRIGHT S.W., CHEN T.Y., FLEBBE L.M., LEI M.G. Monoclonal antibody to mouse lipopolysaccharide receptor protects mice against the lethal effects of endotoxin. *J. Infect. Dis.* 1990, 162, 1063-1068.
NASSAR C.F., SAADEH F.M., AYYASH R.E., KANJ N.M. Effects of aminophylline and terbutaline sulfate on the contractility of feline diaphragm. *Gen. Pharmacol.* 1991, 22, 1191-1197.
OGUNBIYI P.O., BLACK W.D., EYRE P. Parainfluenza-3 virus-induced enhancement of histamine release from calf lung mast cells effect of levamisole. *J. Vet. Pharmacol. Therap.* 1988, 11, 338-344.
OLSON N.C., SALZER W.L., Mc CALL C.E. Biochemical, physiological and clinical aspects of endotoxemia. *Mol. Aspects Med.* 1988, 10, 511-629.
OLSON N.C., JOYCE P.B., FLEISHER L.N. Mono-hydroxyeicosatetraenoic acids during porcine endotoxemia. Effect of a platelet-activating factor receptor antagonist. *Lab. Invest.* 1990a, 63, 221-232.
OLSON N.C, KRUSE-ELLIOTT K.T., JOHNSON L. Effect of LY 171883 on endotoxin-induced lung injury in pigs. *J. Appl. Physiol.* 1990b, 69, 1315-1322.
PACCITI N., BRYSON S.E., McKECHNIE K., RODGER I.W., PARATT J.R. Leucotriene antagonist FPL 57231 prevents the acute pulmonary effects of *Escherichia*

coli endotoxin in cats. *Circ. Shock* 1987, 21, 155-168.
PACIOREK P.M., BURDEN D.T., GATER P.R., HAWTHORNE Y.M., SPENCE A.M., TAYLOR J.C., WATERFALL J.F. Inhibition by Ro 31-6930 of agonist and allergen induced bronchoconstriction in anaesthetised guinea-pigs and cats. *Pulm. Pharmacol.* 1991, 4, 225-232.
PATRIGNANI P., FILABOZZI P., CATELLA F., PUGLIESE F., PATRONO C. Differential effects of dazoxiben, a selective thromboxane-synthase inhibitor, on platelet and renal prostagladin-endoperoxyde metabolism. *J. Pharmacol. Exp. Ther.* 1984, 228, 472-477.
PAVIA D., AGNEW J.E., LOPEZ-VIDRIERO M.T., NEWMAN S.P., CLARKE S.W. The effect of metered dose aerosols on the viscoelastic properties and clearance of bronchial secretions. In : *Metered Dose Inhalers*, Epstein, S.W. (Ed.), Astra, Mississauga, 1984, pp 38-48.
PEARCE H.G., WYBURN R.S., GOULDEN B.E. A clinical evaluation of Bisolvon® for the treatment of some equine respiratory diseases. *N. Z. Vet. J.* 1978, 26, 28-30.
PERSICO F.J. Low molecular weight inhibitors of interleukin 1. In : *Cytokines and Inflammation*, Kimball, E.S. (Ed.), CRC Press, 1991, pp 59-80.
PHILLIPPS G.H. Structure-activity relationships of topically active steroids: the selection of fluticasone propionate. *Respir. Med.* 1990, 84 (Suppl. A), 19-23.
PICAVET T., MUYLLE E., DEVRIESE L.A., GERYL J. Efficacy of tilmicosin in treament of pulmonary infections in calves. *Vet. Rec.* 1991, 129, 400-403.
POTCHOIBA M.J., CARLSON J.R., NOCERINI M.R., BREEZE R.G. Effect of monensin and supplemental hay on ruminal 3-methylindole formation in adult cows after abrupt change to lush pasture. *Am. J. Vet. Res.* 1992, 53,129-133
POUPLARD L., LEKEUX P., DETRY M. Efficacy of ivermectin and levamisole against immature larvae of *D. viviparus* in cattle. *Vet. Rec.* 1986, 118, 557-559.
POVEY R.C. Effect of orally-administered ribavirin on experimental feline calivirus infection in cats. *Am. J. Vet. Res.* 1978, 39, 1337-1341.
RIMAR S., GILLIS C.N. Pulmonary vasodilation by inhaled nitric oxyde after endothelial injury. *J. Appl. Physiol.* 1992, 73, 2179-2183.
ROBINSON N.E. Rôle du système nerveux autonome dans l'obstruction des voies aériennes du cheval. *Ann. Méd. Vét.* 1993, 137, 153-159.
ROBUSCHI M., GAMBARO G., SPAGNOTTO S., VAGHI A., BIANCO S. Inhaled frusemide is highly effective in preventing ultrasonically nebulised water bronchoconstriction. *Pulm. Pharmacol.* 1989, 1, 187-191.
RUBARTELLI A., SITIA R. Interleukin-1 and thioredoxin are secreted through a novel pathway of secretion. *Biochem. Soc. Trans.* 1991, 19, 255-259.
RUOFF W.W. Fungal pneumonia in horses. In Proceedings : 34th Annual Convention of American Association of Equine Practitioners, 1988, p 423.
SANDBERG K., EDBERG K.E., BENTON W., SILBERBERG A., SLADEK M., SUNDELL H.W. Surfactant improves gas mixing and alveolar ventilation in preterm lambs. *Pediatr. Res.* 1991, 30, 181-189.
SASSE H.H.L., HAJER R. Enkele veterinair-klinische ervaringen met het gebruik van een β_2-receptoren stimulerend sympaticomymeticum (NAB 365®) bij paarden met longaandoeningen. *Tijdschr. Diergeneesk.* 1977, 102, 1233-1238.
SAUNDERS R.N., HANDLEY D.A. Platelet-activating factor antagonists. *Annu. Rev. Pharmacol. Toxicol.* 1987, 27, 237-255.
SCHELTZE S., BERKOVIC D., TOMSING O., UNGER C., KRONDE M. Tumor necrosis factor induces rapid production of 1'2' diacylglycerol by a phosphatidylcholine-specific phospholipase. *C. J. Exp. Med.* 1991, 174, 975-978.
SCHRAUFSTATTER I.V., REVAK S.D., COCHRANE C.G. Proteases and oxidants in

experimental pulmonary inflammatory injury. *J. Clin. Invest.* 1984, 73, 1175-1184.
SCHULE R., MULLER M., KALTSCHMIDT C., RENKAWITZ R. Many transcription factors interact synergistically with steroid receptors. *Science* 1988, 242 (4884), 1418-1420.
SCOTT J.S., BERNEY C.E., DERKSEN F.J., ROBINSON N.E. β-Adrenergic receptor activity in ponies with recurrent obstructive pulmonary disease. *Am. J. Vet. Res.* 1991, 52, 1416-1422.
SEEKAMP A., CHERYL L., ZHU D., DEMLING R. Catalase prevents prostanoid release and lung lipid peroxidation after endotoxemia in sheep. *J. Appl. Physiol.* 1988, 65, 1210-1216.
SELMAN I.E., ALLAN E.M., GIBBS H.A., WISEMAN A., YOUNG W.B. Effect of antiprostaglandin therapy in experimental parainfluenza type 3 pneumonia in weaned, conventional calves. *Vet. Rec.* 1984, 4, 101-105.
SHEEHAN K.C., RUDDLE N.H., SCHREIBER R.D. Generation and characterization of monoclonal antibodies that neutralize murine tumor necrosis factors. *J. Immunol.* 1989, 142, 3884-3893.
SHEN T.Y., HWANG S.B., CHANG M.N., DOEBBER T.W., LAM M.H., WU W.S., WANG X., HAN G.Q., LI R.Z. Characterization of a patelet-activating factor antagonist isolated from haifenteng: specific inhibition of in vitro and in vivo platelet-activating factor-induced effects. *Proc. Natl. Acad. Sci.* 1985, 82, 672-676.
SLOCOMBE R.F., MALARK J., INGERSOLL R., DERKSEN F.J., ROBINSON N.E. Importance of neutrophils in the pathogenesis of acute pneumonic pasteurellosis in calves. *Am. J. Vet. Res.* 1985, 46, 2253-2258.
SLUTSKY A.S. Mechanical ventilation. In : *The Lung: Scientific Foundations*, Crystal, R.G., West, J.B. (Eds), Raven Press, New York, 1991, pp 2163-2174.
SNAPPER J.R., HUTCHISON A.A., OGLETREE M.L. Effects of cyclooxygenase inhibitors on the alterations in lung mechanics caused by endotoxemia in the unanesthetized sheep. *J. Clin. Invest.* 1983, 72, 63-76.
SNIDER R.M., CONSTANTINE J.W., LOWE J.A., LONGO K.P., LEBEL W.S., WOODY H.A., DROZDA S.E., DESAI M.C., VINICK F.J., SPECER R.W., HESS H.J. A potent nonpeptide antagonist of the substance P (NK_1) receptor. *Science* 1991, 251, 435-437.
SNYDER D.S., URANUE E.R. Corticosteroids inhibit murine macrophage expression and interleukin 1 production. *J. Immunol.* 1982, 129, 1803-1805.
SOMA L.R., BEECH J., GERBER N.H. Effects of cromolyn in horses with chronic obstructive pulmonary disease. *Vet. Res. Commun.* 1987, 11, 339.
SOUTHORN P.A., POWIS G. Free radicals in medicine II. Involvement in human disease. *Mayo Clin. Proc.* 1988, 63, 390-408.
STRUHAR D., HARBECK R.J. Inhibition of induced acute lung edema by a novel protein-kinase C inhibitor. *FASEB J.* 1987, 1, 116-118.
SVENDSEN U.G., JORGENSEN H. Inhaled nedocromil sodium as additional treatment to high-dose inhaled corticosteroids in the management of bronchial asthma. *Eur. Respir. J.* 1991, 4, 992-999.
TAGARI P., ABRAHAM W.M., McGOLRICK J., CHARLESON S., SOLER M., AHMED A., CORTEZ A., FORD-HUTCHINSON A.W. Increased leukotriene E_4 excretion during antigen-induced bronchoconstriction in allergic sheep. *J. Appl. Physiol.* 1990, 68, 1321-1327.
TOKUYAMA K., LOTVALL J.O., LÖFDAHL C.G., BARNES P.J., CHUNG K.F. Inhaled formoterol inhibits histamine-induced airflow obstruction and airway microvascular leakage. *Eur. J. Pharmacol.* 1991, 193, 35-39.
TOOGOOD J.H. Complications of topical steroid therapy for asthma. *Am. Rev. Respir.*

Dis. 1990, 141, S89-S96.

TRACEY K., FONG Y., HESSE D.G., MANOGUE K.R., LEE A.T., KUO G.C., LOWRY S.F., CERAMI A. Anti-cachectin/TNF monoclonal antibodies prevent septic shock during lethal bacteriemia. *Nature* 1987, 330, 662-664.

TRAVIS J. Oxidants and antioxidants in the lung. *Am. J. Respir. Dis.* 1987, 135, 773-774.

TUMEN J., MEYRICK B., BERRY L., BRIGHAM K.L. Antiproteinases protect cultured, lung endothelial cells from endotoxin injury. *J. Appl. Physiol.* 1988, 65, 835-843.

TURGUT K., SASSE H.H.L. Influence of clenbuterol on mucociliary transport in healthy horses and horses with chronic obstructive pulmonary disease. *Vet. Rec.* 1989, 125, 526-530.

TURK M.A., KLEI T.R. Effect of ivermectin treatment on eosinophilic pneumonia and other extravascular lesions of late *Strongylus vulgaris* larval migration in foals. *Vet. Pathol.* 1984, 21, 87-92.

TWOMEY B.M., DALE M.M. Cyclooxygenase-independant effect of non-steroidal anti-inflammatory drugs on the neutrophil respiratory burst. *Biochem. Pharmacol.* 1992, 4, 413-418.

ULICH T.R., YIN S.M., GUO K.Z., Del CASTILLO J., EISENBERG S.P., THOMPSON R.C. The intratracheal administration of endotoxin and cytokines. III. The interleukin-1 (IL-1) receptor antagonist inhibits endotoxin and IL-1 induced acute inflammation. *Am. J. Pathol.* 1991, 138, 521-524.

VAN ALSTINE W.G., HOFSTAD N.S. Antibiotic aerosolization: the effect on experimentally-induced alcaligenes rhinotracheitis in turkeys. *Avian Dis.* 1984, 29, 159-164.

VANDERMYDE C.R., DIPIETRO J.A., TODD K.S., LOCK T.F. Evaluation of fenbendazole for larvicidal effect in experimentally induced *Parascaris equorum* infections in pony foals. *J. Am. Vet. Med. Assoc.* 1987, 12, 1548-1549.

VANE J.R. Inhibition of prostaglandin synthesis as a mechanism of action of aspirin-like drugs. *Nature* 1971, 231, 232-235.

VENTRESCA G.P., NICHOL G.M., BARNES P.J., CHUNG K.F. Inhaled furosemide inhibits cough induced by low chloride content solutions but not by capsaicin. *Am. Rev. Respir. Dis.* 1990, 142, 143-146.

VOGELMEIER C., BUHL R., HOYT R.F., WILSON E., FELLS G.A., HUBBARD R.C., SCHNEBLI H.P., THOMPSON R.C., CRYSTAL G. Aerosilization of recombinant SLPI to augment antineutrophil elastase of pulmonary epithelium. *J. Appl. Physiol.* 1990, 69, 1843-1848.

WALTHER S., JANSSON I., GUNNARSSON M., LENNQUIST S. Nebulized corticosteroid improves pulmonary function and outcome in experimental porcine septicemia. *Acta Anaesthesiol. Scand.* 1991, 35, 635-641.

WANNER A. Alteration of tracheal mucociliary transport in airway disease. *Chest* 1981, 80, 867-869.

WEISS T., DORROW P., FELIX R. Effects of a β adrenergic drug and a secretolytic agent on regional mucociliary clearance in patients in COPD. *Chest* 1981, 80, 881-884.

WICKERTS C.J., BLOMQVIST H., BERG B., ROSBLAD P.G., HEDENSTIERNA G. Furosemide, when used in combination with positive end-expiratory pressure, facilitates the resorption of extravascular lung water in experimental hydrostatic pulmonary oedema. *Acta Anaesthesiol. Scand.* 1991, 35, 776-783.

WOLFE G. Neue aspekte zur Pathogenese und Therapie der hyperreflektorischen Rhinopathie. *Laryngorhinootologie* 1988, 67, 438-445.

WRIGHT P., ISHIHARA Y., BERNARD R.G. Effects of nitroprusside on lung mechanics and hemodynamics after endotoxemia in awake sheep. *J. Appl. Physiol.* 1988, 64,

2026-2032.

WU K.K., SANDUJA R., TSAI A.L., FERHANOGLU G., LOOSE-MITCHEL D.S. Aspirin inhibits interleukin-1 - induced prostaglandin H syntase expression in cultured endothelial cells. *Proc. Natl Acad. Sci.* 1991, 88, 2384-2387.

YANCEY R.J., KINNEY M.L., ROBERTS B.J., GOOGENOUGH K.R., HAMEL J.C., FORD C.W. Ceftiofur sodium, a broad-spectrum cephalosporin: evaluation in vitro and in vivo in mice. *Am. J. Vet. Res.* 1987, 8, 1050-1053.

ZIEGLER E.J., FISHER C.J., SPRUNG C.L., STRANBE R.C., SADOFF J.C., FOULKE G.E., WORTEL C.H., FINK M.P., DELLINGER R.P., TENG N.N. Treatment of gram negative bacteriemia and septic shock with HA-1A human monoclonal antibody against trial the HA-1A Sepsis Study Group. *N. Engl. J. Med.* 1991, 324, 429-436.

AUTHOR INDEX

SUBJECT INDEX